COGNITIVE NEUROPSYCHIATRY
2010, 15 (1/2/3), 1–13

Routledge
Taylor & Francis Group
LONDON AND NEW YORK

Delusion and confabulation: Overlapping or distinct distortions of reality?

Robyn Langdon[1] and Martha Turner[2]

[1]*Macquarie Centre for Cognitive Science, Macquarie University, NSW, Australia,* [2]*Institute of Cognitive Neuroscience, London, UK*

Delusion is commonly defined as a false belief and associated with psychiatric illness like schizophrenia, whereas confabulation is typically described as a false memory and associated with neurological disorder like amnesia. Yet delusion and confabulation both involve the endorsement of distorted representations of reality, whether about the present or the personal past. Moreover, differences in aetiology need not dictate mutual exclusivity with regard to underlying cognitive mechanisms. In response to the growing interest in commonalities and differences between delusion and confabulation, this Special Issue brings together contributors from diverse fields to consider the relations between these two symptoms. Although approaches and opinions differ, all of our contributors share common aims of clarifying theoretical conceptions and exploring boundaries so as to advance understanding of the cognitive neuropsychiatry of both delusion and confabulation. After introducing each contribution, we highlight some common themes and unanswered questions.

Keywords: Delusion; Confabulation; Belief; Memory; Psychosis; Cognitive neuropsychiatry.

INTRODUCTION

People with psychiatric and/or neurological illness sometimes say and think the most amazing things. They might believe they are dead; claim to see, despite being blind; or "remember" things that never happened. Historical demarcations between academic disciplines dictate that these are distinct clinical phenomena: delusion, anosognosia (commonly conceived as a delusional denial of illness), and confabulation. In this Special Issue we

Correspondence should be addressed to Robyn Langdon, Macquarie Centre for Cognitive Science, Macquarie University, Ryde, NSW 2109, Australia. E-mail: rlangdon@maccs.mq.edu.au

We want to thank all of our contributors for their very helpful suggestions on an earlier version of this manuscript.

DOI: 10.1080/13546800903519095

bring together researchers from diverse fields—memory researchers, clinical neuropsychologists, psychiatrists, cognitive scientists, and philosophers—to consider the extent to which these putatively distinct clinical phenomena overlap. Approaches differ; new data are presented, reviews provided, phenomenological details reported, and more speculative, novel hypotheses mounted. Opinions also differ; some contributors use the term, "confabulation", very generally to refer to false claims, whether these concern belief or memory, and whether they arise in clinical or nonclinical populations, and others focus on pathological conditions, with several contributors advocating an exclusive approach, according to which no symptom qualifies as both delusional and confabulatory. Yet other contributors consider the similarities between delusion and confabulation and explore points of intersection and a common explanatory framework. Despite their differing views and approaches, all of our contributors share the aims of clarifying theoretical conceptions and learning more about underlying mechanisms so as to advance the cognitive neuropsychiatry of delusion and confabulation.

All of the papers in this Special Issue stem from an international, interdisciplinary workshop on "Delusion and Confabulation: Overlapping or distinct psychopathologies of reality distortion", held at the Macquarie Centre for Cognitive Science (MACCS) in Sydney, Australia, 13–14 July 2007, and ongoing collaborative discussions that were prompted by that meeting. This 2007 workshop was itself inspired by an earlier symposium on confabulation and delusion held the year before during the Fourth International Conference on Memory, in Sydney, Australia (see Fotopoulou, 2010 this issue). The aim of the MACCS workshop was to promote innovative, crossdisciplinary approaches to untangling the relations between delusion and confabulation, both of which involve the endorsement of mistaken representations of reality. By testing boundaries between these historically demarcated, although not clearly conceptually demarcated, constructs, we sought to explore the possibility of an overarching theoretical framework for mapping out the shared and distinct conceptual space occupied by all such distortions of reality, or, if no such framework could be agreed upon, we sought to refine conceptual distinctions and highlight new research directions.

CONTRASTING APPROACHES TO DELUSION AND CONFABULATION

Michael Kopelman sets the scene for our Special Issue by introducing the many different forms of false memory and delusion that can be observed in neurological and psychiatric illness. With regard to false memories, he contrasts *spontaneous* and *provoked* confabulations following brain injury, and discusses recovered memories and false confessions, to name but a few. With regard to delusions, he describes the variable contexts, themes, and associated phenomenology of different delusions and raises concern that current models lack the complexity and the flexibility to adequately account for these variations. In considering whether false memories in neurological and psychiatric contexts might reflect common or distinct processes (involving, e.g., pathological memory processes or nonpathological memory processes, which are distorted in delusional contexts), Kopelman suggests that the contrast between spontaneous confabulations and "delusional memories" might be particularly informative. Spontaneous confabulations involve persistent, unprovoked outpourings of mistaken memories in the context of organic amnesia, whereas delusional memories are conceived as either genuine memories, which trigger delusional interpretations, or mistaken memories that are constructed in the context of psychotic illness like schizophrenia. To emphasise specificity in theorising, Kopelman suggests that confabulations, delusions, and delusional memories ought to be kept conceptually distinct, while noting that false beliefs will inevitably become false memories.

The contributions from Gianfranco Dalla Barba and his coauthor, Marie-Françoise Boissé, and from Asaf Gilboa highlight the interests and concerns of memory researchers. Both of these papers focus on memory-related confabulations, which have proven historically challenging to identify and classify. Dalla Barba and Boissé present a new analysis of 284 provoked confabulations and 52 spontaneous confabulations collected from eight confabulating patients with diverse aetiologies. For Dalla Barba and Boissé, the provoked/spontaneous distinction is inadequate to capture the core nature of the majority of these confabulations, which, they suggest, primarily involve general memories, routine habits, and misplacements (e.g., true events misplaced in time and place). They suggest that these more commonplace confabulations are best accounted for by a cognitive abnormality that affects the normal sense of "temporal consciousness" about one's past, present, or likely future. Underpinning normal temporal consciousness, they propose, is the medial temporal lobe (MTL) and, in confabulators, normal functioning of the MTL is disrupted when related brain structures become damaged.

Gilboa also focuses on memory-related confabulation and highlights the role of defective strategic retrieval. He conceives of the core and the constitutional properties of confabulation as involving different types of memory-related monitoring dysfunction that affect: (1) a rapid intuitive "feeling of rightness"; (2) a more deliberative conscious "editor"; and (3) control processes that mediate the initiation of actions based upon retrieved memories. Although Gilboa allows a degree of overlap between delusion and confabulation with regard to the generic influences of stored schemas and emotional biases, he suggests that these core and constitutional properties of confabulation are not integral to delusion.

Aikaterini Fotopoulou adopts a uniquely historical perspective to argue against the traditional academic polarisation between neurocognitive and psychodynamic approaches. She promotes an affective (as well as cognitive) neuropsychology of confabulation and delusion and highlights the importance of emotional and motivational influences in delusion and confabulation—in particular, memory-related confabulation that associates with ventromedial prefrontal lesions and "awareness-related" confabulation that associates with right perisylvian lesions and anosognosia. While acknowledging the important role of stressful life events, Fotopoulou suggests that a pathological exaggeration of otherwise normal emotional biases might, in some delusional people and confabulators, be the direct consequence of neural disturbance; thus emotional and neuroscientific approaches need not be at odds. Despite highlighting commonality with regard to the influence of emotional factors, Fotopoulou nevertheless cautions that underlying mechanisms might differ in different syndromes; like Kopelman, she questions whether a single explanatory framework will be adequate to capture the heterogeneous ways in which emotional factors impact upon different false beliefs and different false memories.

Kasey Metcalf, Robyn Langdon, and Max Coltheart also consider the role of emotional biases in memory-related confabulations. They consider a range of aetiologies, whereas Fotopoulou focuses primarily on the two syndromes mentioned earlier. Metcalf and colleagues adopt Fotopoulou's approach to compare the emotional valence of six patients' confabulations to the patients' actual situations. They then extend this line of research to compare the patients' confabulations about current versus past events. Their findings suggest that positive emotional biases are not universal when diverse aetiologies are considered. Metcalf and colleagues thus propose that the role of emotional biases in confabulations of varying aetiology is best conceived in terms of a need to maintain a consistent self-concept (whether positive or negative). This motivated drive for self-coherence then interacts with the greater ease with which elements of highly familiar, premorbid daily activities and routines come to mind in the context of memory impairment, akin to the observations of Dalla Barba and Boissé.

Ryan McKay and Marcel Kinsbourne continue the focus on emotional biases in false claims, whether these involve confabulation, delusion or anosognosia. They conclude, like Fotopoulou, that the evidence is strongly supportive of a role for motivational factors across domains. They then widen their taxonomy of false claims beyond the pathological to consider the "garden-variety" false claims that are seen in the course of normal cognitive functioning. In doing so, they underscore some of Fotopoulou's and Metcalf's and colleagues' ideas concerning the interplay between normal and abnormal processes in delusion and confabulation, and echo the growing interest in continuity approaches to delusion and a lack of clinical insight (see, e.g., Bell & Halligan, in press; Johns & van Os, 2001).

Akira O'Connor, Colin Lever, and Chris Moulin introduce an entirely different form of false memory, one that highlights the interface between false memory and false belief—déjà vécu. Déjà vécu involves a delusional conviction that one is experiencing events that have happened before, as evidenced by the recollection of those events as having happened before. In contrast, healthy people who experience déjà vu know that no past experience could justify their erroneous sense of familiarity and so reject it. Patients who experience persistent déjà vécu find their false memories so compelling that they are unwilling to engage in related activities such as reading the newspaper; this is because they believe that they have already read these newspaper stories before. O'Connor and colleagues describe a series of cases of frequent déjà vécu and highlight the differences with "healthy" déjà experiences in nonbrain-damaged people. They propose an innovative cognitive neuroscientific hypothesis to account for the generation of déjà vécu experiences—the "encoding-experienced-as-retrieval" hypothesis, according to which normal processes of separating encoding and retrieval modes in the hippocampal memory system become dysfunctional, leading to the mistaken experience of encoding as retrieval.

Vaughan Carr shifts the focus fully onto delusions. He discusses delusions in the context of schizophrenia and provides a wealth of phenomenological details about the early phase of schizophrenic illness, which is a bewildering and disturbing time of vague and disconcerting shifts in the general sense of self and the world (involving, e.g., feelings of alienation, fragmentation, and/or aberrant heightened significance). O'Connor and colleagues hint at a direct and immediate relation in déjà vécu between the mistaken experiencing of novel events as having occurred before and the mistaken believing that these events have occurred before, but Carr describes a more gradual process by which ineffable "protopsychotic anomalous experiences" come to be understood via the "discovery" of what the patient takes to be a unifying meaning. Carr echoes some of Gilboa's ideas, although now with regard to delusion; he argues that the search for meaning in schizophrenia is compromised by reduced prefrontal monitoring, resulting in idiosyncratic associations, and that the discovery of a unifying meaning is accompanied by an aesthetic "sense of rightness". This sense of rightness, he suggests, contributes to the incorrigibility of the delusion (i.e., the resistance to counterevidence and counter-argument).

Rochelle Cox and Amanda Barnier offer another unique contribution in which they review a novel methodology for recreating, examining, and challenging temporary delusions and confabulations in the laboratory: instrumental hypnosis. They illustrate with regard to hypnotic analogues of fantastic delusions like mirrored-self misidentification, somatoparaphrenia (the delusional belief that one's own limb belongs to someone else), alien control, and self-identity delusions. Despite the fantastic belief content, they find that their high-hypnotisable subjects endorse their beliefs with conviction and resist challenge, just like clinically delusional patients. Their results open the door to a new approach for testing theories of delusion and confabulation, although Cox and Barnier caution of possible limitations with regard to generalizing from hypnotised nonclinical people to clinical cases.

William Hirstein also focuses on more fantastic delusional and confabulated content, in particular, Capgras syndrome, which involves the delusional belief that a loved one has been replaced by a visually similar impostor, and asomatognosia, which can be broadly defined as the denial of ownership of one's limb, and sometimes takes the form of somatoparaphrenia. In general, Hirstein conceives of confabulation as a mistaken claim, which is communicated by the patient, whereas delusion is a mistaken belief, which need not be communicated. On his view, these two symptoms are alike conceptually since both conform to a "two error" (Hirstein, 2005) or a "two deficit" (Langdon & Coltheart, 2000) account, according to which the cooccurrence of two different types of error is necessary to fully account for the symptoms—one is a knowledge error, which explains the generation of the specific delusional or confabulated content, and the other is a correction error, which explains the failure to discount the implausible claim. Hirstein goes on to critique current affective responsiveness and personal relatedness theories of Capgras and asomatognosia and proposes, instead, a new mind-reading theory of these phenomena (more on this later).

Max Coltheart, Peter Menzies, and John Sutton differ from Hirstein in thinking that the affective responsiveness theory of Capgras is compelling; this is the view that the Capgras content is triggered by the loss of heightened autonomic response to familiar faces. They use the Capgras example to illustrate a Bayesian, probabilistic account of the abductive inferential process that might generate the delusional content. In the case of Capgras, the hypothesis that a stranger is standing in front of one (the initial seed of the Capgras impostor delusion) is shown to be a rational explanation of the unexpected lack of autonomic response. Their example highlights a number of interesting points with regard to theories of delusion and the role of experience. We emphasise two, the first being that the neuropsychological abnormality, which initially prompts a delusional belief, does not always have a conscious correlate; hence, Coltheart and colleagues think it better to refer to the explanation of abnormal data rather than the explanation of abnormal experience. Their second point is that a person who has lost the normal autonomic response to familiar faces is not irrational to initially entertain the belief that the person she sees in front of her is a stranger. The core indicator of delusional belief, they intimate, is seen when the person, who has lost the autonomic response to familiar faces, is unable to revise her stranger belief. This should occur, for example, when she is confronted with the conflicting views of family members and the medical evidence of her brain injury.

In accord with McKay and Kinsbourne, Robyn Langdon and Tim Bayne note that some authors will use the term, confabulation, to refer to nonpathological excuses that are fabricated unintentionally by healthy people to present other people with a coherent account of what one is up to. However, they set aside these nonpathological processes to focus on three cardinal signs of (pathological) delusions: incomprehensibility (which can be indicated by either fantastic belief content or lack of contextually appropriate supportive evidence), incorrigibility, and unwarranted subjective conviction. After allowing the existence of (quasidelusional) *corrigible* confabulations that will shift under challenge, they propose that incorrigible spontaneous confabulations lie at the "received" end of a "received–reflective" spectrum of delusions; the spontaneous confabulator simply receives into consciousness an apparent, yet implausible, memory experience, which she instantaneously takes to be true. Reflective delusions, in contrast, are more like Carr's examples: The person first reflects upon disquieting and confusing experiences before an explanatory delusional belief gradually emerges. Underlying received delusions, they propose, is: (1) an automatic, normal default to endorse and maintain experiential content (mnemonic or perceptual) as belief (which might be associated with Carr's sense of rightness, or Gilboa's feeling of rightness); coupled with (2) an inability to inhibit the default truth-setting of (mis)perceived realities, which explains the incorrigibility.

Our Special Issue concludes with a contribution from Turner and Coltheart, who comprehensively review the similarities and differences between delusion and confabulation. To some extent, these differences are no greater than the differences between different delusions; that is, in accord with two-error or two-deficit theories, delusion and confabulation clearly differ with regard to the first deficit—the neuropsychological impairment that affects cognitive (perceptual or mnemonic) or affective processing. Yet, common monitoring deficits might still account for similarity with regard to the failure to reject implausible thoughts. These authors begin with, and depart from, Gilboa and colleagues; they agree that disruptions to both unconscious and conscious checking processes are important, but depart from Gilboa in considering whether these monitoring failures might be common to delusion and confabulation. They review possible candidates for these common failures and, in contrast to previous authors, who focus on feelings of rightness, they propose a normal unconscious process of tagging suspect content so that it can be checked by a separate set of deliberative conscious processes. They thus suggest a "doubt tag" (or a feeling of doubt rather than a feeling of rightness), which is absent in some delusional people and confabulators. They also point out that the inclusion of both unconscious and conscious monitoring allows for the explanation of a range of phenomena including, for example: (a) delusional and confabulated content, which arises fully formed in consciousness with a pathological absence of doubt that confers a resistance to revision; (b) delusional and confabulated content, which arises primarily via impairments of conscious monitoring that is initiated to explain ineffable disquieting experiences (the output of these conscious processes may be less resistant to revision); and (c) both plausible and implausible "secondary confabulations" and elaborations (plausible if the conscious checking processes are intact and implausible if they are not).

COMMON THEMES AND UNANSWERED QUESTIONS

Our contributors differ in whether they consider delusion and confabulation to be distinct or overlapping disorders and, if overlapping, to what degree. Despite their differences, however, there are some common themes. One theme, which is approached in different ways, concerns the role of aberrant experience. The contrast between O'Connor and colleagues' paper and that of Carr highlights these differences. Patients with déjà vécu, for example, appear to endorse a mistaken experience of retrieval as genuine and believe that novel events have happened before. In other words, there is an immediate onset of delusional conviction with the onset of a conscious (mistaken) experience of retrieval (a "this has happened before" experience). This sort of immediacy is absent in Carr's description of the role of aberrant experience in the formation of psychotic delusions at early stages of schizophrenia; in the latter case, there appears to be a noticeable gap between the onset of the initial aberrant experience and the onset of the delusional conviction. This distinction is directly addressed in the contributions by Coltheart and colleagues, Langdon and Bayne, and Turner and Coltheart. Langdon and Bayne, for example, propose a received–reflective spectrum of delusions. Received delusions lie at one pole of this spectrum and describe those cases in which experience delivers the delusional content fully formed and fully (mis)believed into consciousness. Reflective delusions lie at the other pole and describe delusions that begin with a vague and disquieting aberrant experience which the person reflects upon, triggering a search for explanation. These different approaches to the role of aberrant experience seem important when considering the similarities and differences between delusion and confabulation, and indeed between different types of delusion and between different types of false memory (e.g., between spontaneous confabulations and Kopelman's delusional memories).

This issue concerning the role of aberrant experience is closely related to another theme concerning unconscious and conscious processes. Dalla Barba and Boisse caution that any theory which highlights unconscious processes runs the risk of falling into the "fallacy of the homunculus" in attributing intentionality to unconscious processes. However some of our other contributors disagree; they think that this fallacy does not apply when one conceives of unconscious processes as directly causative of behaviour, despite their unconscious status. Coltheart, Menzies, and Sutton, for example, explicitly propose that both the abnormality that prompts hypothesis generation and the abductive inferential process that generates the delusional content may be unconscious. Gilboa and Turner and Coltheart also consider the role of both unconscious and conscious monitoring processes in their models.

Three other contributions (Fotopoulou; McKay and Kinsbourne; Metcalf and colleagues) also focus on unconscious processes in delusion and confabulation, in particular, unconscious *emotional* and *motivational* processes. These contributors suggest that emotional factors are potentially just as important as those factors that are traditionally described as cognitive (including, e.g., perceptual and mnemonic processing). Their contributions highlight that the "cognitive" in "cognitive neuropsychiatry" can sometimes be misleading. This is because it is sometimes taken to imply that cognitive neuropsychiatrists are not interested in emotional, affective, or somatic processing, which is far from the truth. Cognitive neuropsychiatrists are concerned with explaining psychiatric symptoms in terms of breakdowns in models of information processing; the processing might be unconscious or conscious and the information might concern the senses, affect, somatic markers, beliefs, or memories.

Langdon and Bayne take a slightly different tack with regard to unconscious and conscious processes; they focus on a temporal dimension. In their view, unconscious processes precede the emergence into consciousness, and concurrent endorsement as veridical, of a received delusion; further along the received–reflective continuum, both conscious and unconscious continue to nuance the final delusional content, after the initial (semiformed) delusional thought first comes to mind. Other contributors likewise hint at the importance of a temporal dimension. Coltheart, Menzies, and Sutton, for example, suggest that frank delusionality is not apparent until the patient fails to revise her belief. The temporal gap between the onset of brain damage and the onset of frank symptoms (which ultimately stem from that brain damage) also seems important; consider a potential Capgras patient who suffers a stroke during the night. This stroke impairs both the patient's belief evaluation/revision system and a heightened autonomic response to familiar faces (for the sake of argument we will focus on a face-specific autonomic responsiveness theory of Capgras: see, e.g., Ellis &

Lewis, 2001). The abnormal data—the unexpected lack of autonomic response—will only register with this person's internal monitor, after she has awoken, gone down to the kitchen to see her spouse, who has turned around to show his face. It cannot be until then, according to the face-specific autonomic responsiveness theory, that the stranger thought can arise. And, if it does arise before then—say on seeing the spouse's body shape and movements before he has turned around, then this face-specific theory cannot be correct; at least it cannot be correct for the person in question. Hirstein's mind-reading account of a difficulty with matching an egocentric representation of the mind of a familiar person with an allocentric representation of that familiar person's physical appearance might, in contrast, still apply. We also offer this example to highlight the importance of detailed phenomenological reports of delusional and confabulating patients.

Another theme concerns feelings of rightness and wrongness. Gilboa, in his contribution, describes a preconscious feeling of rightness, Carr an aesthetic sense of rightness resulting from the discovery of unifying meaning, and Turner and Coltheart refer to a failure to associate delusional and confabulated thoughts with normal sensations of doubt. It remains unclear whether what is signalled is rightness or wrongness, or indeed on what basis this might occur, but this seems an important commonality between delusion and confabulation and one that deserves further attention. One possibility is that the same checking process, likely involving the ventromedial prefrontal cortex (VMPFC) or the orbitofrontal cortex (OFC: see, e.g., Hirstein, 2005), outputs either a right or wrong signal. However, we would caution against assuming a single process that outputs all such signals. The VMPFC is a complex system and one that is involved in both reward and punishment signalling (see, e.g., Moscovitch & Winocur, 2002, who ascribe "acceptance" and "rejection" signals to anterior and posterior parts of the VMPFC, respectively). As such, it is not inconceivable that someone might experience concurrent feelings of rightness and wrongness about the same state of affairs—say feelings of rightness about the truth of a perceived reality, or a memory, or the aesthetic fit of an explanation, and feelings of wrongness about the likely unpleasant consequences of acting too quickly on an out-of-the-ordinary belief (see Langdon & Connaughton, in press, for discussion).

A related issue is whether feelings of rightness or wrongness are pathological. The contributions from Gilboa and from Turner and Coltheart characterise these processes as in some form disordered, whereas Carr suggests that an aesthetic sense of rightness is part of the normal creative process. If so, this raises the question of whether, in the presence of an aberrant perceptual (or affective or mnemonic) experience and a (normal) feeling of rightness, a second error of critical evaluation is necessary to explain the acceptance (rather than rejection) of delusions and confabulations. In other words, do we need a second type of error (say involving critical evaluation) to fully account for delusions and confabulations or would a one-error account suffice? Perhaps future research in this regard will benefit from clearer delineation of three stages: (1) the generation of the delusional or confabulated content; (2) the initial adoption of the content as delusional belief or confabulated memory; and (3) the maintenance of the delusion or confabulation. Two-factor theorists have, thus far, tended to conflate Stages 2 and 3 when they have described the second error or deficit as a failure to reject the implausible thought. However, as Coltheart and colleagues argue, the initial adoption of a delusional belief might, in some cases, be a rational, nonpathological response to a first neuropsychological impairment—that is, no additional pathology (beyond the first neuropsychological deficit) is necessary to explain the initial adoption of the delusional belief. Frank delusionality, they imply, only becomes apparent with incorrigibility. If so, the more critical question for one-error and two-error theorists might be whether nonpathological feelings of rightness or wrongness are sufficient to explain delusional incorrigibility. Carr would likely say "yes"; other contributors would say "no": Hirstein, who conceives of a second-stage correction error; Coltheart, Menzies, and Sutton, who describe a second failure of belief revision; and Langdon and Bayne, who conceive the belief revision failure as a difficulty with inhibiting a belief to reason about it as if it might not be true. Turner and Coltheart, in contrast, allow for degrees of conviction and related incorrigibility with regard to particular combinations of disruptions to unconscious and conscious monitoring. Perhaps, hypnotically induced delusions and confabulations will provide a useful testing ground for evaluating these competing one-error, two-error, or even multiple-error views, as proposed by Cox and Barnier.

We turn now to consider the relation between the pathological and the nonpathological. Although our primary focus in this Special Issue is pathology, delusion-like beliefs and confabulation-like fabrications occur in healthy people (see, e.g., McKay & Kinsbourne's paper). Where and how do we draw the line between the pathological and the nonpathological? One response is that such nonclinical phenomena reflect partial pathology—for example, the presence of a second deficit of belief evaluation in the absence of a first neuropsychological deficit, which would trigger persistent perceptual (or affective or mnemonic) anomalies and hence persistent clinical delusions or confabulations. Alternatively, one might adopt a quasidimensional approach (see, e.g., Claridge, 1994, with regard to the relation between nonclinical schizotypy and clinical schizophrenia), according to which a nonclinical dimension of vulnerability interacts with a disease or injury process to cause a qualitative shift towards the more extreme manifestations that are seen in clinical disorders. This approach is taken by Fotopoulou, who argues that some delusions and confabulations involve pathological exaggerations of otherwise normal emotional biases. Finally, there is the fully dimensional approach, according to which misbeliefs exist along a continuum with clinical delusion and confabulation lying at the extreme end—in this case, there is only quantitative difference (see, e.g., Bell & Halligan, in press, for discussion).

Finally, we consider a common theme of dimensionality; our contributors consider variation along continua of implausibility, bizarreness of (delusional or confabulated) content, conviction, incorrigibility, associated distress, preoccupation, and impact upon daily life. One particularly intriguing dimension relates to the behavioural consequences of delusion and confabulation. Only Gilboa explicitly incorporates into his model control processes that mediate action, although O'Connor and colleagues vividly illustrate the debilitating behavioural consequences of misbelieving in déjà vécu. There appears to be a general assumption operating here; this is that people typically act on their beliefs. For example, it is implicit in the "propositional attitude" approach to belief that beliefs influence people's behaviour since people believe that their beliefs are true (see, e.g., Stephens & Graham, 2004). However, there is variation in the extent to which nonclinical and clinical people act on their beliefs and whether or not a clinical or a nonclinical person acts on her beliefs might be mediated by how much she cares about her belief. (The same point applies to acting on memories.) What a person cares about will normally be influenced by unconscious reward/punishment signals, emotional/motivational factors, and conscious concerns. If so, unusually passive cases of delusion and confabulation (e.g., the Capgras patient who expresses no concern about her missing spouse and fails to contact authorities, despite her conviction about the impostor) might be explained by concurrent pathologies associated with conditions like anhedonia (a lack of enjoyment, which is a common in schizophrenia) or anosodiaphoria (in anosodiaphoria, there is a dissociation between conviction and concern such that a brain-injured patient insightfully acknowledges her disability, while being oddly indifferent to the consequences of her handicap: Babinski, 1914, as cited in Critchley, 1953). The extent to which (mis)beliefs impact upon daily life will also be mediated by preoccupation. This is why clinical psychiatrists typically see delusional people who are distressed and preoccupied by their delusions, which, in turn, interfere with their daily function. It seems that current models of delusion and confabulation will need to be further augmented to incorporate mechanisms that mediate degrees of concern, preoccupation, and acting upon beliefs.[1]

[1] We thank Peter Halligan for helpful discussion of these ideas.

There is no consensus in our Special Issue with regard to fine-grained cognitive models that can account for variations of delusion and confabulation in terms of specific patterns of intact and damaged components. To advance more specific models of this type: Some contributors focus primarily on differences between delusion and confabulation; others propose a common explanatory framework (or taxonomy of processes) to guide future tests of similarity and difference; and yet others propose conceptual intersections between delusion and confabulation and suggest reciprocal usages of methodologies from one field to inform another. Although there is clearly more to learn, the novel hypotheses, theories, and methodologies discussed in this Special Issue highlight promising new directions. We conclude by returning to Kopelman's comment that false beliefs inevitably become false memories. Since beliefs about the present become memories about the past and since memories about the past influence the expectations that shape current perceptions, we think it important that theorising and research on delusion and confabulation be complementary. We hope that this Special Issue will instigate these complementary lines of theorising and research in order to advance the cognitive neuropsychiatry of both delusion and confabulation.

REFERENCES

Bell, V., & Halligan, P. W. (in press). The neural basis of abnormal personal belief. In F. Kruger & J. Grafman (Eds.), *The neural basis of human belief systems.* Hove, UK: Psychology Press.

Claridge, G. (1994). Single indicator of risk for schizophrenia: Probable fact or likely myth? *Schizophrenia Bulletin, 20*, 151–168.

Critchley, M. (1953). *The parietal lobes.* London: Edward Arnold.

Ellis, H. D., & Lewis, M. B. (2001). Capgras delusion: A window on face recognition. *Trends in Cognitive Sciences, 5*, 149–156.

Fotopoulou, A. (2010). The affective neuropsychology of confabulation and delusion. *Cognitive Neuropsychology, 15*(1/2/3), 38–63.

Hirstein, W. (2005). *Brain fiction: Self-deception and the riddle of confabulation.* Cambridge, MA: MIT Press.

Johns, L. C., & van Os, J. (2001). The continuity of psychotic experiences in the general population. *Clinical Psychology Review, 21*, 1125–1141.

Langdon, R., & Coltheart, M. (2000). The cognitive neuropsychology of delusions. *Mind and Language, 15*, 184–218.

Langdon, R., & Connaughton, E. (in press). The neuropsychology of belief formation. In F. Kruger & J. Grafman (Eds.), *The neural basis of human belief systems.* Hove, UK: Psychology Press.

Moscovitch, M., & Winocur, G. (2002). The frontal cortex and working with memory. In D. T. Stuss & R. Knight (Eds.), *Principles of frontal lobe function* (pp. 188–209). New York: Oxford University Press.

Stephens, G. L., & Graham, G. (2004). Reconceiving delusion. *International Review of Psychiatry, 16*, 236–241.

COGNITIVE NEUROPSYCHIATRY
2010, 15 (1/2/3), 14–37

Varieties of confabulation and delusion

Michael D. Kopelman
King's College London, Institute of Psychiatry, London, UK

Introduction. Different types of confabulation or false memory can arise from brain disease. There are competing explanatory theories for the mechanisms underlying confabulation. Recent literature has attempted to relate the notion of delusion to that of confabulation.
Method. A brief review of the literature relating to these ideas.
Results. The varieties of confabulation or false memory that can arise from brain disease are considered. The varieties of delusion and the contexts in which they arise are considered. Comparisons are made between the characteristics of spontaneous confabulation and those of delusional memory.
Conclusion. It is suggested that global theories purporting to account for both confabulation and delusions, in whatever circumstances they arise, can have only limited explanatory power. On the other hand, there are resemblances between confabulation and delusional memory, and the similarities and differences between these phenomena deserve further empirical investigation.

Keywords: Confabulation; False memory; Delusion; Delusional memory.

INTRODUCTION

In this paper, I will give a brief outline of the varieties of confabulation and delusion, which can arise in neurological or psychiatric disorders. Questions arise concerning whether false memories occurring in these different contexts represent the same or differing phenomena, and whether they reflect common underlying dysfunctions or deficits. In considering these issues, I will focus upon a comparison of "spontaneous confabulation" and "delusional memory".

Correspondence should be addressed to Professor Michael Kopelman, Academic Unit of Neuropsychiatry, 3rd Floor, Adamson Centre, South Wing, St. Thomas's Hospital, Lambeth Palace Road, London SE1 7EH, UK. E-mail: michael.kopelman@kcl.ac.uk

 DOI: 10.1080/13546800902732830

CONFABULATION

Types of confabulation

Confabulation broadly refers to false or erroneous memories arising in the context of neurological disease. The memories may be either false in themselves or "real" memories jumbled in temporal context and retrieved inappropriately.

Following Berlyne (1972), I distinguished between "spontaneous" confabulation and "momentary" or "provoked" confabulation (Kopelman, 1987b). In spontaneous confabulation, there is a persistent, unprovoked outpouring of erroneous memories. By contrast, in momentary or provoked confabulation, fleeting intrusion errors or distortions arise in response to a challenge to memory, such as a memory test. Others have argued (e.g., Gilboa et al., 2006) that the distinction between spontaneous and provoked confabulations is not always clear-cut. For example, in normal conversation, a question might arise which provokes a confabulation—should this be called "spontaneous" or "provoked"? However, I would maintain that, difficult though it is to draw a precise boundary, the conceptual distinction is valuable—not only because the extreme forms of spontaneous confabulation are qualitatively quite distinct from simple intrusion errors or distortions, but also because there may have differing underlying mechanisms.

Further to this distinction between spontaneous and provoked confabulations, Schnider (Schnider, von Däniken, & Gutbrod, 1996; Schnider, 2003) attempted to tighten the definition of spontaneous confabulations by requiring that patients should have actually acted upon them, a tighter but more restrictive definition than Kopelman's. Berlyne (1972) used the term "spontaneous" interchangeably with "fantastic", whereas others have viewed bizarre or fantastic confabulations as a specific subtype of spontaneous confabulation, involving an additional dysfunction (Burgess & Shallice, 1996a).

Spontaneous confabulation

> RJ's confabulation [was] not limited to test situations. He confabulated in interacting with therapists, fellow patients, and his family. For example, one weekend while at home with his family he sat up in bed and turned to his wife, asking her, "Why do you keep telling people we are married?" His wife explained that they were married and had children, to which he replied that children did not necessarily imply marriage. She then took out the wedding photographs and showed them to him. At this point he admitted that the person marrying her looked like him but denied that it was he. (Baddeley & Wilson, 1986)

> AB was a 43-year-old hospital employee, who was admitted to the Accident and Emergency department with Wernicke's encephalopathy (confusion opthalmoplegia, ataxia, and nystagmus), and she was found to have a half empty bottle of vodka in her handbag. Despite high doses of multivitamins, the patient continued to confabulate floridly, and subsequently cancer of the cervix was diagnosed. She confabulated in episodic memory, saying that she had been admitted for measles, and that her parents were visiting her regularly, despite the fact that they had been dead for 4 and 20 years respectively. She talked about being employed in the hospital, but identified the wrong hospital. She said that her brother was a doctor living on the 22nd floor, when her ward was on the top floor (the 12th). She also confabulated in semantic memory, saying that Stanley Baldwin was still the Prime Minister, and that Robert Maxwell (the newspaper proprietor) had been shot. (Kopelman, Ng, & van den Brouke, 1997)

> BS was a 61-year-old man, who had been found collapsed on a pavement by a neighbour. He was confused and disorientated, and he showed pronounced nystagmus. He was also very ataxic, and he could stand only with support. At admission, he admitted to consuming a bottle of whisky a day. He was "stuck" in the 1970s or early 1980s, thinking that Margaret Thatcher was Prime Minister and Richard Nixon was President of the United States. He confabulated in episodic memory, thinking that he had recently taken a girlfriend home to his parents at Christmas, and that he was still serving in the airforce (as he had done in the 1970s). He also confabulated in personal semantic memory, thinking that his brother had emigrated to Canada, when the brother was in fact visiting on a weekly basis, and also in semantic memory, thinking that the Pope had recently been assassinated. (Kopelman, unpublished)

These three patients exhibited pronounced examples of spontaneous confabulation. Spontaneous confabulation most commonly occurs in autobiographical memory (Dalla Barba, 1993a; Dalla Barba, Cappelletti, Signorini, & Denes, 1997), but it can occur in semantic memory as well (Dalla Barba, 1993b; Kopelman et al., 1997; Moscovitch & Melo, 1997). Spontaneous confabulation has usually been attributed to executive dysfunction, resulting from frontal lobe pathology (Baddeley & Wilson, 1986; Kapur & Coughlan, 1980; Luria, 1976; Moscovitch & Melo, 1997; Stuss, Alexander, Liberman, & Levine, 1978), but confusional states and/or metabolic disturbance can also produce executive dysfunction and confabulation (DeLuca & Cicerone, 1991; Kopelman et al., 1997).

More recently, on the basis of lesion and/or functional imaging studies, spontaneous confabulation has been attributed more precisely to pathology within either ventromedial frontal cortex and orbitofrontal cortex (Gilboa et al., 2006; Gilboa & Moscovitch, 2002; Toosy et al., 2008; Turner, Cipolotti, Yousry, & Shallice, 2008) or in orbitofrontal cortex alone (Schnider, 2008; Schnider, Treyer, & Buck, 2005).

Theories of spontaneous confabulation can be broadly subdivided into those emphasising (1) context memory confusions or a source monitoring deficit; (2) trace specification/verification (strategic retrieval) deficits; (3) motivational theories, or (4) interactionist accounts.

Context confusions/source monitoring deficits

These accounts go back to Korsakoff (1889/1955, p. 404), who argued that many of his patients confused "old recollections with present impressions":

> In telling of something about the past, the patient would suddenly confuse events and would introduce the events related to one period into the story about another period. . . . Telling of a trip she had made to Finland before her illness and describing her voyage in fair detail, the patient mixed into the story her recollections of the Crimea, and so it turned out that in Finland people always eat lamb and the inhabitants are Tartars.

Korsakoff placed emphasis upon such temporal confusions in the genesis of confabulation, rather than on complete fabrications in memory, and subsequent writers in the clinical literature also made this observation (Moll, 1915; Talland, 1965; van der Horst, 1932; Victor, Adams, & Collins, 1971).

In a series of neat experiments, Schnider (Schnider, Ptak, von Daniken, & Remonda, 2000; Schnider et al., 1996) demonstrated that spontaneous confabulators (defined in terms of their having acted upon their confabulations) could be differentiated from other amnesic patients and from healthy controls on the basis of their errors on a temporal context memory task, but not on other memory and executive tasks. Moreover, this very specific deficit subsided as the confabulation improved. Although the experimental data on which he bases his argument remain essentially the same, Schnider (2003, 2008) now interprets this dysfunction more generally as a failure in "reality monitoring", resulting from the malfunctioning of a very rapidly acting (200–300 ms) filter, located within the orbitofrontal cortex, which sets the "cortical format" for subsequent memory encoding. However, Gilboa et al. (2006) found that other difficult discriminations (unrelated to temporal context) can also produce a high rate of false positive identifications by confabulators; and in preliminary observations, Bajo, Fleminger, and Kopelman (2008) showed that most (83%), but not all, confabulators produce the predicted pattern of performance on Schnider's task.

Somewhat related is Dalla Barba's (1993a; Dalla Barba et al., 1997) variant of this hypothesis. Dalla Barba has argued that so-called "temporal consciousness" is intact in confabulating patients, but it is malfunctioning. These patients are aware of a past, present, and future (unlike severely amnesic patients), but, in making memory judgements, they employ only the most stable elements from their long-term memory stores. They tend to be "stuck" in the past, and this usually (but not always) means their early memories. Consequently, asked what they did today or what they will do tomorrow, confabulating patients reply with the well-established memories from their pasts, however irrelevant these memories may be to their present situation. Dalla Barba has investigated this deficit in patients with Korsakoff's syndrome, other amnesic patients, and Alzheimer patients. (See also Dalla Barba & Boissé, 2010 this issue.)

Trace specification and verification deficits

Moscovitch (1989) postulated a deficit in the strategic component of retrieval processes, such that loose rules of plausibility and association are left to guide memory retrieval, and the resulting "memories" are not edited or suppressed in a normal fashion. Somewhat similarly, Conway and Tacchi (1996) postulated a failure in the executive evaluation of accessed memories during confabulation, and Kopelman (1987b, p. 1482) attributed spontaneous confabulation to "the extremely incoherent and context-free retrieval of memories and associations".

Burgess and Shallice (1996a) postulated deficits in a description process, an editor process, and a mediator process, which all contributed differently to the clinical phenomena of confabulations. The "descriptor" produced a specification of the type of trace that would satisfy the demands of a retrieval task, and "noisy" specification would increase the chance of an inappropriate representation being produced as a candidate memory. The "editor" checked that the output of a long-term storage system fitted with previously retrieved memory elements, and also with the overall task requirement. When the "editor" was impaired, confabulators would respond to a question without giving it adequate consideration or without checking and self-correcting themselves, somewhat similar to a previous hypothesis which had been proposed by Mercer, Wapner, Gardner, and Benson (1977). The "mediator" controlled cognitive (strategic and problem-solving) operations concerning the adequacy or plausibility of retrieved memory elements under strategic control. Impairment of this module resulted in reasoning errors and produced bizarre or fantastic responses.

Schacter, Norman, and Koutstaal (1998) proposed a general "constructive memory framework", emphasising both encoding operations (initial binding of the distributed features of an episode together as a coherent trace with sufficient pattern separation of similar episodes) and retrieval processes (formation of a sufficiently focused retrieval description with which to probe memory stores, plus postretrieval monitoring and verification). If episodes were not stored in a manner that allowed them to be accessed separately at retrieval, *or* if retrieval cues were not specific or focused enough, *or* if criterion setting were lax, memory distortion or confabulation would be likely to result.

Moscovitch and Melo (1997) postulated that confabulation was the product of impaired cue-retrieval (cues can be ambiguous, resulting in retrieval errors in normal subjects, but especially if memory is impaired), faulty strategic search (producing misleading cues and, thereby, inappropriate memories), and defective monitoring (the resulting errors would not be edited out). More recently, Gilboa et al. (2006) have modified this theory a little, suggesting that a failure in strategic retrieval and postretrieval monitoring, related to ventromedial and orbitofrontal pathology, is critical for spontaneous confabulation to arise. They argued that postretrieval monitoring has at least two components: an early, rapid, preconscious component, impairment of which is sufficient to cause confabulation, and a conscious elaborate monitoring of retrieval content for inconsistencies, conflicting evidence, and compatibility with task requirements. They argued that a failure to make fine-grained distinctions within memory could account for Schnider's observations.

Finally Metcalf, Langdon, and Coltheart (2007), taking as their starting-point Langdon and Coltheart's (2000) model of delusional belief, argued that two deficits are likely in most cases of spontaneous confabulation—an executive retrieval deficit and an evaluation deficit. In addition, they postulated that a specific personal bias may influence the content of confabulation.

Motivational hypothesis

Conway and Tacchi (1996) had earlier argued that a person's current preoccupations and motivations can strongly influence the content of confabulation. Conway and Tacchi (1996, p. 333) gave a graphic account of how their patient used her confabulations to transform "the present into a time of harmony and comfort rather than distress" in a manner not dissimilar from Blanche Dubois in *A Streetcar Named Desire.* They explained the patient's confabulation in terms of a combination of a failure of the executive editing of memories and of motivational biases.

Following this line of argument, Fotopoulou and colleagues (Fotopoulou, Conway, Griffiths, Birchall, & Tyrer, 2007; Fotopoulou, Conway, & Solms, 2007; Fotopoulou, Conway, Solms, Tyrer, & Kopelman, 2008; Fotopoulou, Solms, & Turnbull, 2004) have demonstrated that the content of confabulations are more likely to include pleasant experiences or positive self-representations than the corresponding "reality". Confabulating patients are also more likely to identify incorrectly pleasant autobiographical memories as currently relevant. (See Fotopoulou, 2010 this issue; also Turnbull, Jenkins, & Rowley, 2004).

In this connection, Jaspers's (1913/1974) distinction between the "content" or "theme" of abnormal mental phenomena (including motivational factors) and their "form" (relating to an underlying deficit or dysfunction) needs to be drawn.

Interaction accounts

Johnson and colleagues (Johnson, 1991; Johnson, Hashtroudi, & Lindsay, 1993) argued that confabulation might result from a wide range of source (context) or reality monitoring deficits (differentiating "real" memories from the imagined) which, in turn, could be secondary to impairments in encoding, retrieval, motivation, or judgement processes. However, Johnson, O'Connor, and Cantor (1997) failed to show that a severely confabulating patient differed from three other patients with frontal lesions in terms of performance on several measures of source monitoring. Hence, they concluded that confabulation might reflect an interaction between three factors—a vivid imagination, an inability to retrieve autobiographical memories systematically, and source monitoring deficits.

Somewhat similarly, Kopelman et al. (1997), following a detailed analysis of a severely confabulating patient's errors, suggested that many confabulations (particularly in episodic memory) result from the conflation and inappropriate retrieval of "real" memory fragments out of temporal sequence, but that other confabulations result from perseverations (particularly in semantic memory), or from the patient giving instantaneous, ill-considered, and unchecked responses to immediate environmental and social cues.

Momentary confabulation

The fleeting intrusion errors or distortions made by patients in memory tests (e.g., story recall) resemble those made by healthy subjects in many contexts. As Bartlett (1932, 175 [1995 reissue]) wrote of story recall:

> Epithets are changed into their opposites; incidents and events are transposed; names and numbers rarely survive intact ... opinions and conclusions are reversed. ...At the same time, the subjects may be very well satisfied with their efforts believing themselves to have passed on all important features with little or no change. ...Condensation, elaboration and invention are common features of ordinary remembering.

Consistent with this, Hammersley and Read (1986) found that healthy subjects were more vulnerable to interference effects from misleading information when recalling a story at 1 week's delay than at immediate recall, and that misleading information was most likely to produce errors if it was presented shortly before the recall of a story. Similar intrusions and distortions by both adults and children have been demonstrated in other experimental tasks (Lindsay & Read, 1994; Read & Lindsay, 1997; Schacter et al., 1998).

Kopelman (1987b) deliberately compared the recall of amnesic patients with that of healthy controls at a prolonged delay. The recall of Logical Memory passages by Korsakoff and Alzheimer patients at immediate recall and 45 minutes' delay was compared with that of healthy controls at a 1-week delay. This design reduced the overall level of the healthy participants' recall scores to nearer that of the amnesic patients, and 47% of the healthy participants showed some evidence of momentary confabulation at the 1-week delay compared with 50% of the Korsakoff patients and 44% of the Alzheimer group at immediate or 45 minutes' delay. Moreover, there were qualitative similarities between the intrusion errors produced by each group. Consequently, Kopelman concluded that momentary or provoked confabulation in patients reflects "normal" mechanisms that occur when memory is "weak".

Although "momentary confabulations" are usually a "normal" phenomenon arising when memory is poor, and do not imply any underlying pathology, Turner et al. (2008) have recently argued that, in patients with ventromedial or orbitofrontal pathology, both spontaneous and provoked confabulations can arise.

Summary

In summary, spontaneous confabulation can be profuse, bizarre, preoccupying, and held with absolute conviction. Spontaneous confabulations appear to result from ventromedial or orbitomedial neuropathology. They may reflect faulty trace specification and verification (monitoring) of retrieved memories, confusions in temporal context, perseverations especially in semantic memory, an unchecked response to social or environmental cues, and/or underlying motivational and emotional biases. By contrast, momentary or provoked confabulations are fleeting distortions or intrusion errors. These can be seen in healthy subjects when their memory is "weak", and so do not necessarily imply any underlying pathology, although Turner et al. (2008) have recently suggested that ventro- or orbitomedial frontal pathology can also give rise to these confabulations.

OTHER FORMS OF FALSE MEMORY

Kopelman (1999) described other instances in which false memory can arise, some of which are not necessarily related to overt neurological damage.

The false recognition syndrome

Patients with frontal lesions have been described who show a high rate of false recognition responses on cognitive testing, not necessarily related to "extensive" spontaneous confabulation (Delbecq-Derouesné, Beauvois, & Shallice, 1990; Parkin, Bindschaedler, Harsent, & Metzler, 1996; Schacter, Curran, Galluccio, Milberg, & Bates, 1996). In two of these patients (Parkin et al., 1996; Schacter et al., 1996), the pathological false recognition appeared to be particularly evident when novel material was presented from previously studied semantic categories, but it was also present in response to nonstudied words, pseudowords, faces, and environmental sounds. It was suggested that false alarms arose when the test items were "generally" (Schacter et al.) or "incidentally" (Parkin et al.) consistent with the class, category, or characteristics of a study list, and that the patients failed to recollect the identity of particular items. In such instances, both patients seemed to show an overreliance on familiarity judgements. However, unlike confabulating patients, these patients showed a relative preservation of recall for everyday experiences. It remains unclear whether such cases provide a "model" for one particular component of spontaneous confabulation, or whether theirs is a qualitatively distinct disorder.

Recovered memory for childhood sexual abuse

This hugely controversial topic has been extensively reviewed elsewhere (e.g., Conway, 1997; Read & Lindsay, 1997). It has been claimed that many apparently recovered memories of childhood sexual abuse are likely to be false, particularly if retrieved after a long delay or in response to leading questions by therapists. Although cases of forgetting of traumatic experiences, including childhood sexual abuse, have certainly been reported (Loftus, Polonsky, & Fullilove, 1994), and empirical evidence of recovery of such memories has also been described (Brewin, 2007; Schooler, Ambadar, & Bendiksen, 1997), it seems likely that at least some recovered memories are false. Shimamura (1997) documented evidence that highly emotional or traumatic experiences can enhance memory storage transiently but in a fragmented form, in which "free floating" memory fragments are poorly located in temporal and spatial context, particularly in the absence of memory rehearsal. On the basis of what is known about frontal and medial-temporal mechanisms in memory, Shimamura argued that such memory fragments would be especially vulnerable both to forgetting and to distortions and augmentations such that, if memory were reinstated, it would be very unlikely to be either accurate or complete. A somewhat similar argument was proposed by Schacter (1996; Schacter, Norman, & Koutstaal,

1997). In addition, the genesis of such erroneous memories almost certainly cannot be understood independently of the social contexts in which they arise (Kopelman, 1997).

Confabulation in schizophrenia

Nathaniel-James and Frith (1996) described "confabulation" in schizophrenic patients. They required their patients to recall a fable/story, and then to identify the correct moral from it. They found a significantly increased rate of intrusion errors or confabulations in schizophrenic patients' recall compared with healthy participants. This remained true even after attempting to control for the level of recall performance, and it appeared to be correlated with performance on an executive test (the Hayling; Burgess & Shallice, 1996b). The authors argued that these patients' confabulations were qualitatively different from those made by healthy subjects in that they tended to introduce irrelevant or unrelated material into the stories, and, in a subsequent investigation, Nathaniel-James, Foong, and Frith (1996) showed that the schizophrenic patients were unable to distinguish plausible from implausible stories or to correct their errors after listening to a tape-recording of their own recall. However, Kopelman (1999) argued that it remained possible that the "confabulations" of schizophrenic patients are simply momentary intrusion errors and distortions, resulting from the impaired memory which has been previously described in such patients, coloured by their preoccupying delusional beliefs (see later).

False confessions

Gudjonsson (2003) has described the various circumstances in which people come to make false confessions on a voluntary basis (see also Gudjonsson & MacKeith, 1988), which he labels "confabulations". For example, Gudjonsson, Kopelman, and MacKeith (1999) described a case of false confession in a 17-year-old man who was eventually released from prison 25 years later. He was a man of low self-esteem and high suggestibility who, during the course of a police interview lasting 48 hours (in the absence of a lawyer or doctor) in which he was in a distressed and aroused state, progressed from thinking "It might have been me" to "I don't know if I killed her or not. I keep seeing her", through "I must have done it because I can see a picture of her" to "I am sure I killed her ... I know I did it." One of the factors that contributes to false confessions is source amnesia (Johnson et al., 1993), which gives rise to a form of "memory distrust", such that interviewees become confused concerning whether "memories" have been generated internally or from external sources of information (source memory errors).

The false confessions which result may then become internalised, in which case Gudjonsson describes them as "confabulations"; in a series of investigations, Gudjonsson and colleagues have investigated the circumstances and correlates of such false confessions.

Pseudologia fantastica

Occasional patients are seen who create a web of fantasies, lies, and untruths around themselves, almost compulsively, and Fish (1967) classified this phenomenon as a form of confabulation. This tends to occur in people who are of low IQ or self-esteem, but who do not have known brain disease or frontal lobe dysfunction. Kopelman (1999) reported a young man, poorly educated and not very bright, who talked endlessly about being a pop star, about the other stars he knew, and about his show business activities, despite the fact that it soon became clearly apparent that he had led a fairly mundane life in South London. He had given himself a derivation of a famous pop star's name, and he claimed that he was "world-wide famous in Streatham". Such activity is not necessarily harmless. In the case of R. v. O'Brien and others, 1999 (also known as the "Cardiff 3"), the Court of Appeal established that Mr H's confession to the murder of a milkman 12 years' earlier (which had resulted in his imprisonment and that of two acquaintances) was likely to have been a fabrication. Mr H had lied about many things during his childhood and adolescence, claiming (for example) to have been a successful rugby football player (he was crippled following a series of operations for two club feet). One of the most persuasive pieces of evidence in court came from his former solicitor, who described how Mr H had confessed to a previous offence, which he could not have done because he was being interviewed by the police for something else at the time that that alleged offence had taken place!

Summary

In brief, false memories can arise in many situations, which are not necessarily related to overt neurological damage. Hence, Kopelman (1999) put forward a model which incorporated input from the social environment. It also incorporated a personal semantic belief system which biased retrieval from autobiographical memory, into which I have now incorporated prevailing preoccupations, mood state, and personal fantasy to take account of the motivational biases within a person's confabulation (Figure 1). Some forms of false memory are a direct consequence of neurological damage, e.g., spontaneous confabulation as a result of damaged control or "filter" systems within the ventromedial and orbitomedial frontal regions, or the false

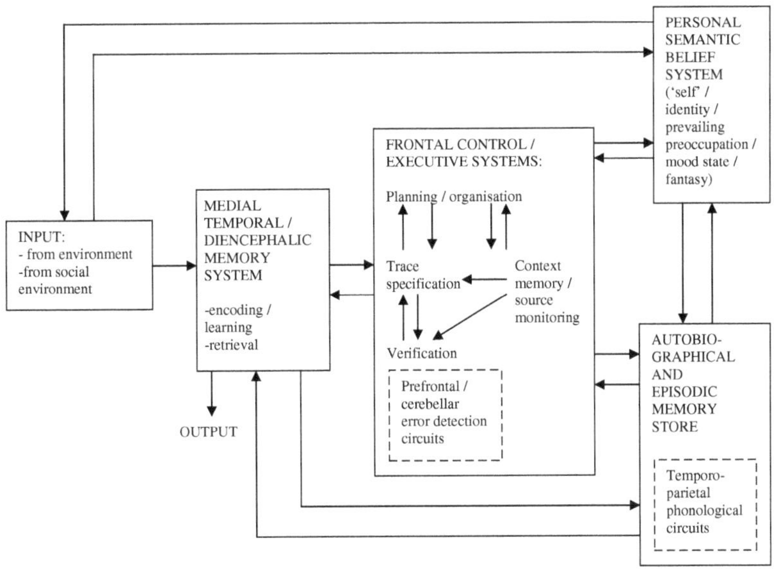

Figure 1. Social, personal, and biological (brain) systems involved in producing confabulations, false recognitions, and false memories.

recognition syndrome arising from dysfunction in Schacter et al.'s (1996) postulated prefrontal/cerebellar error detection circuits. Other forms of false memory derive from a combination of psychosocial input, prevailing emotional preoccupations, mood state, and/or personal fantasies biasing the frontal control mechanisms, and giving rise to, e.g., source memory errors and internalised confabulations in false confession or the "confabulations" of schizophrenia.

DELUSIONS

A delusion is a false belief, held as an absolute conviction, not amenable to argument, not culturally explicable, often bizarre, and usually preoccupying (Clare, 1976; Kopelman, 1994; Mullen, 1986).

The content and character of delusions may take many forms (Cutting, 1997; Gelder, Gath, & Mayou, 1983; Mellor, 1970; Mullen, 1986; Schneider, 1959). Among the so-called first-rank symptoms of schizophrenia are delusions of control (relating to actions, affect, or volition) and delusions concerning thoughts (thought insertion, thought withdrawal, or thought diffusion/"broadcasting"). Grandiose delusions may occur in mania or in frontal lobe disease. By contrast, depression may give rise to delusions of worthlessness or guilt, hypochondriacal/somatic delusions, or nihilistic delusions including Cotard's syndrome. Religious delusions may occur in a variety of syndromes, including epilepsy. Delusions of reference and persecutory delusions may occur in many psychiatric and neurological disorders, including alcohol- or substance- induced psychoses. Sexual, amorous, or jealous delusions also occur in various contexts, particularly alcohol abuse. Delusions of being burgled are characteristic of dementia. Delusions of misidentification, e.g., the Capgras syndrome, can occur in either neurological or psychiatric disorder; in the former, they tend to be associated with combined right parietal and frontal pathology (Alexander, Stuss, & Benson, 1979; Ellis & Young, 1990).

Furthermore, delusions arise in differing circumstances (Cutting, 1997; Mullen, 1986; Schneider, 1959). For example, delusions can occur apparently "out of the blue" (primary or autochthonous delusions), or they may emerge from a particularly perplexed psychological state (known as "delusional mood" or "delusional atmosphere"), in which a sense of perplexity, foreboding, dread, and anxiety precedes the occurrence of frank delusions. Alternatively, delusions can arise secondarily to a "real" perception (as in the misleadingly called "delusional perception" or in somatic passivity experiences), or as a consequence of hallucinations (e.g., auditory hallucinations expressing derogatory or persecutory ideas). Delusions can also emerge secondarily to an affective state (mania, depression), or in consequence of an acute medical disorder (e.g., confusion, delirium tremens) or chronic neurological disease (e.g., temporal lobe epilepsy, dementia). As already mentioned, there is a somewhat different flavour to delusions in these different situations, and any comprehensive theory of delusions needs to account for this.

Cognitive theories of delusions will be the major topic of some of the other papers in this volume. Amongst these theories, Maher (1992) has argued that delusions or false beliefs arise as rational responses to abnormal perceptual experiences. Ellis and Young (1990; Ellis, Young, Quayle, & de Pauw, 1997) attributed the Capgras delusion to disrupted signalling of the emotional or affective significance of a face in the two-route model of face processing (Bauer, 1984; Bruce & Young, 1986); and they attributed the Fregoli delusion to dysfunction in the person identity nodes and the cognitive system of that model. Similarly, Young, Robertson, Hellawell, de Pauw, and Pentland (1992) attributed the Cotard delusion to an underlying lack of feelings of familiarity, resulting in a sense of unreality (compare Leafhead & Kopelman, 1997). Frith and Corcoran (1996) attributed persecutory delusions in part to abnormal "theory of mind" experiences, and Bentall (2003) to an abnormal pattern of attributions, protecting the individual against chronic feelings of low-self esteem. The latter might also relate to Garety and Freeman's (1999) finding that psychotic patients tend to jump to conclusions on probabilistic reasoning tasks. Coltheart and colleagues (e.g., Davies & Coltheart, 2000; Langdon & Coltheart, 2000; McKay, Langdon, & Coltheart, 2005, 2007) have argued in favour of (1) a primary perceptual/affective deficit, which distorts or makes anomalous current sensory information, semantic or autonomic input, or emotional experience; and (2) an abnormality in belief evaluation, which causes the uncritical acceptance/maintenance of an implausible hypothesis or belief. In addition, there may be personal attributional biases which nuance the favoured explanations that are generated to account for the anomalous experience.

There are two points that can be made here. First, it is not clear that any of these theories can account for the entire variety of delusional beliefs, the differing circumstances in which they can arise, and for why particular delusions characterise specific disorders/age groups. In order to explain such phenomena, the present very general theories have to be stretched in diverse directions. Bell, Halligan, and Ellis (2006) have made a related point, whilst distinguishing between theories which explain delusions as a breakdown of normal belief formation, those which explain only the pathology, and those approaches which view delusions as one end of a continuum of anomalous mental phenomena. Figure 2 attempts to incorporate some of these factors into the Langdon and Coltheart (2000) model. Hence, it indicates that the prevailing psychological state, hallucinations, mood state (compare Cutting, 1997; Mullen, 1986; Turnbull & Solms, 2007), or somatic disease can precipitate delusion formation, whether by promoting a perceptual anomaly and/or by producing a deficit in belief evaluation. Likewise, the age and sex of an individual, not to mention his/her underlying clinical condition (as discussed above) can influence the content and character of the specific delusions which arise. This model leaves to be clarified whether delusions always result from a perceptual anomaly or whether they can occur "out of the blue" or secondary to a "real/true" perception, as traditional theory postulates (Jaspers, 1923/1963; Schneider, 1959).

Second, unlike confabulation, delusions are not in themselves necessarily a memory phenomenon, although they become incorporated into memory. For example, relatively common delusions—for instance, that one's thoughts are being controlled or that one has a special religious mission, or that spies are lining up outside the house—do not necessarily have a memory component, but instead may result from an anomalous perceptual experience, abnormal attentional biases, or from a dysfunctional belief evaluation system.

By contrast, delusional memories clearly are a memory phenomenon, although it should be noted that delusions are common in psychiatric patients whereas delusional memories are rare.

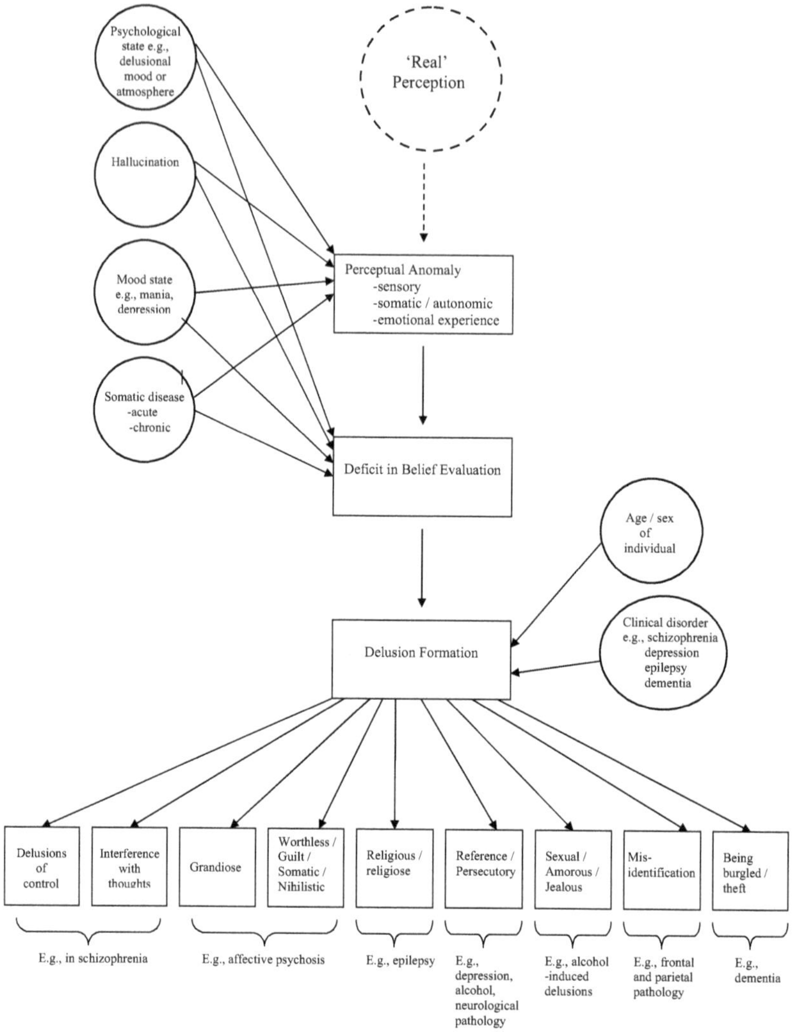

Figure 2. Modified model of delusion formation incorporating precipitating factors to delusion formation and factors influencing the content or theme of a particular delusion.

DELUSIONAL MEMORIES

Definitions

In the literature on psychiatric phenomenology, differing definitions of delusional memory are given, well summarised by Buchanan (1991). For example, Mullen (1986) described delusional memory as "a delusional insight [which] occurs not as an intuition about the world or as a change in knowledge of or about the world but in the form of a memory". Buchanan argued that this definition of delusional memory is analogous to Jaspers's (1923/1963) concept of a "delusional idea". By contrast, Gelder et al. (1983) stated that: "It is not the memory that is delusional but the interpretation that has been applied to it." Buchanan (1991, 472) stated that this definition is much more analogous to Jaspers's (1923) concept of "delusional perception" (a "real" perception giving rise to delusional interpretation). Buchanan pointed out that Schneider (1959) incorporated both definitions: "If a special meaning is subsequently attached to a remembered percept, then this becomes a delusional perception with two component parts. ... A similar belief can also be held as a delusional intuition [idea] if, for example, it comes into someone's head that he [she] had supernatural gifts as a child." In other words, a delusional memory can be akin to either a delusional perception or a delusional idea (intuition).

This duality of description led Kopelman (1997) to define delusional memory as consisting of *either* a true memory that gives rise to a deluded interpretation *or* (perhaps more commonly) a false memory arising in the context of a psychosis.

Case examples

DL was a 33-year-old man, first seen in 1981, 7 years after a high profile murder in London. Lord Lucan had disappeared after his children's nanny was found battered to death at the family's Belgravia home, and Lady Lucan had also been viciously beaten up. To this day, Lord Lucan has never been found, although sightings have been reported intermittently in various parts of the world. DL gave a graphic account of having being hired to carry out the attempted killing of Lady Lucan, claiming that he had been introduced to Lord Lucan at a nightclub, where the plan had been put to him and Lady Lucan had been pointed out to him. He recalled that he had indeed assaulted Lady Lucan, and that he had killed both Lord Lucan and the couple's nanny, and he described in detail both the meeting at which he had been hired and the killings. The account was so convincing that I was wondering about telephoning the police until the patient told me about the "angels" on the bonnet of his car. There was no evidence of any neurological or medical condition, but this "memory" occurred in the context of other "first-rank" symptoms of schizophrenia (the patient's first episode). Following treatment with a neuroleptic medication (thioridazine), these delusional preoccupations were substantially ameliorated, although, as commonly occurs in such cases, the "memory" was never completely abolished. (Kopelman, 1997)

WM was a 47-year-old clerical worker, who was studying part time for a PhD in English Literature, and she was extremely articulate about Chaucerian and Shakespearian literature. However she claimed that, in 1970, she had been working on a fruit-picking farm during the summer in East Anglia, when she encountered an internationally famous orchestral conductor, who also happened to be fruit-picking there. No words were exchanged between them, but she claimed that, subsequently, he traced her, and he followed her in London, and that her friends had challenged him about this. She reported that she retreated to a rural town, where her parents were then living, but the musician followed her there. She believed that he was in love with her, and she said that she was prepared "to meet him half way". She claimed that he had recently been divorced, and he was psychologically unsettled at that time. Subsequently, he stopped pursuing her, and they have exchanged only a few words since, when she waited for him outside stage doors. However, she had written to him on a regular basis, although never receiving a reply. On one occasion, he was sent a final demand by an expensive London store after she had purchased a wedding dress and had arranged for the bill to be sent to him. On another occasion, she deposited her suitcases outside his flat, intending to move in. Although being of apparently very sober, sensible demeanour, this patient also described "first-rank" symptoms of schizophrenia, including thought insertion, thought diffusion, and controlled actions. All her abnormal beliefs appeared to derive from her "memory" of meeting the conductor on a fruit farm, and there is no evidence that that meeting ever took place. (Kopelman, Guinan, & Lewis, 1995)

FJ, an Irishman, had been 39 when he was charged with killing his employer and friend in an arson attack at the friend's newspaper store in 1976. The testimony against him came from two Irish acquaintances, who were arrested and charged with the murder shortly after it happened, and who turned evidence against him. When seen by psychiatrists 3 months before the trial, FJ was described as truculent, irritable, and difficult but not psychotic and fit to plead. However, during the course of the trial, FJ started to believe that the prison officers were poisoning his drinking water, that gas was being piped through a hole in the wall into his Old Bailey cell, and that there was a conspiracy against him involving the prosecution lawyers, the Judge, and ultimately his own lawyers. Consequently, FJ fired his own lawyers, carried out his own defence and, perhaps not surprisingly, he was convicted of the murder. Twenty-five years later, FJ had not developed any new psychotic symptoms in the intervening period, but he retained his abnormal beliefs as absolute convictions, and they had now become delusional memories. His conviction was overturned as "unsafe" in 2002 when he was 65, i.e., 26 years after his arrest. (Kopelman, unpublished)

Patient P was a 24-year-old PhD student at a well-known university. He had been abused by his stepfather when aged 12, and the stepfather was subsequently convicted of abusing someone else. During his teenage years and early twenties, P coped with the situation by consuming lots of alcohol and cannabis. P had had one brief homosexual relationship and a number of girlfriends. Following a difficult time in his life (involving the break-up of a relationship and unforeseen difficulties in his research which were not P's fault), he started to feel very stressed, and he went to see a staff counsellor. He talked about the abuse in early adolescence, and about his alcohol and cannabis consumption. He then started to talk about his father having abused him, and he confronted his father about this. Over the next few days, the accusations multiplied, involving claims of sexual abuse by his aunt, mother, and grandparents. A few days after this, P became overtly psychotic, believing that his therapist was in a conspiracy with his father. He was treated with a neuroleptic (trifluoperazine), and his delusional beliefs subsided over the next 2 to 3 weeks. At that point, there were still dim "memory fragments" but, eventually, he came to believe that only his stepfather had abused him, and indeed there was no evidence of abuse by any other relative. It appeared that these delusional memories emerged as an elaboration of one "real" memory in the context of a psychotic disorder, possibly alcohol and cannabis precipitated. (Kopelman, unpublished)

Delusional memory and spontaneous confabulation

In three of the above examples (DL, WM, P), the delusional memories appeared to arise spontaneously as false memories in the context of psychosis. In the fourth example (FJ), the delusional memories were not "true memories giving rise to a deluded interpretation" but consisted of false memories of "events" still being given a deluded interpretation (i.e., that they really did happen). Although it might be argued that, in this sense, any memory of an "old" delusion could be interpreted as a delusional memory, the difference is that FJ was still experiencing these memories with absolute ("delusional") conviction and the desire to act upon them, whereas he was no longer experiencing any other hallucinations or delusions in his current everyday life, and he had not done so since his conviction 25 years earlier.

In any event, delusional memory is by definition a memory phenomenon, and it is the closest analogue in psychiatric patients of spontaneous confabulation in neurological cases. By definition, a delusional memory is held as an absolute conviction, not amenable to argument, and not culturally explicable. Moreover, delusional memories are usually intensely preoccupying and often bizarre. Similar features have been described in spontaneous confabulation by Baddeley and Wilson (1986), who pointed to closely similar characteristics in the confabulations of a patient with bilateral frontal damage following a traumatic head injury. Hence, the clinical phenomena of delusional memories can closely resemble those of spontaneous confabulations.

However, there appear to be certain respects in which delusional memories differ from spontaneous confabulations. The first is that they may be more elaborate and systematised, and sometimes they occur in people who are otherwise functioning normally without obviously abnormal behaviour (Baddeley, Thornton, Chua, & McKenna, 1996; Kopelman, 1999; Kopelman et al., 1995). This was true of the first two examples given earlier, and also of the third man when he was seen in 2002. Second, but related to this first point, delusional memory patients are often cognitively intact, whereas patients exhibiting spontaneous confabulation almost invariably show impairment on standard tests of executive function and are often profoundly amnesic. In the Kopelman et al. (1995) case, WM had a verbal IQ of 131, and she did not show any evidence of executive or anterograde memory impairment. Patient P had a NART-R IQ of 113, and he scored in the normal or superior range on Logical Memory, immediate and delayed, the Recognition Memory Test for words and faces, the Autobiographical Memory Interview, the Modified Card-Sorting test, cognitive estimates, and Trailmaking B. Similarly, David and Howard (1994) reported that four patients with delusional memories showed normal performance on the cognitive estimates test (Shallice & Evens, 1978); and Baddeley et al. (1996) concluded that the delusional memories and delusional beliefs of schizophrenic patients, although often bizarre, did not simply reflect a breakdown in executive function or autobiographical memory.

In summary, although delusional memories share many characteristics with spontaneous confabulation, they differ in that delusional memories appear to be thematic and unrelated to executive dysfunction, whereas confabulations are usually fluctuating and multifaceted as well as virtually always related to executive dysfunction (Baddeley et al., 1996; Kopelman et al., 1995; but see Burgess & McNeil, 1999).

However, the similarities and differences between delusional memories and spontaneous confabulation deserve further investigation. Moreover, although I am arguing that they should (at least for the present) be kept conceptually distinct, it must be acknowledged that, occasionally, certain specific forms of delusion, such as delusional misidentification, can coincide with or evolve from spontaneous confabulations, because of common underlying (frontal) pathology (Benson & Stuss, 1990; Box, Laing, & Kopelman, 1999; Mattioli, Miozzo, & Vignolo, 1999).

CONCLUSION—THE REQUIREMENTS FOR THEORY

Any comprehensive theory of false memories needs to take account of the very different situations in which false memories arise. Most existing theories focus purely upon spontaneous confabulation in brain disease. Kopelman (1999) considered various tentative possibilities. In spontaneous confabulation, ventromedial and orbitofrontal damage affect trace specification and verification systems, whereas momentary confabulation appears to result from a "normal" response to a "weak" memory trace. In delusional memory, Kopelman suggested that there may be anomalous processing of input modulated by personal self-beliefs, mental state, and expectations. In false confession, source memory errors occur, usually in the context of low self-esteem and/or depression and social coercion. In pseudologia fantastica, there may be anomalous, biased, or selective retrieval from autobiographical memory. Some of these phenomena may arise from a combination of factors, e.g., the absence of rehearsal and a particular social context in cases of false memories for child abuse. In others, an interaction between social and biological factors may be important, e.g., the confabulations produced by brain-damaged patients in very stressful or extreme situations. These possibilities were interpreted within a very general model of memory and executive function, where social factors and a notion of "self" were incorporated (Kopelman, 1999), but they need to be explored further. Cognitive models need to accommodate the full range of contexts in which false memories can arise.

Second and similarly, any theory of delusions needs to take account of all the circumstances, primary and secondary, in which delusions arise, and the fact that they can have very different characteristics and content across these different contexts. It is not entirely clear that the existing models are able to do this, except in very general terms, but Figure 2 attempts to incorporate (in a preliminary fashion) some of the pertinent factors that can precipitate a delusion and/or determine its particular content or theme.

Third, confabulations, delusions, and delusional memories, in my view, need to be kept conceptually distinct. Although confabulations and delusional memories are, by definition, memory phenomena, other delusions may primarily reflect abnormal perceptual, attentional, or interpretative (belief) phenomena, even though they come to be incorporated into memory subsequently.

Although spontaneous confabulation and delusional memories share many characteristics, they differ in that confabulations tend to be fluctuating and multifaceted, as well as virtually always related to executive dysfunction, whereas delusional memories appear to be thematic and unrelated to executive dysfunction. However, specifying the characteristics and underlying psychopathology of these two memory phenomena remains an issue for further empirical investigation.

REFERENCES

Alexander, M. P., Stuss, D. T., & Benson, D. F. (1979). Capgras syndrome: A reduplicative phenomenon. *Neurology, 29*, 334–339.

Baddeley, A. D., Thornton, A., Chua, S. E., & McKenna, P. (1996). Schizophrenic delusions and the construction of autobiographical memory. In D. C. Rubin (Ed.), *Autobiographical memory* (2nd ed.). Cambridge, UK: Cambridge University Press.

Baddeley, A. D., & Wilson, B. (1986). Amnesia, autobiographical memory, and confabulation. In D. C. Rubin (Ed.), *Autobiographical memory* (pp. 225–252). Cambridge, UK: Cambridge University Press.

Bajo, A. Fleminger, S., & Kopelman, M. D. (2008, September). *Ongoing reality monitoring versus mood state in determining confabulation*. Poster presented at the first meeting of the Federation of European Neuropsychological Societies.

Bartlett, F. C. (1932). *Remembering: A study in experimental and social psychology*. Cambridge, UK: Cambridge University Press.

Bauer, R. M. (1984). Autonomic recognition of names and faces in prosopagnosia: A neuropsychological study. *Neuropsychologia*, *22*, 457–469.

Bell, V., Halligan, P. W., & Ellis, H. D. (2006). Explaining delusions: A cognitive perspective. *Trends in Cognitive Sciences*, *10*(5), 219–226.

Benson, D. F., & Stuss, D. T. (1990). Frontal lobe influences on delusions: A clinical perspective. *Schizophrenia Bulletin*, *16*, 403–411.

Bentall, R. P. (Ed.). (2003). *Madness explained: Psychosis and human nature*. London: Penguin.

Berlyne, N. (1972). Confabulation. *British Journal of Psychiatry*, *120*, 31–39.

Box, O., Laing, H., & Kopelman, M. D. (1999). The evolution of spontaneous confabulation, delusional misidentification and a related delusion in a case of severe head injury. *Neurocase*, *5*, 251–262.

Brewin, C. R. (2007). Autobiographical memory for trauma: Update on four controversies. *Memory*, *15*(3), 227–248.

Bruce, V., & Young, A. W. (1986). Understanding face recognition. *British Journal of Psychology*, *77*, 305–327.

Buchanan, A. (1991). Delusional memories: First-rank symptoms? *British Journal of Psychiatry*, *159*, 472–474.

Burgess, P. W., & McNeil, J. E. (1999). Content-specific confabulation. *Cortex*, *35*, 163–182.

Burgess, P. W., & Shallice, T. (1996a). Confabulation and the control of recollection. *Memory*, *4*, 359–411.

Burgess, P. W., & Shallice, T. (1996b). Response suppression, initiation and strategy use following frontal lobe lesions. *Neuropsychologia*, *34*, 263–273.

Clare, A. (1976). *Psychiatry in dissent: Controversial issues in thought and practice*. London: Tavistock.

Conway, M. A. (Ed.). (1997). *Recovered memories and false memories*. New York: Oxford University Press.

Conway, M. A., & Tacchi, P. C. (1996). Motivated confabulation. *Neurocase*, *2*, 325–339.

Cutting, J. (1997). *Principles of psychopathology*. Oxford, UK: Oxford Medical Publications.

Dalla Barba, G. (1993a). Confabulation: Knowledge and recollective experience. *Cognitive Neuropsyschology*, *10*, 1–20.

Dalla Barba, G. (1993b). Different patterns of confabulation. *Cortex*, *29*, 567–581.

Dalla Barba, G., & Boissé, M. F. (2010). Temporal consciousness and confabulation: Is the medial temporal lobe "temporal"? *Cognitive Neuropsychiatry*, *15*(1/2/3), 95–117.

Dalla Barba, G., Cappelletti, J. Y., Signorini, M., & Denes, G. (1997). Confabulation: remembering "another" past, planning "another" future. *Neurocase*, *3*, 425–436.

David, A. S., & Howard, R. (1994). An experimental phenomenological approach to delusional memory in schizophrenia and late paraphrenia. *Psychological Medicine*, *24*, 515–524.

Davies, M., & Coltheart, M. (2000). Introduction: Pathologies of belief. In M. Coltheart & M. Davies (Eds.), *Pathologies of belief* (pp. 1–46). Malden, MA: Blackwell Publishers.

Delbecq-Derouesné, J., Beauvois, M. F., & Shallice, T. (1990). Preserved recall versus impaired recognition. *Brain*, *113*, 1045–1074.

DeLuca, J., & Cicerone, K. D. (1991). Confabulation following aneurysm of the anterior communicating artery. *Cortex*, *27*, 417–423.

Ellis, H. D., & Young, A. W. (1990). Accounting for delusional misidentifications. *British Journal of Psychiatry*, *157*, 239–248.

Ellis, H. D., Young, A. W., Quayle, A. H., & de Pauw, K. W. (1997). Reduced autonomic responses to faces in Capgras delusion. *Proceeding of the Royal Society of London: Biological Sciences*, *B264*, 1085–1092.

Fish, F. (1967). *Clinical psychopathology: Signs and symptoms in psychiatry.* Bristol, UK: John Wright & Sons.

Fotopoulou, A. (2010). The affective neuropsychology of confabulation and delusion. *Cognitive Neuropsychiatry, 15*(1/2/3), 38–63.

Fotopoulou, A., Conway, M., Griffiths, P., Birchall, D., & Tyrer, S. (2007). Self-enhancing confabulation: Revisiting the motivational hypothesis. *Neurocase, 13*, 6–15.

Fotopoulou, A., Conway, M. A., & Solms, M. (2007). Confabulation: Motivated reality monitoring. *Neuropsychologia, 45*, 2180–2190.

Fotopoulou, A., Conway, M. A., Solms, M., Tyrer, S., & Kopelman, M. D. (2008). Self-serving confabulation in prose recall. *Neuropsychologia, 46*, 1429–1441.

Fotopoulou, A., Solms, M., & Turnbull, O. (2004). Wishful reality distortions in confabulation: A case study. *Neuropsychologia, 42*(6), 727–744.

Frith, C., & Corcoran, R. (1996). Exploring "theory of mind" in people with schizophrenia. *Psychological Medicine, 26*, 521–530.

Garety, P. A., & Freeman, D. (1999). Cognitive approaches to delusions: A critical review of theories and evidence. *British Journal of Clinical Psychology, 38*, 113–154.

Gelder, M., Gath, D., & Mayou, R. (1983). *Oxford textbook of psychiatry.* Oxford, UK: Oxford University Press.

Gilboa, A., Alain, C., Stuss, D. T., Melo, B., Miller, S., & Moscovitch, M. (2006). Mechanisms of spontaneous confabulations: A strategic retrieval account. *Brain, 129*, 1399–1414.

Gilboa, A., & Moscovitch, M. (2002). The cognitive neuroscience of confabulation: A review and a model. In A. D. Baddeley, M. D. Kopelman, & B. A. Wilson (Eds.), *The handbook of memory disorders* (2nd ed., pp. 315–342). Chichester, UK: Wiley.

Gudjonsson, G. H. (2003). *The psychology of interrogations and confessions: A handbook.* Chichester, UK: Wiley.

Gudjonsson, G. H., Kopelman, M. D., & MacKeith, J. A. C. (1999). Unreliable admissions to homicide: A case of misdiagnosis of amnesia and misuse of abreaction technique. *British Journal of Psychiatry, 174*, 455–459.

Gudjonsson, G. H., & MacKeith, J. A. C. (1988). Retracted confessions: Legal, psychological and psychiatric aspects. *Medicine, Science and the Law, 28*, 187–194.

Hammersley, R., & Read, J. D. (1986). What is integration? Remembering a story and remembering false implications about the story. *British Journal of Psychology, 77*, 329–341.

Jaspers, K. (1974). Causal and "meaningful" connections between life history and psychosis. In S. R Hirsh & M. Shepherd (Eds.), *Themes and variations in European psychiatry* (pp. 81–93). Bristol, UK: John Wright & Sons. (Original work published 1913)

Jaspers, K. (1923). *Allgemeine Psychopathologie* (3rd ed.). Berlin: Springer. [Translated (1963) by J. Hoenig & M. W. Hamilton, Manchester University Press.]

Johnson, M. K. (1991). Reality monitoring: Evidence from confabulation in organic brain disease patients. In G. P. Prigatano & D. L. Schacter (Eds.), *Awareness of deficit after brain injury: Clinical and theoretical issues* (pp. 176–197). New York: Oxford University Press.

Johnson, M. K., Hashtroudi, S., & Lindsay, D. S. (1993). Source monitoring. *Psychological Bulletin, 114*, 3–28.

Johnson, M. K., O'Connor, M., & Cantor, J. (1997). Confabulation, memory deficits, and frontal dysfunction. *Brain and Cognition, 34*, 189–206.

Kapur, N., & Coughlan, A. K. (1980). Confabulation and frontal lobe dysfunction. *Journal of Neurology, Neurosurgery and Psychiatry, 43*, 461–463.

Kopelman, M. D. (1987a). Amnesia: Organic and psychogenic. *British Journal of Psychiatry, 150*, 428–442.

Kopelman, M. D. (1987b). Two types of confabulation. *Journal of Neurology, Neurosurgery and Psychiatry, 50*, 1482–1487.

Kopelman, M. D. (1994). Structured psychiatric interview: Psychiatric history and assessment of the mental state. *British Journal of Hospital Medicine, 52*, 93–98.

Kopelman, M. D. (1997). Anomalies of autobiographical memory: Retrograde amnesia, confabulation, delusional memory, psychogenic amnesia, and false memories. In J. D. Read & D. S. Lindsay (Eds.), *Recollections of trauma: Scientific research and clinical practice* (pp. 273–303). New York and London: Plenum Press.

Kopelman, M. D. (1999). Varieties of false memory. *Cognitive Neuropsychology, 16*, 197–214.

Kopelman, M. D., Guinan, E. M., & Lewis, P. D. R. (1995). Delusional memory, confabulation, and frontal lobe dysfunction: A case study in de Clerambault's syndrome. *Neurocase, 1*, 71–77.

Kopelman, M. D., Ng, N., & van den Brouke, O. (1997). Confabulation extending across episodic memory, personal and general semantic memory. *Cognitive Neuropsychology, 14*, 683–712.

Korsakoff, S. S. (1955). Psychic disorder in conjunction with peripheral neuritis (Trans. and repub. by M. Victor & P. I. Yakovlev). *Neurology, 5*, 394–406. (Original work published 1889)

Langdon, R., & Coltheart, M. (2000). The cognitive neuropsychology of delusions. *Mind and Language, 15*(1), 183–216.

Leafhead, K. M., & Kopelman, M. D. (1997). Face memory impairment in the Cotard delusion. In A. Parkin (Ed.), *Case studies in the neuropsychology of memory* (pp. 195–177). Hove, UK: Lawrence Erlbaum Associates Ltd.

Lindsay, D. S., & Read, J. D. (1994). Psychotherapy and memories of childhood sexual abuse: A cognitive perspective. *Applied Cognitive Psychology, 8*, 281–338.

Loftus, E. F., Polonsky, S., & Fullilove, M. T. (1994). Memories of childhood sexual abuse: Remembering and repressing. *Psychology of Women, 18*, 67–84.

Luria, A. R. (1976). *The neuropsychology of memory.* New York: Wiley.

MacKay, R., Langdon, R., & Coltheart, M. (2005). "Sleights of mind": Delusions, defences and self-deception. *Cognitive Neuropsychiatry, 10*, 305–326.

MacKay, R., Langdon, R., & Coltheart, M. (2007). The defensive function of persecutory delusions: An investigation using the implicit association test. *Cognitive Neuropsychiatry, 12*, 1–24.

Maher, B. A. (1992). Delusions: Contemporary etiological hypotheses. *Psychiatric Annals, 22*, 260–268.

Mattioli, F., Miozzo, A., & Vignolo, L. A. (1999). Confabulation and delusional misidentification: A four year follow-up study. *Cortex, 35*, 413–422.

Mellor, C. S. (1970). First-rank symptoms of schizophrenia. *British Journal of Psychiatry, 117*, 15–23.

Mercer, B., Wapner, W., Gardner, H., & Benson, D. (1977). A study of confabulation. *Archives of Neurology, 34*, 429–433.

Metcalf, K., Langdon, R., & Coltheart, M. (2007). Models of confabulation: A critical review and new framework. *Cognitive Neuropsychology, 24*(1), 23–47.

Moll, J. M. (1915). The amnesic or Korsakoff's syndrome with alcoholic aetiology: An analysis of 30 cases. *Journal of Mental Science, 61*, 423–437.

Moscovitch, M. (1989). Confabulation and the frontal system: Strategic versus associative retrieval in neuropsychological theories of memory. In H. L. Roediger & F. I. Craik (Eds.), *Varieties of memory and consciousness: Essays in honour of Endel Tulving* (pp. 133–160). Hillsdale, NJ: Lawrence Erlbaum Associates, Inc.

Moscovitch, M., & Melo, B. (1997). Strategic retrieval and the frontal lobes: Evidence from confabulation and amnesia. *Neuropsychologia, 35*, 1017–1034.

Mullen, P. E. (1986). The mental state and states of mind. In P. Hill, R. Murray, & A. Thorley (Eds.), *Essentials of postgraduate psychiatry.* London: Grune & Stratton.

Nathaniel-James, D. A., Foong, J., & Frith, C. D. (1996). The mechanisms of confabulation in schizophrenia. *Neurocase, 2*, 475–483.

Nathaniel-James, D. A., & Frith, C. D. (1996). Confabulation in schizophrenia: Evidence of a new form? *Psychological Medicine, 26*, 391–399.

Parkin, A. J., Bindschaedler, C., Harsent, L., & Metzler, C. (1996). Pathological false alarm rates following damage to the left frontal cortex. *Brain and Cognition, 32*, 14–27.

Read, J. D. & Lindsay, D. S. (Eds.). (1997). *Recollections of trauma: Scientific research and clinical practice*. New York: Plenum Press.

Schacter, D. L. (1996). *Searching for memory: The brain, the mind, and the past*. New York: Basic Books.

Schacter, D. L., Curran, T., Galluccio, L., Milberg, W. P., & Bates, J. F. (1996). False recognitions and the right frontal lobe: A case study. *Neuropsychologia, 34*, 793–808.

Schacter, D. L., Norman, K. A., & Koutstaal, W. (1997). The recovered memories debate: A cognitive neuroscience perspective. In M. A. Conway (Ed.), *Recovered memories and false memories* (pp. 63–99). New York: Oxford University Press.

Schacter, D. L., Norman, K. A., & Koutstaal, W. (1998). The cognitive neuroscience of constructive memory. *Annual Review of Psychology, 49*, 289–318.

Schneider, K. (1959). *Clinical psychopathology*. New York: Grune & Stratton.

Schnider, A. (2003). Spontaneous confabulation and the adaptation of thought to ongoing reality. *Nature Reviews Neuroscience, 4*, 662–671.

Schnider, A. (2008). *Confabulations and memory's reality*. Oxford, UK: Oxford University Press.

Schnider, A., Ptak, R., von Däniken, C., & Remonda, L. (2000). Recovery from spontaneous confabulations parallels recovery of temporal confusion in memory. *Neurology, 55*, 74–83.

Schnider, A., Treyer, V., & Buck, A. (2005). The human orbito-frontal cortex monitors outcomes even when no reward is at stake. *Neuropsychologia, 43*, 316–323.

Schnider, A., von Däniken, C., & Gutbrod, K. (1996). The mechanisms of spontaneous and provoked confabulations. *Brain, 119*, 1365–1375.

Schooler, J. W., Ambadar, Z., & Bendiksen, M. (1997). A cognitive corroborative case study approach for investigating discovered memories of sexual abuse. In J. D. Read & D. S. Lindsay (Eds.), *Recollections of trauma: Scientific evidence and clinical practice* (pp. 379–388). New York: Plenum Press.

Shallice, T., & Evens, M. E. (1978). The involvement of the frontal lobes in cognitive estimates. *Cortex, 14*, 294–303.

Shimamura, A. P. (1997). Recollection: Perspectives on reinstated memory and child trauma. In J. D. Read & D. S. Lindsay (Eds.), *Recollections of trauma: Scientific evidence and clinical practice* (pp. 253–272). New York: Plenum Press.

Stuss, D. T., Alexander, M. P., Liberman, A., & Levine, H. (1978). An extraordinary form of confabulation. *Neurology, 28*, 1166–1172.

Talland, G. A. (1965). *Deranged memory*. New York: Academic Press.

Toosy, A. T., Burbridge, S. E., Pitkanen, M., Loyal, A. S., Akanuma, N., Laing, H., et al. (2008). Functional imaging correlates of fronto-temporal dysfunction in Morvan's syndrome. *Journal of Neurology, Neurosurgery and Psychiatry, 79*, 734–735.

Turnbull, O. H., Jenkins, D., & Rowley, M. L. (2004). The pleasantness of false beliefs: An emotion-based account of confabulation. *Neuropsycholoanalysis, 6*, 5–16.

Turnbull, O. H., & Solms, M. (2007). Awareness, desire and false beliefs: Freud in the light of modern neuropsychology. *Cortex, 43*, 1083–1090.

Turner, M. S., Cipolotti, L., Yousry, T. A., & Shallice, T. (2008). Confabulation: Damage to a specific inferior prefrontal system. *Cortex, 44*, 637–648.

Van der Horst, L. (1932). Über die psychologie des Korsakow syndroms. *Monatsschrift für Psychologie und Neurologie, 83*, 65–84.

Victor, M., Adams, R. D., & Collins, G. H. (1971). *The Wernicke-Korsakoff syndrome*. Philadelphia: F. A. Davis Co.

Young, A. W., Robertson, I. H., Hellawell, D. J., de Pauw, K. W., & Pentland, B. (1992). Cotard delusion after brain injury. *Psychological Medicine, 22*, 799–804.

COGNITIVE NEUROPSYCHIATRY
2010, 15 (1/2/3), 38–63

The affective neuropsychology of confabulation and delusion

Aikaterini Fotopoulou

Institute of Cognitive Neuroscience, University College London, London, UK

The paper reviews the history of the scientific understanding of the role of emotion in confabulation and delusion. I argue that the significance of emotion in the pathogenesis of these symptoms was obscured by academic polarisation between psychodynamic and neurocognitive traditions and was also often obfuscated by rigid distinctions between psychogenic and neurogenic explanations. This tradition of epistemic dualism was implicitly maintained in the fields of cognitive neuropsychology and cognitive neuropsychiatry. This paper focuses on memory-related confabulation following ventromedial frontal lobe lesions, awareness-related confabulation following right perisylvian lesions, and delusions of various aetiologies. Ambiguity regarding the definition and taxonomy of symptoms renders direct comparison difficult, but certain overriding principles are becoming discernible. Recent findings suggest that emotion and motivation influence both confabulation and delusion. These influences may be instigated directly by neural dysfunction or indirectly by life changes and altered social circumstances, or by a combination of these. Importantly, the rejection of epistemic dualism in the conceptualisation of both symptoms can allow us to study them in parallel and draw conclusions about the relation between cognition and emotion. Specifically, confabulation and delusion can be described as faulty attempts to balance the conflicting demands of accurate and self-serving reality representation.

Keywords: Confabulation; Delusion; Emotion; Motivation; Reality monitoring.

Correspondence should be addressed to Aikaterini (Katerina) Fotopoulou, Institute of Cognitive Neuroscience, University College London, Alexandra House, 17 Queen Square, London WC1N 3AR, UK. E-mail: a.fotopoulou@ucl.ac.uk

I would like to thank the organisers of the Symposium on Confabulation and Delusion, Max Coltheart, Robyn Langdon, and Martha Turner. I am grateful to Ryan McKay, and all other presenters of the symposium, for their inspiring presentations and for helping me shape my thoughts on these issues. I would also like to thank Martin Conway for his support in organising a similar symposium during the fourth international conference on Memory in Sydney and all the participants of that symposium.

 DOI: 10.1080/13546800903250949

INTRODUCTION

Until recently, research on emotion was limited in both cognitive science and neuroscience. Emotion was considered too elusive to be studied in the laboratory, despite the pivotal role ascribed to it by great nineteenth-century scholars such as William James, Sigmund Freud, and John Hughlings Jackson. This neglect penetrated neurology, psychiatry, and their relationship during most of the twentieth century. In this paper, I will focus on the role of emotion in confabulation and delusion, as this role was conceptualised in neurology and psychiatry. I will argue that the influence of affective processes in false memories and beliefs was deemphasised due to rigid distinctions between psychogenic and neurogenic explanations. I will further discuss how this tradition of epistemic dualism was implicitly maintained in the fields of cognitive neuropsychology and cognitive neuropsychiatry. Subsequently, I will present recent approaches to confabulation and delusion that take emotions into account and I will review supportive empirical evidence. These perspectives can be heuristically labelled as *the "affective neuropsychology" of confabulation and delusion.*

Defining delusions, confabulations, and their relation

Delusions are considered a critical clinical manifestation of psychosis and are of determining importance in the diagnosis of schizophrenia. Notwithstanding their diagnostic significance, defining delusions has proven a persistent, rarefied challenge. Delusions are typically described by diagnostic manuals as firmly sustained false beliefs, which are resistant to correction and are not shared by members of the same sociocultural group. Yet the utility of these characteristics is repeatedly questioned. Characteristically, even the notion that delusions represent beliefs has incited considerable objections (see Bayne & Pacherie, 2005, for review). Some scholars have concluded that delusions are context-dependent, multidimensional, and impossible to adequately define (David, 1999). Others have proposed heuristic definitions. For example, Oltmanns (1988) suggested that the presence of delusions can be verified by checking the presence of a number of different characteristics, without assuming any of them is necessary or sufficient for defining delusions.

The term "confabulation" was first used at the turn of the twentieth century, substituting Korsakoff's term "pseudoreminiscences" (Korsakoff, 1889/1996), to describe the false recollections of amnesic patients. Amnesic confabulatory behaviour is nowadays considered pathognomonic of Wernicke-Korsakoff's syndrome, and is reported in many other neuropathologies (see Johnson, Hayes, D'Esposito, & Raye, 2000, for a meta-analysis). In this memory-related use of the term, confabulations are understood as false memories produced without conscious knowledge of their falsehood. Relative consensus surrounds this definition (Dalla Barba, 1993; Johnson et al., 2000; Moscovitch, 1989). Less agreement exists regarding the subtypes and characteristics of memory-related confabulation, but some evidence suggests that spontaneous confabulations may be distinct phenomena from provoked memory errors (see, for review, Kopelman, 2010 this issue; Schnider, 2003). Typically, confabulatory content is operationally described as disorganised, polythematic, and fleeting (Baddeley & Wilson, 1986). However, organised, content-specific, and persistent confabulations have also been reported (Baddeley & Wilson, 1986; Burgess & McNeil, 1999).

Furthermore, the term confabulation is also used to describe the false statements of patients in many other memory-independent neurological syndromes, such as Anton's syndrome (unawareness of blindness), unawareness of hemiplegia, and cerebral disconnection syndromes (DeLuca, 2000; Feinberg & Roane, 1997; Hirstein, 2005). In these syndromes, patients' general memory abilities are not typically compromised. However, their ability to perceive and draw correct inferences about themselves and their environment is defective. Thus, they can unintentionally produce erroneous statements about their condition, or their abilities ("awareness-related confabulation"). For example, cortically blind patients with Anton's syndrome may deny any subjective experience of visual loss. However, it should be noted that the behaviour which constitutes confabulation in these patients is not identical across studies of even the same syndrome. For example, in anosognosia for hemiplegia one may designate as a confabulation patients' general erroneous assessment of their bodily state (e.g., "There is nothing wrong with my arm, I can move it"; Davies, Davies, & Coltheart, 2005), or one can refer only to instances of "illusory limb movements" (e.g., when the patient claimed he moved his arm as instructed by the examiner at that particular moment; Feinberg, Roane, & Ali, 2000), or just to associated somatoparaphrenic beliefs (e.g., this arm belongs to my niece) and false memories (e.g., false events and excuses, e.g., I went walking yesterday and I am tired now).

In an attempt to clarify the use of the term confabulation across domains, some authors distinguish between its various applications (e.g., DeLuca, 2000; Feinberg & Roane, 1997; Fotopoulou & Conway, 2004). For instance, Feinberg and Roane (1997) distinguish between "neutral" and "personal" confabulation. Neutral confabulation relates to an underlying deficit (e.g., cortical blindness) in any sensory domain and it is usually confined to that domain. By contrast, personal confabulation includes self-referential content that is not restricted to any sensory domain, is held with delusional conviction, and is refractory to correction. Unfortunately, these distinctions are not consistently used in the literature. In the remainder of the paper,

I will use the term confabulation to refer to two syndromes: namely "memory-related confabulation" following damage to the ventromedial frontal lobe (VFL) and "awareness-related confabulation" as it occurs following perisylvian lesions to the right hemisphere and in relation to anosognosia for hemiplegia (unawareness of paralysis). Although one may observe that at the level of individual symptoms, VFL patients may also produce some confabulations that relate to unawareness of deficit and patients with right perisylvian lesions (RPL) may also produce some confabulations about past events, the terms "awareness-related confabulation" and "memory-related confabulation" will be used here to refer to these two different neuropathological syndromes, which are marked primarily by one or other type of confabulation and which are associated with RPL versus VFL damage, respectively.

Given the aforementioned ambiguity about the defining characteristics and subtypes of both delusion and confabulation, the relation between the two phenomena is not clearly delineated. Thus far, no single criterion has been proposed as sufficient or necessary to distinguish between them (Gilleen & David, 2005; Kopelman, 1999). Although confabulations have diagnostic use mainly within neurology and delusions within psychiatry, delusions also occur following acquired brain injury or disease (e.g., Feinberg & Roane, 1997). For example, some authors describe anosognosia for hemiplegia as a delusion (e.g., Davies et al., 2005). Similarly, memory-related confabulation is reported in the context of schizophrenia (e.g., Nathaniel-James & Frith, 1996). Some studies distinguish delusions from confabulations in the same patient population (Baddeley, Thornton, Chua, & McKenna, 1996; Lee et al., 2007; Mattioli, Miozzo, & Vignolo, 1999), but the criteria for such distinctions seem arbitrary and are rarely used in more than a handful of studies. Others claim that they represent different facets of the same underlying aetiology. For example, Hirstein (2005) argues that confabulations, delusions, and the false memories of healthy individuals can be defined along a continuum of self-deception. Attempting to disentangle and to clarify the overall relation between the two concepts goes beyond the scope of this paper. Here I will consider each symptom as it has been addressed within its respective field and I will focus on the role of emotion in both phenomena.

EMOTION IN CONFABULATION

Classic views: Memory-related confabulation as deficit, compensation, or defence

Memory-related confabulation was first described by Korsakoff (1889/1996) as a symptom of a specific memory disorder caused by "multiple neuritis, which is an extensive inflammation and degeneration of nerves throughout the body" (p. 2). Given this neurological background, various early authors attempted to differentiate "organic" confabulations from other forms of false memories and beliefs (e.g., "delusional memories") that were encountered in disorders without a known "organic" aetiology (for review, see Markova & Berrios, 2000). Similar distinctions between organic and nonorganic explanations of symptoms (e.g., motor paralysis) were more widely established. Progressively, the divide between psychiatry and neurology grew deeper. Memory-related confabulation fell on the neurological side of the division and thus it was considered a "neurogenic" memory failure. Not surprisingly, the primary focus of studies on memory-related confabulation in the first half of the twentieth century was on specifying its neurological aetiology and its relation to amnesia.

By contrast, describing memory-related confabulation as motivated was synonymous with negating its neurogenic nature and indeed some authors did (see next section). Emotion and motivation were seen as the mark of psychogenic processes and thus their role in organic disease could only be conceptualised as secondary. Thus, for those neurologists and psychiatrists who were convinced by the clear neurological onset of memory-related confabulation, potential observations of motivational factors had to be deemphasised. For instance, in one of Talland's (1961) case descriptions he noted that "motivational influences undoubtedly played their part in producing her glib evasive answers as well as her obstinate adherence to a past image of herself, but the mechanism by which such influences interacted with the amnesic derangement could not be determined" (p. 376). Several other authors recognised motivational factors in confabulating patients. Given however the more general assumption of a rigid distinction between cognitive deficits (as impairments to functions directly subserved by brain processes) and emotional consequences (as secondary reactions to a new psychological reality, essentially unrelated to the damaged brain structures and functions) it was hard to assume a direct interaction between a memory dysfunction and emotion. Hence, Talland concluded his influential review with this frequently quoted statement: "Confabulation serves no other purpose, is motivated in no other way than factual information based on genuine data" (p. 393).

At the other extreme, some authors proposed that memory-related confabulation is not "neurogenic", but is instead caused by some psychogenic compensatory mechanisms. The "embarrassment hypothesis" proposed that memory-related confabulation occurs as a purposive act contrived by the patient to spare him from the embarrassment of not being able to remember the events of his life (see Talland, 1961, for review). This perspective explained confabulation as the result of some compensatory motivational mechanism, which is essentially unrelated to normal memory processes and the neurocognitive deficits leading to their impairment. This view was criticised as patients seemed genuinely unaware of their memory errors (anosognosic) and many confabulating patients did not show a tendency to increase their confabulation rate when they were confronted with questions to which they did not know the answer (see Schnider, 2008, for review).

The incoherent and at times wishful quality of memory-related confabulation was frequently compared to the recollective quality of dreams and this led some psychodynamic authors to suggest that the individual's wishes guided memory-related confabulation in the same way as they controlled dream fantasy (reviewed by Berlyne, 1972). More generally, several early authors attributed the occurrence of memory-related confabulation, at least in part, to tendencies inherent in the patient's premorbid personality structure, such as increased suggestibility, or denial coping strategies (see Berlyne, 1972; Fotopoulou, 2009; Schnider, 2008, for reviews). Notwithstanding these descriptions, psychodynamic interpretations of memory-related confabulation were relatively scarce. The hypothesis that confabulation is a form of "psychological denial", i.e., a compensatory coping mechanism instigated by excessive anxiety, was mostly advanced in the work of Weinstein and colleagues (for review, see Weinstein, 1996). They observed that the patients most likely to show confabulation and denial of deficit were the ones characterised by their relatives as premorbidly stubborn, introverted with regard to their feelings, and prestige- and power-seeking. In addition, these patients had premorbidly been using coping mechanisms such as denial and minimisation when confronted with other health issues. Their theory emphasised that although confabulations frequently involve references to past events, they are to some degree, symbolic representations, or dramatisations of some current personal preoccupation or disability. These symbolic functions are based on kernels of awareness of deficit, i.e., confabulations implicitly express illness preoccupations and anxieties, which the patient is not capable of fully appreciating (see also Feinberg & Roane, 1997). Finally, Weinstein (1996) observed that during the narration of confabulations, patients become engrossed in detail, lose their previous irritability, and then appear utterly relaxed. He thus argued that memory-related confabulation seems to have an ultimate adaptive role.

Although these views highlighted potential positive aspects of memory-related confabulation, there was little experimental evidence in their support. In a study on senile dementia, Gainotti (1975) found that 75% of the tested confabulating patients were described by their relatives as having a strong tendency to seek prestige and domination and to deny, ignore, or rationalise illness prior to their brain disease. However, these coping mechanisms were considered independent of the specific neuropathological features of the syndromes they aimed to explain. Thus, their explanatory power with regards to the syndromes themselves was limited. Indeed, Weinstein (1996) acknowledged that these descriptions were less likely to be relevant to spontaneous confabulation with vivid imagery, as reported in patients with anterior communicative artery aneurysms and anterior cingulectomies. Nevertheless, not all psychodynamic authors considered emotional mechanisms in isolation. Instead, some regarded the emotional manifestations of confabulation as the direct consequence of cognitive dysfunctions. For instance, Betlheim and Hartman (1924/1951) argued that the characteristic amnesic derangement of the Korsakoff syndrome caused a lack of cognitive restraint. This, in turn, allowed the normally implicit effect of primitive, emotion-based forms of cognition to become more explicit and colour recollection even under controlled experimental conditions. Thus, memory-related confabulation is regarded as the direct result of an organically caused dysfunction of the normal mechanisms of remembering.

Yet in the following decades this perspective received little experimental attention. Instead, the more simple "embarrassment" or "defence" explanations were established as the motivational hypotheses, only to be deemphasised and largely dismissed as more sophisticated neurocognitive models of memory-related confabulation came to the foreground (see next section). This dominance of "cooler" cognitive explanations coincided with a more general and at times rather passionate academic rejection of the once prevalent field of psychoanalysis. Although the criticisms were often validated and substantiated by solid empirical data, it has more recently become apparent that some psychodynamic ideas may be worth investigating and possibly integrating with current neuroscientific knowledge (e.g., Kaplan-Solms & Solms, 2000; McKay, Langdon, & Coltheart 2005).

Modern views: The cognitive neuropsychology of memory-related confabulation

Consistent with the tradition of cognitive neuropsychology, research on memory-related confabulation in the last decades has predominately approached confabulation as a useful symptom from which one can infer neurocognitive models of normal memory function (e.g., Dalla Barba, 1993; Gilboa et al., 2006). In this tradition, two main classes of theories have been put forward: explanations that focus on impaired temporality or reality monitoring (Dalla Barba, 1993; Johnson et al., 2000; Schnider, 2003) and explanations that emphasise deficits in the control of memory retrieval (Burgess & Shallice, 1996; Gilboa et al., 2006; Moscovitch, 1989). With regard to the first main class of theories, confabulating patients are conceived to misattribute experiences of a given time to events that occurred at another time, or to confuse the order of experienced events (Dalla Barba, 1993;

Talland, 1961; Schnider, 2003). In a similar vein, it has been suggested that confabulating patients are unable to distinguish between real and imagined events (Johnson et al., 2000), or alternatively that they are unable to distinguish between events that are currently relevant and those that are not (Schnider, 2003; but see Gilboa et al., 2006).

With regard to the second main class of theories, memory-related confabulation has been explained as a deficit in the control of memory retrieval. Memory-related confabulation can concern both experiences encoded and stored before the onset of brain damage as well as experiences that occur subsequent to the brain damage. Thus, memory-related confabulation seems to be associated more with retrieval rather than encoding or storage difficulties. In the "strategic" or "generative" retrieval accounts, confabulation is explained as a deficit in the strategic processes that are required during the organised and accurate retrieval of memories (Burgess & Shallice, 1996; Conway & Tacchi, 1996; Moscovitch, 1989). According to these models, when memories are not elicited directly or automatically by a cue, a number of control processes, including memory search and monitoring processes, are called for to guide recollection. Memory-related confabulation represents a failure of one or more of these processes.

These models have undoubtedly increased our understanding of memory-related confabulation. Given the recent technological sophistication of neuroimaging, these studies have also been able to specify the sites necessary for these higher order memory functions, such as the orbitofrontal cortex and the ventromedial prefrontal cortex (e.g., Schnider, 2003; Turner, Cipolotti, Yousry, & Shallice, 2008). However, the emotional facets of memory-related confabulation seem to have been neglected by cognitive neuropsychologists even more than they were previously deemphasised by neurologists and psychiatrists. With the marked exception of a case study by Conway and Tacchi (1996), no study on memory-related confabulation published in the 1980s or 1990s focuses on the emotional content of confabulation (although see Feinberg & Roane, 1997, and Kopelman, 1999, for clinical and theoretical considerations). It is of note that the role of emotion in memory-related confabulation was not empirically tested and rejected on the grounds of negative findings. Instead, until the twenty-first century the emotional content of memory-related confabulation was for the most part left outside the scope of empirical investigations of confabulation.

The affective neuropsychology of memory-related confabulation: The return of the emotional

Fotopoulou and colleagues (reviewed by Fotopoulou, 2008), motivated by the clinical descriptions of Conway and Tacchi (1996) and Solms (2000), aimed to systematically assess the role of emotion in memory-related confabulation. The main hypothesis put forward by these investigators was that the false recollections of confabulating patients should show a self-serving bias that is greater than that typically encountered in the memory distortions of healthy volunteers (Walker, Skowronski, & Thompson, 2000). Of course, the vicissitudes of human motivation extend far beyond self-serving biases. However, this operationalisation was considered a useful first step to the challenge of systematically studying the role of emotion in memory-related confabulation. Moreover, this exaggeration of self-serving biases in memory was not seen as an exaggeration of motivation per se (a psychogenic explanation). Instead, it was conceptualised as the direct outcome of reduced executive control over memory. There seems to be a trade-off between the influence of cognitive inhibition and motivational influences on memory (Conway, 2005). For example, although emotion typically enhances memory, trying to suppress the emotional impact of an event may lead to worse memory for the event (Gross, 2002). Consequently, impairment in one aspect (retrieval control and inhibition) may generate exaggeration in the other (excessive influence of emotion on memory). Specifically, when irrelevant memory representations are not inhibited and memories are not retrieved in an appropriate manner (as the various neurocognitive theories support; see earlier), motivational factors may acquire a greater role in determining which memories are selected for retrieval and accepted as true. This lack of affective regulation in memory was expected due to the typically reported damage to the ventromedial frontal cortex in memory-related confabulation, which is more generally thought to be responsible for affective regulation (e.g., Bechara, Damasio, & Damasio, 2000) and particularly the inhibition and extinction of previously rewarded responses (Elliott, Friston, & Dolan, 2000). Thus, damage to these areas may also lead to a failure of extinction or inhibition of rewarding representations in the domain of personal memory. Therefore, personally "rewarding" representations may be preferentially selected over other, less positive candidate thoughts and memories, irrespective of their low pertinence to reality.

Consistent with this hypothesis, a number of single-case and group studies on memory-related confabulation (e.g., Fotopoulou, Conway, Tyrer, et al., 2008; Fotopoulou, Solms, & Turnbull, 2004) found that the content of spontaneous confabulations contains mostly positive and wishful descriptions (to a degree greater than that found in the memory distortions of healthy volunteers). A positive bias has also been observed in the provoked confabulations, elicited during an autobiographical memory interview, in another patient with memory-related confabulation (Fotopoulou, Conway, Griffiths, Birchall, & Tyrer, 2007). In the latter study, the patient's confabulations portrayed a self-representation that was more positive than that depicted in his real memories and those depicted in the memories of matched healthy controls. A further case series ($N = 4$) showed that patients with memory-related confabulation were more likely to make reality monitoring errors, accepting false or temporally irrelevant information as part of their recent past, when the information was pleasant rather than unpleasant (Fotopoulou, Conway, & Solms, 2007). For example, a patient was significantly more likely to falsely claim that he actually remembered winning the lottery recently than to falsely claim that he remembered losing his job. Finally, in a recent prose recall study, patients with memory-related confabulation ($N = 15$) showed a strong selective bias in recalling negative self-referent stories, in that they recalled such information in a manner which portrayed a more positive image of themselves (Fotopoulou, Conway, Solms, Tyrer, & Kopelman, 2008). This positive bias was not present in stories that were not encoded in a self-referent manner, and was significantly greater than that observed in the recall of healthy volunteers and amnesic nonconfabulating patients. This study shows that patients with memory-related confabulation do not have a difficulty in processing negative emotions in general. Instead, they show a specific self-related motivational bias in their memory.

In the studies reviewed here, patients frequently described themselves as being in familiar surroundings, and as performing professional or leisure activities, instead of being at the hospital (see also Turnbull, Berry, & Evans, 2004). Patients also often minimised their current disabilities and attributed them to premorbid traits and attitudes (e.g., "I could never remember names"). Moreover, some patients persistently denied the death of close relatives and other unpleasant events of the remote or recent past and they were noted to inflate their abilities, exaggerate their previous professional skills, and overstate their social and financial position (Fotopoulou, Conway, Griffiths, et al., 2007). Given the close link between autobiographical memory and personal identity (Conway, 2005; McAdams, 2001), we have conceptualised these tendencies in the content of memory-related confabulation as serving at least two functions: self-enhancement (embellishment of one's self-image) and self-coherence (adherence to one's premorbid self-image) (Fotopoulou, 2008). In the first case, patients' confabulations point to a tendency to inflate one's current or past self-identity; in the second case patients' confabulations seem to establish a sense of self-continuity with one's past (premorbid) identity. Both tendencies have been noted in the autobiographical distortions of healthy volunteers (see Conway, 2005, for review).

More generally, social psychology has provided considerable evidence that people are motivated to view their current self favourably and engage in considerable memory distortion in order to maintain such a view (e.g., Walker et al., 2000). This is particularly evident in older adults who show a strong self-serving positivity bias in their autobiographical recollections and this seems to have positive effects on their mood and well-being (for review, see Mather & Carstensen, 2005).

Normally aging adults and patients with memory-related confabulation show deterioration and dysfunction respectively in prefrontal brain regions (Hedden & Gabrieli, 2004). We therefore have claimed that the resulting deterioration of executive memory processes may be causing the observed exaggeration of self-enhancement and self-coherence in the memory of both normally aging adults and patients with memory-related confabulation (Fotopoulou, Conway, Solms, et al., 2008). This proposal is consistent with recently emerging models of memory-related confabulation that include personal goals and wishful ideation among the critical factors that may determine the retrieval of false memories in confabulating patients (Gilboa et al., 2006; Johnson et al., 2000; Kopelman, 1999; Metcalf, Langdon, & Coltheart, 2007). Acknowledging the role of emotion in memory-related confabulation has also pivotal clinical consequences (see Fotopoulou, 2008, for review). It thus seems that at least some authors have recognised that emotion may have a determining role in memory-related confabulation and that a total psychological picture of the syndrome requires consideration of the interaction between neurocognitive factors and emotion.

I have thus far emphasised that memory-related confabulation may not result from the exaggeration of psychological motivation per se, but rather from an exaggeration (due to neurocognitive impairment) of the organically predetermined influence of motivation on memory formation. It is, however, plausible that given the self-threatening situation patients find themselves in after brain damage, the psychological need to avoid recalling negative self-referent information may be exaggerated (a secondary, indirect effect of brain damage). Furthermore, certain patients may be premorbidly more inclined than others to hold a positive self-regard and distort memories in self-enhancing ways, depending on their previous coping strategies, social role, and other psychosocial characteristics. Thus, potential individual differences should not be excluded from the understanding of memory-related confabulation without further study.

Awareness-Related Confabulation and Negative Emotions

The Dalla Barba confabulation battery (1993) was used to measure the propensity to confabulate about personal facts, personal past episodes, knowledge of famous facts and famous people, and orientation in time and place in a consecutive series of 15 patients with right perisylvian lesions (RPL) resulting in anosognosia for hemiplegia (AHP) (Fotopoulou, 2005; Fotopoulou & Conway, 2004). We found an increased propensity to confabulate on the battery in five of these individuals (Fotopoulou, 2005; Fotopoulou, unpublished data). Specifically, although these five patients with RPL confabulated less on average than 15 patients with VFL lesions and memory-related confabulation recruited in the same period (Fotopoulou, Conway, Tyrer, et al., 2008), they confabulated more than amnesic nonconfabulatory patients, nonconfabulating controls with RPL, and healthy controls. Four of these patients with RPL and awareness-related confabulation were also clearly attempting to act upon their confabulations, e.g., one patient "secretly" called her lawyer to say that she was healthy but nevertheless held in hospital against her will. There was no obvious neuroanatomical difference between the lesions of patients with RPL and AHP who showed awareness-related confabulation and those who did not.

The patients with RPL and awareness-related confabulation appeared better oriented in time and place than the patients with VFL damage and memory-related confabulation and they also performed better on tests of executive functions, and episodic and autobiographical memory (Fotopoulou, 2005; Fotopoulou & Conway, 2004). Despite these relatively preserved abilities, patients with awareness-related confabulation produced false statements about their bodily and mental integrity and their direct everyday-living implications. Unlike the memory-related confabulations of patients with VPF lesions, awareness-related confabulations rarely extended to the remote past. Emotional differences between the two confabulation syndromes were also noted. The valence of anosognosic false statements in patients with RPL was mostly positive (e.g., "I am not paralysed. There is nothing wrong with me"). However, the majority of the associated false memories and beliefs (indirectly linked to patient's disabilities) were predominately negative, often "paranoid" or self-scolding in content. For example, one patient frequently believed that certain members of staff were trying to kill her. At times she described specific murder attempts. We used the same method we had used previously to measure the valence of memory-related confabulation in patients with VFL lesions (Fotopoulou et al., 2004; Fotopoulou, Conway, Tyrer, et al., 2008) to measure the emotional valence of awareness-related confabulation in the first three of the confabulating patients with RPL. Indeed, we confirmed that the emotional content of awareness-related confabulation was negative on average across the three patients and individually (Fotopoulou, 2005).

We have interpreted these unpleasant false statements in awareness-related confabulation as misattributions (either internalisations or, externalisations) of unpleasant emotions that relate to "implicit" or occasional awareness of one's disability (Fotopoulou & Conway, 2004; see also Feinberg & Roane, 1997). For example, a patient with an RPL and AHP expressed intense anger towards the hospital staff because they had "amputated" her left arm and "put it into a mincemeat maker, remoulded it and put it back on". These bizarre beliefs and the related accusations of staff may have been influenced by paralysis-related negative feelings (implicit emotional awareness), despite the patient's explicit unawareness of her paralysis. The presence of this "implicit" awareness of deficits in AHP has been experimentally documented (Nardone, Ward, Fotopoulou, & Turnbull, 2007); however, the issue of whether these misattributions are motivated is the subject of ongoing debate. At the one extreme, a psychogenic hypothesis is that awareness-related confabulation reflects defence mechanisms against anxiety and depression, not much different to memory-related confabulation (Weinstein, 1996). At the other extreme, some authors have suggested that all features of AHP can be explained on the basis of specific neurocognitive deficits (e.g., deficits in forward motor planning; Heilman, Barret, & Adair, 1998) and thus awareness-related confabulation is unrelated to other syndromes of confabulation. Challenging the rigidity of the distinction between psychogenic and neurogenic factors in these explanations, a number of authors have recently proposed intermediate, more parsimonious explanations.

Some have remarked that AHP is the consequence of abnormal affective regulation (Turnbull, Owen, & Evans, 2005), or a deficient affective drive to respond to uncertainties about current bodily states (Vuilleumier, 2004). Damage to right hemisphere areas responsible for affective evaluation and novelty detection might play a determining role in such deficits (Ramachandran, 1995). Alternatively, damage to subcortical circuits (e.g., basal ganglia) that are involved both in motivation and in detection of "errors" might lead to an inability to revise beliefs based on novel perceptual experience (Vuilleumier, 2004). Marcel et al. (2004) recently argued that right brain damage may alter emotional and attitudinal processes implicated in self-attribution (versus external attribution) of perceptual experiences (Marcel, Tegnér, & Nimmo-Smith, 2004). Interestingly, we assessed three patients with RPL and awareness-related confabulation on the prose recall experiment outlined earlier (Fotopoulou, Conway, Solms, et al., 2008). We found that their performance was similar to that of patients with VPL lesions and memory-related confabulation; they remembered the self-referent unpleasant stories as significantly less negative (i.e., in more self-serving ways) than other-referent unpleasant stories (Fotopoulou, 2005).

Thus, although the emotional valence of awareness-related confabulation is predominately negative, this syndrome may still reveal the exaggeration of self-serving emotional mechanisms similar to those discussed in relation to memory-related confabulation. Moreover, as in the case of memory-related confabulation, it is plausible to assume that neurocognitive deficits disrupt the existing neural mechanisms by which cognition controls and inhibits emotion. For example, some people may find it difficult to initially accept negative news, such as the diagnosis of a serious illness, or the dangers of smoking. They may instead misattribute these unpleasant facts to the incompetence of doctors, or the intentions of health campaigners, respectively. Progressively, however, they may manage to appreciate the situation in more realistic terms. In the event of stroke to the critical right-hemisphere areas, these denial copying strategies may be exaggerated due to the dysfunction of those basic cognitive mechanisms (required for body awareness) that allow one to appreciate the situation in realistic terms and control the related emotions. AHP and awareness-related confabulation may therefore not represent "defences" in the psychodynamic sense. Rather they seem to be *neurological equivalents* of these defences, i.e., the premorbid tendencies of an individual are exaggerated due to a specific neurocognitive deficit. In Ramachandran's terms, "what one is really seeing in these patients is an amplified version of Freudian defense mechanisms caught in *flagrante delicto*; mechanisms of precisely the same sort that we all use in our daily lives. However, since the defenses are grotesquely exaggerated, studying them might give us, for the first time, an *experimental handle* on defense mechanisms" (Ramachandran, 1994, p. 26, original emphasis).

In summary, both neurocognitive and emotional factors seem to play a role in awareness-related confabulation. However, it appears that different cognitive deficits, combined with different direct and indirect emotional influences, lead to the two confabulation syndromes discussed here, namely awareness-related and memory-related confabulation.

EMOTION IN DELUSIONS

Classic views

The conceptualisation of delusions is closely linked to the history of the study of psychosis. Initially psychosis was considered a subcategory of the wider class of neuroses, but it eventually came to be regarded as distinct from neuroses. The meaning of this distinction took many different forms during the twentieth century and was marked by the development of the equally variable distinction between functional and organic explanations (see Beer, 1996, for review). At the end of the nineteenth century the neurologist Freud argued that all mental phenomena, including neurosis and psychosis, have psychological determination (Freud, 1924/1961). He further envisioned that his psychological observations would be linked to neurochemical findings in the future (as opposed to the neuroanatomical explanations of his time). Nevertheless, most psychiatrists at the time viewed psychosis as unrelated to psychological mechanisms. This view was crystallised in the writings of Karl Jaspers (1963), who distinguished "affective illness from madness proper" on the basis that the first is meaningful to the healthy and allows empathy, whereas the second is not understandable, i.e., it is not psychologically meaningful. This distinction between neurosis and psychosis took many other forms and varied among countries; however, it gradually became accepted that neurotic and psychotic behaviours are of different aetiology (Roth, 1963). These clinical observations were systematised by others, notably Kurt Schneider, and became embedded in psychiatric classification systems.

In this epistemological context, delusions, as one of the hallmarks of schizophrenia, were separated from the study of "psychological factors", such as mood and motivation. Characteristically, Jaspers (1963) distinguished between primary delusions (delusions proper), which were uniquely bizarre and nonunderstandable, and secondary delusions (delusion-like ideas), which stem understandably from normal emotional states (see Eilan, 2000, for a critical review). This distinction seems to have informed the currently prevailing distinction between mood-incongruent delusions that have been mostly associated with schizophrenia and mood-congruent delusions that are mostly related to affective psychosis. Yet there has been little and inconclusive empirical investigation of the relationship between affect and delusion across diagnostic categories (e.g., Oulis et al., 2000). Crucially, delusions have been mostly studied in the context of schizophrenia and the possible emotions conveyed have been considered as the mere noise of the pathological mechanism that produced them. As a consequence, the possible psychosocial and motivational aspects of delusions were, until recently, neglected (for critical reviews see Freeman & Garety, 2003; McKay et al., 2005).

In brief, the mainstream study of delusions at the end of the twentieth century inherited two epistemological principles from the sharp distinction between neurosis (as functional disorders) and psychosis (as organic with known or unknown causes): (1) delusions should be studied as pathological phenomena, i.e., essentially unrelated to "normal" psychological states; and (2) delusions should be studied as emotionally meaningless phenomena, i.e., essentially unrelated to normal emotional and motivational processes (see Freeman & Garety, 2003; McKay et al., 2005, for reviews).

Modern views: The cognitive neuropsychiatry of delusions

In the last few decades, there has been a change in the conceptualisation of delusion with relation to the above two principles. Clinical psychologists, encouraged by evidence that psychological treatment can reduce delusions and hallucinations (e.g., Drury, Birchwood, Cochrane, & Macmillan, 1996), endeavoured to understand the symptoms of psychosis in psychological terms (see later). In parallel, the study of delusions has been significantly influenced by the tradition of cognitive neuropsychiatry. This tradition, using the methods of cognitive neuropsychology, addresses psychiatric symptoms as resulting from impairments to processes implicated in normal models of neurocognitive function (David, 1993).

Cognitive neuropsychiatric theories can be divided into two main categories: "perceptual" and "cognitive" theories (see Davies, Coltheart, Langdon, & Breen, 2001, for review). Perceptual models, as outlined by Maher (1974), assume that delusions are explanations of abnormal perceptual experience derived via normal reasoning processes, while cognitive accounts propose that delusions reflect cognitive and reasoning biases or abnormalities. A number of candidate biases have been put forward, including probabilistic reasoning bias, attributional biases, and attentional biases (see Gilleen & David, 2005, for review). Other cognitive theories postulate that patients with delusions have reality monitoring deficits (Johnson et al., 2000), i.e., there is impairment of the higher order cognitive ability to distinguish between internal and external representations. Alternatively, delusions have been considered as resulting from impairments of "theory of mind", the cognitive processes that enable individuals to reflect upon and take appropriate account of the mental states of others (Frith, 1992).

The so-called "two-factor" theories of delusions consider both perceptual and cognitive factors and were developed mainly to explain monothematic (vs. polythematic) and circumscribed (vs. elaborated) delusions (Davies et al., 2001; Stone & Young, 1997). Whereas Maher's perceptual theory suggests that abnormal perception is sufficient to cause delusions (one-factor theory), two-factor theories postulate that perceptual aberrations may be necessary to explain how delusions, in particular bizarre delusions, are generated but are not sufficient to explain why the delusions are adopted and maintained in the face of implausibility and contrary evidence (Davies et al., 2001; Langdon & Coltheart, 2000). A second factor, such as some of the cognitive biases and deficits described by cognitive theories, is required which leads to the adoption of the delusional belief and prevents the individuals from revising their beliefs in light of strong evidence against them. This "two-factor" approach to delusions has more recently been applied to all monothematic delusion other positive symptoms (Coltheart, Langdon, & McKay, 2007). Thus, this approach claims that although bizarre, monothematic delusions are aetiologically heterogeneous (they are caused by different "first-factor" pathologies), they share a neurocognitive homogeneity (they are caused by a combination of two neurocognitive factors).

The psychoanalytic position: Delusion as defence

As in the case of confabulation, the first motivational theories of delusion stemmed from the psychodynamic tradition. Contrary to mainstream psychiatry, psychoanalytic theories proposed that the content of delusions, although it may appear incomprehensible to the observer, is of great personal meaning to the patient. In Freudian thought, delusions are formed as a second, derivative step in the pathogenesis of psychosis (Freud, 1924/1961). According to Freud, psychosis involves a pathological disruption of normal perception, memory and judgement (cognition) due to the overwhelming conflict between the person's motivation and the demands of external reality. Delusions are formed as subsequent substitutions of the appropriate contents of cognition by representations that are more compatible to the subject's wishes and drives. In this sense, delusions are regarded as motivated phenomena serving "defensive", self-protecting functions; delusions are formed and maintained as attempts to relieve or protect individuals from the psychological pain or distress accompanying psychological conflict. Nevertheless, it is important to emphasise that Freud regarded delusions as mostly unsuccessful attempts to protect the individual from anxiety. He noted that the initial cognitive disruption necessarily leads to illness. The representation of reality "cannot be remolded in satisfying forms" and thus leaves the individual with false memories, beliefs, and perceptions that "are of a most distressing character and [are] bound up with a generation of anxiety" (1924/1961 p. 186).

Although the concept of "defence" is central to psychoanalytic theory, its meaning has not been consistent throughout the years and varies greatly between different psychodynamic theories (Laplance & Pontalis, 1973). As in the case of confabulation, different psychoanalytic hypotheses have been proposed to account for the defensive function of delusions. Initial proposals emphasised the role of inhibited sexual desires and other unconscious wishes, whereas subsequent models seemed to focus more on which self-protective functions delusions served and which "mechanisms of defence" were employed in each case. This heterogeneity, coupled with the lack of empirical investigation, has contributed to the discrediting of the psychoanalytic approach to delusions in the second half of the twentieth century (e.g., see McKay et al., 2005, for review). These criticisms coincided with more general doubts over the scientific validity of psychoanalysis. Nevertheless, as aforementioned, a number of scientists have, more recently, suggested that certain of the insights of psychoanalytic theory may be worth empirically assessing and integrating with current neuroscientific knowledge. Most relevant to the present paper are the recent theories that consider the role of emotion in delusion (e.g., Bentall, Corcoran, Howard, Blackwood, & Kinderman, 2001). These models are reviewed next.

The affective neuropsychiatry of delusion: The return of the emotional

The recent effort to understand the symptoms of psychosis in psychological terms, brought about by the traditions of clinical psychology and cognitive neuropsychiatry, have also opened the door to the study of the relation between emotion and false beliefs. Consistent with the psychodynamic notion of projection as a mechanism of externalisation of internal unconscious conflict, Bentall et al. (2001) have postulated that patients with paranoid delusions make excessive external attributions of blame in order to protect a vulnerable self-esteem. However, recent experimental and neuroimaging studies of the predictions of this model have produced mixed results (see Bentall, Fernyhough, Morrison, Lewis, & Corcoran, 2007, for review). Moreover, although an association between low self-esteem, depression, and paranoia is well-established (see Freeman, 2007, for a review), the causal direction of this association is debated.

As Freud had supported (see earlier), it is plausible that paranoid thoughts themselves may be affecting one's mood and self-esteem (see also Bentall et al., 2001). Indeed, Freeman and Garety (2003) have argued that persecutory delusions are a direct reflection of emotional concerns, so that the content of delusions shares the main themes of emotions. Delusions are viewed as attempts to explain (not explain away, as in Bentall's view) anomalous experiences by using emotionally laden, preexisting beliefs about the self and the world. Trower and Chadwick (1995) have argued that one function of paranoia is defensive ("Poor Me Paranoia"); another may be a direct reflection of intense negative emotions ("Bad Me Paranoia") (but see Bentall et al., 2007). Evidence that can unequivocally decide between these alternatives (defensive vs. direct role of affect in delusion) is yet to be put forward. It is also possible that emotions have both roles in the formation of delusions. Whichever is the case, there is now sufficient evidence that low mood, low self-esteem, and negative self-beliefs have a role in the development of paranoid thoughts and perhaps even in other delusions (Garety, Bebbington, Fowler, Freeman, & Kuipers, 2007).

More generally, there is now increasing recognition that emotion can contribute to the development of psychotic symptoms (see Garety et al., 2007, for review). Nevertheless, current motivational accounts of delusions differ with respect to the degree with which they can integrate emotional with neurocognitive factors. Indeed, the multifactorial models of delusions, developed mostly based on research on persecutory delusions (e.g., Bentall et al., 2001; Garety et al., 2007), rarely point to direct aetiological interactions between the cognitive and emotional factors they incorporate. By contrast, some other models have endeavoured to draw direct links between cognitive deficits and emotional factors.

McKay et al. (2005) have incorporated motives in the "two-factor" model of Coltheart and colleagues (described earlier) by proposing that motives are important doxastic (relating to belief) forces. Emotions and desires may affect both perceptual input (the first factor) and belief evaluation (the second factor). For example, in AHP covert awareness of one's disability (Nardone et al., 2007) and the motive to defend one's self-esteem may lead one to avoid perceptual input relating to the facts of the disability (first stage). In addition, one may be motivated to accept as correct the beliefs that satisfy one's desire not to be disabled, thus reducing the significance of contrary evidence (second stage). This hypothesis remains to be tested. McKay and colleagues also used Ramachandran's (1995) view of the right hemisphere, as a "discrepancy detector", to argue that right hemisphere lesions or abnormalities may underlie the faulty belief evaluation in all delusions. I have outlined the benefits of such integrative, nondualistic hypotheses in the previous sections on memory-related confabulation and awareness-related confabulation. However, the consistency-checking functions of the right hemisphere have not been empirically confirmed (Fotopoulou, Tsakiris, et al., 2008), and this explanation cannot account for delusions associated with subcortical or left-hemisphere lesions (see Kunert, Norra, & Hoff, 2007, for review).

Gibbs and David (2003) proposed a theory that locates the formation and maintenance of mood-congruent delusions in emotion-based memory biases. A substantial body of work shows that affect biases encoding, enhances consolidation, and facilitates the retrieval of mood-congruent memories. These processes can lead to the persistence of biased recall of mood-congruent memories and beliefs. Neuroimaging studies have demonstrated limbic abnormalities in patients with schizophrenia and bipolar affective disorder, including the amygdala and the hippocampus (see Kunert et al., 2007, for review). According to this model (Gibbs & David, 2003), memory of imagined events could be enhanced by inappropriate conjunction of affective tone, mediated by limbic structures, leading to delusions by way of adding misleading contextual information. In more detail, the misuse of contextual information may be facilitated by the reduced ability of the prefrontal cortex to appropriately filter out and inhibit inappropriate affective responses. Thus, enhanced emotional and sensory characteristics of imagined events could lead patients to reality monitoring confusion and acceptance of these imagined events as real (see also Fotopoulou, Conway, & Solms, 2007). Further episodes of strong affect may lead to a re-remembering of these ideas, thus further enforcing their abnormal emotional-tagging and granting them persistent reality status.

This hypothesis brings the conceptualisation of mood-congruent delusion closer to that of memory-related confabulation. It is also consistent with the views of Freeman and Garety (2003), who conceive a direct relation between emotion and delusional content. Furthermore, it tallies with recent evidence showing that pharmacological or psychological treatment of comorbid mood disorder reduces delusions (e.g., Drury et al., 1996; Seretti, Lattuada, Zanardi, Franchini, & Smeraldi, 2000) and increases insight (Spalletta, Ripa, Bria, Caltagirone, & Robinson, 2006). However, this model has not as yet been empirically tested and it cannot easily be used to explain mood-incongruent delusions and monothematic delusions. In addition, although the role of mood in memory is well-documented, personal goals and motives are also known to be important in memory formation and to serve similar memory and reality-monitoring biasing roles (see Conway & Pleydell-Pearce, 2000, for review). Thus, the role of mood in this model can be extended to include motives, preoccupations, and goals of the individual. This kind of extension would be consistent with the explanation of motivated memory-related confabulation outlined earlier, according to which ventromedial frontal lobe damage enhances the influence of motivation on reality monitoring and memory retrieval (Fotopoulou, Conway, & Solms, 2007; Fotopoulou, Conway, Solms, et al., 2008). Moreover, such an extension to include motives, preoccupations, and goals could provide a potential way of using the same framework to explain mood-incongruent delusions. In a recent study on memory-related confabulation (Fotopoulou, Conway, Tyrer, et al., 2008), we found that the more depressed the patients' mood in a self-reported questionnaire, the more positive the content of their confabulations. Although this finding is preliminary, it is consistent with the idea that some delusions may directly reflect one's mood as Gibbs and David (2003) argue, but others may serve a defensive function (e.g., regulating one's mood) as Bentall and colleagues have argued (see also Trower & Chadwick, 1995).

CONFABULATION AND DELUSION: TOWARDS A SYNTHESIS

This paper outlined the history of research on the role of affect and related processes in confabulation and delusion. I have argued that the significance of emotion in the pathogenesis of these symptoms has been obscured by academic polarisation between psychodynamic and neurocognitive traditions and often obfuscated by rigid distinctions between psychogenic and neurogenic explanations. However, recent research on both confabulation and delusion has brought emotion and motivation to the forefront of academic interest. A number of difficulties and ambiguities regarding the definition and taxonomy of symptoms render direct comparison difficult, but certain overriding principles are beginning to be discernible. Crucially, appropriate directions of future cross-disciplinary research can be envisioned.

Confabulation and delusion can both be described as pathologies involving conflicting demands in memory construction and belief formation (see also Fotopoulou, 2008). Neisser (1988) proposed that remembering is both an act of "utility" (using the past in the service of the present) and "verity" (retracing what took place in the past). Conway (2005) suggested that autobiographical memory is faced with two opposing demands. On the one hand, memories may be altered and even fabricated in order to make the past consistent with current goals and self-images (the demand of "coherence"). On the other hand, memories should, up to a degree, correspond to past experience, irrespective of current concerns (the requirement of "reality correspondence"). Similarly, Stone and Young (1997), following Fodor, have suggested that the belief formation system entails a permanent tension between two principles in potential conflict: Beliefs should tally with the existing web of belief (conservatism); and beliefs should adhere to the deliverances of current perception (observational adequacy). Confabulation and delusion, as well as "normal" false memories and unusual beliefs, can be described as faulty attempts to manage the balance between these conflicting demands of reality representation.

The studies reviewed here provide evidence that emotion and motivation are of determining importance in how this balanced is achieved (see also McKay et al., 2005). Moreover, the current paper has argued that outdated conceptualisations of emotion and motivation as exclusively psychogenic processes should be rejected. The influence of affect and related processes on confabulation and delusion may be instigated by: (1) neural damage or dysfunction to predetermined mechanisms of interaction between emotion and cognition; (2) hard-wired individual differences in these mechanisms; (3) life changes and social circumstances that influence the emotional and cognitive state of individuals; and (4) any combination of these. Importantly, because of this variety, the parallel study of emotional influences and detectable neurocognitive dysfunction can elucidate the nature of the interaction between the two.

For example, in memory-related confabulation poor reality filtering and weak control of recollection due to anterior limbic damage seem to lead to self-serving biases in recall and motivated reality monitoring (Fotopoulou, Conway, & Solms, 2007). It would be of interest to use some of the experimental and neuroimaging paradigms developed in the study of memory-related confabulation (e.g., Schnider, 2003) to verify whether the same reality monitoring deficits and anterior limbic abnormalities underlie delusion formation in affective psychosis, as hypothesised by some authors (Gibbs & David, 2003). Similarly, findings, experimental procedures and hypotheses from the study of awareness-related confabulation may be used in the study of related idiopathic delusions and vice versa. For example, given the typical explicit unawareness and emotional flatness or lability in patients with awareness-related confabulation, it would be interesting to investigate implicit self-esteem and external attribution biases in these patients.

In addition, the role of emotion in clinical confabulation and delusion can be seen in a continuum with the role of emotion in normal memory and reality distortions in healthy and subclinical populations (see Freeman & Garety, 2003, for discussion). For example, memory-related confabulation seems to share some characteristics with the motivated memory distortion of normal autobiographical memory (Conway & Pleydell-Pearce, 2000). Similarly, awareness-related confabulation may be conceived as an exaggeration of the denial healthy individuals show in circumstances of great anxiety or loss (Moyer & Levine, 1998). These conceptualisations may allow the study of clinical confabulations and delusions to inform models of normal motivated cognition and vice versa. To these "continuity" perspectives, one may also add a neurodevelopmental dimension. For example, it is plausible that the emotional processes implicated in delusions may have their origin in early adverse experiences that create an enduring cognitive vulnerability (Garety et al., 2007). Indeed, a different line of research within mainstream psychiatry suggests that psychosis represents the endpoint of abnormal developmental pathways which may begin early in life (for review, see Bentall et al., 2007).

Approaches to confabulation and delusion that take emotion and motivation into account seem to have direct applicability to clinical practice (Fotopoulou, 2008; Freeman & Garety, 2003). Such applicability not only has pragmatic significance and potential for translational research but it also opens up the possibility of investigating the effects of psychological and pharmacological treatment on the evolution of symptoms.

By highlighting the these similarities between confabulations and delusions, I do not mean to deemphasise their differences. On the contrary, I reviewed both memory-related confabulation and awareness-related confabulation to emphasise that different mechanisms, by which emotion and motivation may influence cognition, seem to be affected in these symptoms. As I have argued here, the differences between these two confabulation syndromes seem to outweigh the similarities and thus are better explained as related, yet separate pathologies. The same may apply to the relation of confabulation and delusion. It thus seems that a potential effort to establish a neurocognitive homogeneity (even if relative) between all types of confabulations and delusions and form a single explanatory formula may not tally with the rich heterogeneity of confabulations and delusions. Instead, separate theories for different categories of false remembering and false believing, incorporating different motivational and neurocognitive factors and interacting principles, may enhance the sophistication, testability, and pragmatic value of theories.

REFERENCES

Baddeley, A., & Wilson, B. (1986). Amnesia, autobiographical memory and confabulation. In D. C. Rubin (Ed.), *Autobiographical memory* (pp. 225–252). New York: Cambridge University Press.

Baddeley, A. D., Thornton, A., Chua, S. E., & McKenna, P. (1996). Schizophrenic delusions and the construction of autobiographical memory. In D. C. Rubin (Ed.), *Remembering our past: Studies in autobiographical memory* (pp. 384–428). New York: Cambridge University Press.

Bayne, T. J., & Pacherie, E. (2005). In defense of the doxastic conception of delusions. *Mind and Language*, *20*, 163–188.

Bechara, A., Damasio, H., & Damasio, A. R. (2000). Emotion, decision making and the orbitofrontal cortex. *Cerebral Cortex*, *10*, 295–307.

Beer, M. D. (1996). The dichotomies: Psychosis/neurosis and functional/organic: A historical perspective. *History of Psychiatry*, *7*, 231–255.

Bentall, R. P., Corcoran, R., Howard, R., Blackwood, N., & Kinderman, P. (2001). Persecutory delusions: A review and theoretical integration. *Clinical Psychology Review*, *21*, 1143–1192.

Bentall, R. P., Fernyhough, C., Morrison, A. P., Lewis, S., & Corcoran, R. (2007). Prospects for a cognitive-developmental account of psychotic experiences. *British Journal of Clinical Psychology*, *46*, 155–173.

Berlyne, N. (1972). Confabulation. *British Journal of Psychiatry*, *120*, 31–39.

Betlheim, S., & Hartmann, H. (1951). On parapraxes in the Korsakow psychosis. In D. Rapaport (Ed.), *Organisation and pathology of thought* (pp. 289–307). New York: Columbia University Press. (Original work published 1924)

Burgess, P. W., & Shallice, T. (1996). Confabulation and the control of recollection. *Memory*, *4*, 359–411.

Burgess, P. W., & McNeil, J. E. (1999). Content-specific confabulation. *Cortex*, *35*, 163–182.

Coltheart, M., Langdon, R., & McKay, R. (2007). Schizophrenia and monothematic delusions. *Schizophrenia Bulletin*, *33*(3), 642–647.

Conway, M. A. (2005). Memory and the self. *Journal of Memory and Language*, *53*, 594–628.

Conway, M. A., & Pleydell-Pearce, C. W. (2000). The construction of autobiographical memories in the self memory system. *Psychological Review*, *107*, 261–288.

Conway, M. A., & Tacchi, P. C. (1996). Motivated confabulation. *Neurocase*, *2*, 325–338.

Dalla Barba, G. (1993). Confabulation: Knowledge and recollective experience. *Cognitive Neuropsychology*, *10*, 1–20.

David, A. S. (1993). Cognitive neuropsychiatry? *Psychological Medicine*, *23*, 1–5.

David, A. S. (1999). On the impossibility of defining delusions. *Philosophy, Psychiatry and Psychology*, *6*, 17–20.

Davies, M., Coltheart, M., Langdon, R., & Breen, N. (2001). Monothematic delusions: Towards a two-factor account. *Philosophy, Psychiatry and Psychology*, *8*, 133–158.

Davies, M., Davies, A. A., & Coltheart, M. (2005). Anosognosia and the two-factor theory of delusions. *Mind and Language*, *20*(2), 209–236.

DeLuca, J. (2000). A cognitive perspective on confabulation. *Neuro-Psychoanalysis*, *2*(2), 119–132.

Drury, V., Birchwood, M., Cochrane, R., & Macmillan, F. (1996). Cognitive therapy and recovery from acute psychosis: A controlled trial. I. Impact on psychotic symptoms. *British Journal of Psychiatry*, *169*, 593–601.

Eilan, N. (2000). On understanding schizophrenia. In D. Zahavi (Ed.), *Exploring the self: Philosophical and psychopathological perspectives on self-experience* (pp. 97–113). Amsterdam: John Benjamins.

Elliott, R., Friston, K. J., & Dolan, R. J. (2000). Dissociable neural responses in human reward systems. *Journal of Neuroscience*, *20*, 6159–6165.

Feinberg, T. E., & Roane, D. M. (1997). Anosognosia, completion and confabulation: The neutral-personal dichotomy. *Neurocase*, *3*, 73–85.

Feinberg, T. E., Roane, D. M., & Ali, J. (2000). Illusory limb movements in anosognosia for hemiplegia. *Journal of Neurology, Neurosurgery and Psychiatry*, *68*, 511–513.

Fotopoulou, A. (2005). *Confabulation: Constructing motivated memories*. Unpublished PhD thesis, University of Durham, Durham, UK.

Fotopoulou, A. (2008). False-selves in neuropsychological rehabilitation: The challenge of confabulation. *Neuropsychological Rehabilitation*, *18*(5 and 6), 541–565.

Fotopoulou, A. (2009). Distentangling the motivational theories of confabulation. In W. Hirstein (Ed.), *Confabulation: Views from neuroscience, psychiatry, psychology and philosophy*. Oxford: Oxford University Press.

Fotopoulou, A., & Conway, M. A. (2004). Confabulations pleasant and unpleasant. *Neuropsychoanalysis, 6*(1), 26–33.

Fotopoulou, A., Conway, M. A., Griffiths, P., Birchall, D., & Tyrer, S. (2007). Self-enhancing confabulation: Revising the motivational hypothesis. *Neurocase, 13*, 6–15.

Fotopoulou, A., Conway, M. A., & Solms, M. (2007). Confabulation: Motivated reality monitoring. *Neuropsychologia, 45*, 2180–2190.

Fotopoulou, A., Conway, M. A., Solms, M., Tyrer, S., & Kopelman, M. (2008). Self-serving confabulation in prose recall. *Neuropsychologia, 46*(5), 1429–1441.

Fotopoulou, A., Conway, M. A., Tyrer, S., Birchall, D., Griffiths, P., & Solms, M. (2008). Positive emotional biases in confabulation: An experimental study. *Cortex, 44*(7), 764–772.

Fotopoulou, A., Solms, M., & Turnbull, O. (2004). Wishful reality distortions in confabulation: A case report. *Neuropsychologia, 42*, 727–744.

Fotopoulou, A., Tsakiris, M., Haggard, P., Vagopoulou, A., Rudd, A., & Kopelman, M. (2008). The role of motor intention in motor awareness: An experimental study on anosognosia for hemiplegia. *Brain, 131*(12), 3432–3442.

Freeman, D. (2007). Suspicious minds: The psychology of persecutory delusions. *Clinical Psychology Review, 27*, 425–457.

Freeman, D., & Garety, P. A. (2003). Connecting neurosis and psychosis: The direct influence of emotion on delusions and hallucinations. *Behaviour Research and Therapy, 41*, 923–947.

Freud, S. (1961). The loss of reality in neurosis and psychosis. In *The standard edition of the complete psychological works of Sigmund Freud, Vol. XIX (1923–1925): The ego and the id and other works* (pp. 181–188). (Original work published 1924)

Frith, C. D. (1992). *The cognitive neuropsychology of schizophrenia*. Hove, UK: Lawrence Erlbaum Associates Ltd.

Gainotti, G. (1975). Confabulation of denial in senile dementia: An experimental study. *Psychiatria Clinica, 8*, 99–108.

Garety, P. A., Bebbington, P., Fowler, D., Freeman, D., & Kuipers, E. (2007). Implications for neurobiological research of cognitive models of psychosis: A theoretical paper. *Psychological Medicine, 37*, 1377–1392.

Gibbs, A. A., & David, A. S. (2003). Delusion formation and insight in the context of affective disturbance. *Epidemiologia e Psychiatria Sociale, 12*(3), 167–174.

Gilboa, A., Alain, C., Stuss, D. T., Melo, B., Miller, S., & Moscovitch, M. (2006). Mechanisms of spontaneous confabulations: A strategic retrieval account. *Brain, 129*(6), 1399–1414.

Gilleen, J., & David, A. S. (2005). The cognitive neuropsychiatry of delusions: From psychopathology to neuropsychology and back again. *Psychological Medicine, 35*, 5–12.

Gross, J. J. (2002). Emotion regulation: Affective, cognitive, and social consequences. *Psychophysiology, 39*, 281–291.

Hedden, T., & Gabrieli, J. D. E. (2004). Insights into the ageing mind: A view from cognitive neuroscience. *Nature Reviews Neuroscience, 5*, 87–96.

Heilman, K. M., Barret, A. M., & Adair, J. C. (1998). Possible mechanisms of anosognosia: A defect in self awareness. *Philosophical Transactions of the Royal Society of London, Series B: Biological Sciences, 353*, 1903–1909.

Hirstein, W. (2005). *Brain fiction: Self-deception and the riddle of confabulation*. Cambridge, MA: MIT Press.

Jaspers, K. (1963). *General psychopathology* (J. Hoening & M. Hamilton, Trans.). Manchester, UK: Manchester University Press.

Johnson, M. K., Hayes, S. M., D'Esposito, M., & Raye, C. (2000). Confabulation. In F. Boller & J. Grafman (Eds.), *Handbook of neuropsychology: Vol. 2. Memory and its disorders* (2nd ed., pp. 383–407). Amsterdam: Elsevier Science.

Kaplan-Solms, K. L., & Solms, M. (2000). *Clinical studies in neuropsychoanalysis: Introduction of a depth neuropsychology.* London: Karnac Books.

Kopelman, M. D. (1999). Varieties in false memory. *Cognitive Neuropsychology, 16*(3/4/5), 197–214.

Kopelman, M. D. (2010). Varieties of confabulation and delusion. *Cognitive Neuropsychiatry, 15*(1/2/3), 14–37.

Korsakoff, S. S. (1996). Medico-psychological study of a memory disorder. *Consciousness and Cognition, 5*, 2–21. (Original work published 1889)

Kunert, H. J., Norra, C., & Hoff, N. (2007). Theories of delusional disorders: An update and review. *Psychopathology, 1*(40), 191–202.

Langdon, R., & Coltheart, M. (2000). The cognitive neuropsychology of delusions. *Mind and Language, 15*(1), 184–218.

Laplanche, J., & Pontalis, J. B. (1973). *The language of psychoanalysis* (D. Nicholson-Smith, Trans.). New York: W. W. Norton.

Lee, E., Akanuma, K., Meguro, M., Ishii, H., Yamaguchi, S., & Meguro, K. (2007). Confabulations in remembering past and planning future are associated with psychiatric symptoms in Alzheimer's disease. *Archives of Clinical Neuropsychology, 22*(8), 949–956.

Maher, B. A. (1974). Delusional thinking and perceptual disorder. *Journal of Individual Psychology, 30*, 98–113.

Marcel, A. J., Tegnér, R., & Nimmo-Smith, I. (2004). Anosognosia for plegia: Specificity, extension, partiality and disunity of bodily unawareness. *Cortex, 20*, 19–40.

Markova, I. S., & Berrios, G. E. (2000). Insight into memory deficits. In G. E. Berrios & J. R. Hodges (Eds.), *Memory disorders in psychiatric practice* (pp. 204–233). Cambridge, UK: Cambridge University Press.

Mather, M., & Carstensen, L. L. (2005). Aging and motivated cognition: The positivity effect in attention and memory. *Trends in Cognitive Sciences, 9*(10), 496–502.

Mattioli, F., Miozzo, A., & Vignolo, L. A. (1999). Confabulation and delusional misidentification: A four year follow-up study. *Cortex, 35*(3), 413–422.

McAdams, D. P. (2001). The psychology of life stories. *Review of General Psychology, 5*(2), 100–122.

McKay, R., Langdon, R., & Coltheart, M. (2005). "Sleights of mind": Delusions, defences and self-deception. *Cognitive Neuropsychiatry, 10*(4), 305–326.

Metcalf, K., Langdon, R., & Coltheart, M. (2007). Models of confabulation: A critical review and a new framework. *Cognitive Neuropsychology, 24*(1), 23–47.

Moscovitch, M. (1989). Confabulation and the frontal system: Strategic versus associative retrieval in neuropsychological theories of memory. In H. L. Roediger & F. I. M. Craik (Eds.), *Varieties of memory and consciousness: Essays in honour of Endel Tulving* (pp. 133–160). Hillsdale, NJ: Lawrence Erlbaum Associates, Inc.

Moyer, A., & Levine, E. G. (1998). Clarification of the conceptualization and measurement of denial in psychosocial oncology research. *Annals of Behavioral Medicine, 20*, 149–160.

Nardone, I. B., Ward, R., Fotopoulou, A., & Turnbull, O. E. (2007). Attention and emotion in anosognosia: Evidence of implicit awareness and repression. *Neurocase, 13*(5), 438–445.

Nathaniel-James, D. A., & Frith, C. D. (1996). Confabulation in schizophrenia: Evidence of a new form? *Psychological Medicine, 26*(2), 391–399.

Neisser, U. (1988). Five kinds of self-knowledge. *Philosophical Psychology, 1*, 35–59.

Oltmanns, T. F. (1988). Approaches to the definition and study of delusions. In T. F. Oltmanns & B. A. Maher (Eds.), *Delusional beliefs* (pp. 3–12). New York: Wiley.

Oulis, P., Lykouras, L., Gournellis, R., Mamounas, J., Hatzimanolis, J., & Christodoulou, G. N. (2000). Clinical features of delusional beliefs in schizophrenic and unipolar mood disorder: A comparative study. *Psychopathology, 33*, 310–313.

Ramachandran, V. S. (1994). Phantom limbs, neglect syndromes, repressed memories, and Freudian psychology. *International Review of Neurobiology, 37*, 291–333.

Ramachandran, V. S. (1995). Anosognosia in pariental lobe syndrome. *Consciousness and Cognition, 4*, 22–51.

Roth, M. (1963). Neurosis, psychosis and the concept of disease in psychiatry. *Acta Psychiatrica Scandinavia, 39*, 128–145.

Schnider, A. (2003). Spontaneous confabulation and the adaptation of thought to ongoing reality. *Nature Reviews Neuroscience, 4*, 662–671.

Schnider, A. (2008). *The confabulating mind: How the brain creates reality.* New York: Oxford University Press.

Seretti, A., Lattuada, E., Zanardi, R., Franchini, L., & Smeraldi, E. (2000). Patterns of symptom improvement during antidepressant treatment of delusional depression. *Psychiatry Research, 94*, 185–190.

Solms, M. (2000). A psychoanalytic perspective on confabulation. *Neuro-psychoanalysis, 2*, 133–143.

Spalletta, G., Ripa, A., Bria, P., Caltagirone, C., & Robinson, R. G. (2006). Response of emotional unawareness after stroke to antidepressant treatment. *American Journal of Geriatric Psychiatry, 14*(3), 220–227.

Stone, T., & Young, A. W. (1997). Delusions and brain injury: The philosophy and psychology of belief. *Mind and Language, 12*, 327–364.

Talland, G. A. (1961). Confabulation in the Wernicke-Korsakoff syndrome. *Journal of Nervous and Mental Disease, 132*, 361–381.

Trower, P., & Chadwick, P. (1995). Pathways to defense of the self: A theory of two types of paranoia. *Clinical Psychology: Science and Practice, 2*, 263–278.

Turnbull, O. H., Berry, H., & Evans, C. E. Y. (2004). A positive emotional bias in confabulatory false beliefs about place. *Brain and Cognition, 55*(3), 490–494.

Turnbull, O. H., Owen, V., & Evans, C. E. Y. (2005). Negative emotions in anosognosia. *Cortex, 41*, 67–75.

Turner, M. S., Cipolotti, L., Yousry, T. A., & Shallice, T. (2008). Confabulation: Damage to a specific inferior medial prefrontal system. *Cortex, 44*(6), 637–648.

Vuilleumier, P. (2004). Anosognosia: The neurology of false beliefs and uncertainties. *Cortex, 40*(1), 9–17.

Walker, W. R., Skowronski, J. J., & Thompson, C. P. (2000). Life is pleasant—and memory helps to keep it that way. *Review of General Psychology, 7*(2), 203–210.

Weinstein, E. A. (1996). Symbolic aspects of confabulation following brain injury: Influence of premorbid personality. *Bulletin of the Menninger Clinic, 60*, 331–350.

COGNITIVE NEUROPSYCHIATRY
2010, 15 (1/2/3), 64–94

The role of personal biases in the explanation of confabulation

Kasey Metcalf[1], Robyn Langdon[2], and Max Coltheart[2]

[1]*Brain Injury Rehabilitation Unit, Liverpool Hospital, Sydney, Australia, and* [2]*Macquarie Centre for Cognitive Sciences, Macquarie University, Sydney, Australia*

Introduction. Previous research has demonstrated that motivational forces play an important role in determining the content of confabulation. In particular the content of confabulation has been shown to contain a positive emotional bias. This study investigated the role of personal biases in the confabulations of six patients with diverse aetiologies.

Method. Confabulations were elicited with a series of structured interviews. We then compared the patients' confabulations to their actual situations. Further analyses compared confabulations about current (i.e., the postmorbid period) and past (i.e., premorbid events and general life circumstances) events.

Results. Group analysis confirmed a general bias to recall events that were more positive than the reality. However, examination of individual cases revealed that positive biases were not universal. Confabulations about current circumstances showed the positive bias, whereas an emotional bias was not evident in past confabulations.

Conclusion. We conclude that motivational forces play a role in determining the content of confabulations but conceive of this role primarily in terms of a need to maintain a consistent self-concept (whether positive or negative) overlaid upon the ease with which an individual can retrieve familiar premorbid daily activities and routines.

Keywords: Autobiographical memory; Confabulation; Delusions.

Correspondence should be addressed to Kasey Metcalf, Liverpool Brain Injury Rehabilitation Unit, Liverpool Hospital, Locked Bag 7103, Liverpool BC NSW 1871, Australia. E-mail: kasey.metcalf@sswahs.nsw.gov.au

We would like to thank the patients and families for their participation in this project. We would also like to thank Kate Martin and Thea Hamieh, Clinical Neuropsychologists at the Royal Rehabilitation Centre, Sydney, who were responsible for recruitment and advice concerning the patients. Thanks also to Dr. Kristina Prelog for reviewing patient brain scans and Dr. Aikaterini Fotopoulou for her helpful comments on an earlier draft on this manuscript.

DOI: 10.1080/13546800902767703

Confabulation has been a phenomenon of interest since the early 1900s (Bonhoeffer, 1904, cited in Talland, 1965), but as yet there is no formally accepted definition (Nedjam, Devouche, & Dalla Barba, 2004). The phenomenon was initially described by Berlyne (1972, p. 33) as a "falsification of memory occurring with clear consciousness in association with an organically derived amnesia". For the purposes of this paper we define confabulation as statements or actions that involve distortions or misinterpretations of memories without the conscious intention to deceive (for review on definition see Gilboa & Moscovitch, 2002; Metcalf, Langdon, & Coltheart, 2007; Moscovitch, 1989). Despite numerous attempts over the years to explain the presence of confabulation, research is only just beginning to focus on the factors that determine the content of individual confabulations (Burgess & McNeil, 1999; Conway & Tacchi, 1996; Fotopoulou, Conway, & Solms, 2007; Fotopoulou, Solms, & Turnbull, 2004; Turnbull, Berry, & Evans, 2004). A full account of confabulation, just like a full account of delusion, needs to explain not only the presence of confabulations but also the variable content. With this aim in mind, Metcalf et al. (2007) have recently proposed an explanatory framework for confabulation that borrows from the Langdon and Coltheart (2000a, 200b) two-deficit model of delusional belief formation.

Langdon and Coltheart (2000a, 2000b) originally proposed that the cooccurrence of two neuropsychological deficits is necessary to explain the presence and the content of bizarre monothematic delusions. More recently, this idea has evolved into a more general, two-factor approach, which might be applicable to the genesis of all delusions, whether the aetiology is "organic" or "functional", and whether the delusional content is bizarre or mundane (Coltheart, 2007; Coltheart, Langdon, & McKay, 2007; Davies, Coltheart, Langdon, & Breen, 2001; Langdon, McKay, & Coltheart, 2008). In current descriptions of the two-factor approach, the first factor, which accounts for the delusional content, is most often a primary perceptual/affective deficit that distorts current sensory experience, particularly when delusional content is bizarre. The second factor is an impairment of normal belief evaluation which causes the uncritical acceptance of the implausible thought that first springs to mind in response to the primary perceptual/affective anomaly. This second impairment is broadly hypothesised to result from right-hemisphere damage, most likely right-frontal damage (Coltheart et al., 2007; Langdon et al., 2008). The original two-deficit model of Langdon and Coltheart also included personal attributional biases, which were conceived in terms of premorbid explanatory biases (rather than a deficit) and which nuanced the content of favoured explanations that are generated to explain an anomalous experience. In other words, these biases were originally seen as factor-one processes.

In their application of the two-deficit approach to the explanation of "spontaneous confabulation", which might be likened to bizarre delusion (see

Figure 1 and Kopelman (2010 this issue), for discussion of the distinction between spontaneous and provoked confabulations), Metcalf and colleagues hypothesised that the first deficit (Deficit A in Figure 1) is an impairment of the executive control processes required for normal retrieval (Burgess & Shallice, 1996; Conway & Fthenaki, 2000; Moscovitch, 1989, 1995). This primary deficit is thought to result in an impaired search and retrieval of memories from the autobiographical episodic memory store, although it is acknowledged that disrupted storage or access to the autobiographical memory base may, in some cases, be the first deficit. The second deficit (Deficit B in Figure 1) was then hypothesised to be a disturbance of normal belief or memory evaluation. That is, confabulating patients were conceived as unable to critically evaluate the material generated from their autobiographical memory store causing them to simply accept the (mis)recalled output as a genuine memory. This theoretical framework is similar to the approach of other theorists who also advocate a combination of impairments to explain confabulation (e.g., Burgess & Shallice, 1996; Gilboa et al., 2006; Gilboa & Moscovitch, 2002; Kopelman, 1999).

Metcalf and colleagues also suggested that personal biases preferentially bias the selection of memories. Such biases, they argued, may be influenced

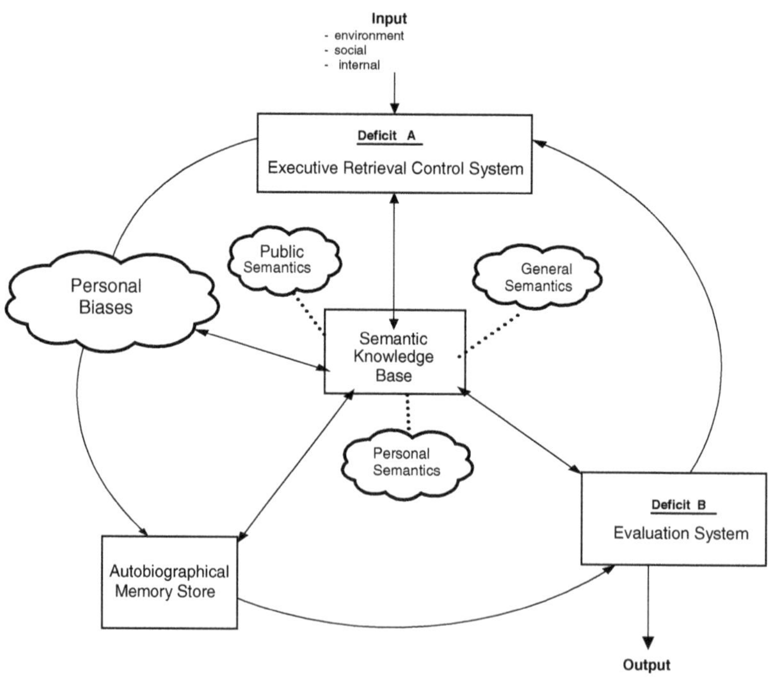

Figure 1. Proposed cognitive-neuropsychological model of confabulation (Metcalf et al., 2007).

by motivations to maintain consistency between an individual's memories and that individual's concept of self (see, e.g., Conway & Tacchi, 1996) and/or to positively enhance the individual's self-image (see, e.g., Fotopoulou, 2010 this issue). Moreover, and consistent with Conway and Tacchi (1996) and Shimamura (2002), it was proposed that memories are retrieved, constructed, and evaluated in cycles. This cyclical process only ceases in healthy individuals when no further information can be retrieved from the autobiographical memory store, either due to diminished access or the evaluation system's final acceptance.

The current study focuses on the role that personal biases play in nuancing the content of individual confabulations. Conway and Tacchi (1996) were among the first to argue that the role of motivation needs to be more fully considered in explaining confabulatory content. Conway and colleagues focused on the motivational role of "the self". In Conway's (Conway, 1996; Conway, Collins, Gathercole, & Anderson, 1996; Conway & Rubin, 1993) constructional model of autobiographical memory—termed the Self Memory System (Conway & Pleydell-Pearce, 2000; Conway, Singer, & Tagini, 2004)—and also in Kopelman's (1999) model of false memories/confabulation, "the self" was regarded as an important constraint on memory retrieval. Conway (1996) and Kopelman both emphasised that retrieved memories need to be concordant with the concept of the self in order to be accepted.

More recently, research has begun to focus on the presence of an *emotional* bias in confabulatory output (Fotopoulou, Conway, Birchall, Griffiths, & Tyer, 2007; Fotopoulou, Conway, & Solms, 2007; Fotopoulou, Conway, Solms, Tyer, & Kopelman, 2008; Fotopoulou, Conway, Tyer, et al., 2008; Fotopoulou et al., 2004). In the initial report in this series of studies, Fotopoulou and colleagues (2004) described patient ES, who began confabulating following removal of a meningioma. ES's confabulations were rated by observers as more pleasant than the actual corresponding situation and the authors suggested that ES was retrieving "wishful thoughts" from his damaged memory system. They agreed with Conway's (1996) notion that autobiographical memory retrieval needs to be in line with concepts of the self, but also suggested that ES's personal goals and emotions may have been particularly salient in his retrieval system and that this information was therefore retrieved with greater ease.

An alternate interpretation of the 2004 findings of Fotopoulou and colleagues became apparent when one considers that the actual real-world situation most confabulators face is dismal. (We will consider more recent work from Fotopoulou and colleagues that addresses this issue later.) Many patients who confabulate are clinically amnesic, have severe executive dysfunction and cannot return to independent lives. Their situation can only be regarded as negative. Therefore, when confabulatory output is compared to the usually unpleasant reality, the content could be seen to be skewed in the positive direction.

The current study focused on the role of emotional biases in confabulation and took as its starting point the approach of Fotopoulou and colleagues (2004). Thus, in our first analysis, we compared the content of patients' confabulations to their actual situations. We expected the content to show a general positive emotional bias (i.e., at a group level), as has been consistently found in the recent research (Fotopoulou, 2010 this issue). We then went on to adopt a single-case study approach, which is the hallmark methodology of cognitive neuropsychology—the forerunner of cognitive neuropsychiatry. Although theories clearly need support from group studies, we hold the view that theories ought also to be able to adequately account for individual patients' patterns of data. We hence investigated these biases in each individual patient so as to gauge whether the positive emotional biases are universal. Six confabulating patients, who were an unselected group of presentations to a rehabilitation hospital, were investigated. Our approach thus differed from previous investigations that have used stringent selection criteria. For example, Fotopoulou, Conway, and Solms (2007) excluded patients who had previous psychiatric history or were currently on medication with known effects on mood or cognition, and other studies have focused exclusively on patients with anterior communicating artery aneurysms (Ciramelli & Ghetti, 2007; Ciaramelli, Ghetti, Frattarelli, & Ladavas, 2006; Gilboa et al., 2006). We adopted, instead, a cognitive neuropsychological approach to focus on the symptom of confabulation, regardless of aetiology. This primarily phenomenological approach has also been advocated by Dalla Barba and Boissé (2010 this issue). In our study, therefore, even patients with atypical neuropathologies and lesion sites which might not fit with the most "typical" damage seen in confabulation were included. Patients were also not excluded on the basis of current medications or past mood disorders.

Additional analyses were then carried out since much recent work has countered the view that the positive bias in confabulation is simply a consequence of the relative dismal state of the patients' current circumstances. Across several studies, and with well-designed control measures that have eliminated the need for direct comparison between confabulations and actual events, Fotopoulou and colleagues have provided evidence that confabulations generally show a predominance of positive emotional, wishful content (see Fotopoulou, 2010 this issue, for a comprehensive review). Fotopoulou (2010 this issue) has suggested that these emotional biases reflect the exaggerated influence of motivational forces in a damaged memory retrieval system. Thus, material that is disproportionately motivated by drives for self-enhancement and positive self-regard come to be retrieved when dysfunction occurs in the normal retrieval process. This disproportionate influence of motivational biases is attributed to a lack of affective regulation caused by damage to the ventromedial frontal cortex, which is common in confabulating patients. Therefore, it is possible that these emotional biases may not be evident in confabulating patients without specific damage to this area.

Thus motivational factors in confabulation are seen to be similar to motivational factors in normal memory retrieval but are exaggerated because of a lack of affective regulation. This view is consistent with Conway (2005) who, in his review, commented that research into normal autobiographical memory has demonstrated a generalised distortion when retelling negative events; for example, healthy people, particularly older adults (see Kennedy, Mather, & Carstensen, 2004; Mather & Carstensen, 2005), are biased to recall memories that maintain a positive self-regard and a stable self-identity.

In the present study, we addressed this issue in a second set of analyses by examining whether positive emotional biases extend to confabulations that concern all periods of a patient's life. If positive biases in confabulation generally reflect a lack of affective regulation and are not simply due to the contrast between default, well-rehearsed memories, which more easily come to mind, and the patient's relatively dismal current circumstances, one might expect such biases to be present in all confabulations, regardless of the time period to which they refer (i.e., whether about the patients' current life circumstance or their premorbid past).

CASE REPORTS

The following six case reports contain details of patients' backgrounds and situations at the time of testing. Our selection criteria included; confabulation identified by naturalistic observation (e.g., family and/or staff reports), not currently in a delirium, able to sustain attention for at least half an hour during neuropsychological testing and sufficient English language comprehension/ expression to order to complete tasks. As the patients were selected on the basis of naturalistic observation, the confabulations they produced took several forms. Four of the six patients assessed (AP, DL, SD, and TW) could be regarded as *spontaneous* confabulators, as defined by Schnider, von Daniken, and Gutbrod (1996). These authors indicated that patients can *only* be given the spontaneous confabulator label if they have acted on their confabulations. One patient (GM) met the spontaneous confabulator label as defined by Kopelman (1987). That is, the patient confabulated without apparent prompting, but the patient was not known to act on his confabulations. Finally, one patient (LF) was included as she confabulated about her past, daily life, and current situation, but did not confabulate without some prompting (e.g., to questions during formal interview or to direct questions during informal conversation). Neuropsychological task performances are summarised in Table 1 and data from the Autobiographical Memory Interview (AMI: Kopelman, Wilson, & Baddeley, 1990) are shown in Table 2.

Patient AP

AP, a 51-year-old right-handed man, suffered a severe hypoxic brain injury secondary to hypertrophic obstructive cardiomyopathy. Prior to his illness he owned and operated his own small business and lived with his wife. He had two children, aged 13 and 22, and had completed a Bachelor's degree in

TABLE 1
Neuropsychological functioning

Test	*AP*	*DL*	*SD*	*GM*	*TW*	*LF*
WTAR	101		104			105
WAIS-III						
FSIQ	75	85	70		64	81
Verbal Comprehension	70	94	88	70	65	103
Perceptual Organisation	89	88	65		76	69
Working Memory	86	94	59	73		75
Processing Speed	84	69	57		60	69
D-KEFS						
Letter Fluency	3	9	10	3	6	5
Category Fluency	1	8	1	6	3	6
Stroop-Inhibition	1		7		4	13
Tower Achievement	5		4		1	5
Trails–Letter Number	1	2	1			
WMS-III						
Auditory Immediate	55	77	56	56		59
Visual Immediate	57	75	57		61	49
Immediate Memory	45	71	47			45
Auditory Delayed	55	86	55	56		52
Visual Delayed	59	65	56		63	56
Auditory Recognition Delayed	55	100	55	60		60
General Memory	47	78	45			45
RAVLT (*z*-scores)						
Total (Trial I–V)	−4.76	−1.37	−3.89		−2.59	−2.58
Intrusions (Trial I–V)	0.79	−0.79	−9.66		−0.54	−1.22
Del Recall (Trial VII)	−4.55	−2.15	−4.73		−2.83	−5.13
Cognitive Estimates Test	6/11	10/11	11/11	8/11	4/11	8/11

The scores reported for WTAR (Wechsler, 2001), WAIS-III (Wechsler, 1997a) and WMS-III (Wechsler, 1997b) are age-adjusted scores ($M = 100$, $SD = 15$). D-KEFS (Delis, Kaplan, & Kramer, 2001) scores are age-scaled scores ($M = 10$, $SD = 3$). Rey Auditory Verbal Learning Test (RAVLT; Senior, 1999) are z-scores. Australianised cognitive estimates test (Shallice & Evans, 1978) is a raw score.

TABLE 2
Schedules from Autobiographical Memory Interview

Subject	*Childhood*	*Early Adult*	*Recent Life–Preinjury*	*Recent Life–Postinjury*	*Total*
(a) Personal semantic schedule					
AP	15/21	6/21	1/13	1/8	23/63
DL	15.5/21	13.5/21	5/13	3/8	37/63
SD	13.5/21	8/21	1/11	5/10	27.5/63
GM	5/21	8.5/21	—	4/21	17.5/63
TW	9/21	11/21	4.5/13	4/8	28.5/63
LF	17/21	16.5/21	8/13	6/8	47.5/63
(b) Autobiographical incident schedule					
AP	1/9	1/9	1/6	0/3	3/27
DL	5/9	9/9	1/6	1/6	16/27
SD	6/9	4/9	1/3	3/6	14/27
GM	0/9	0/9	—	2/9	2/27
TW	2/9	1/9	0/9	1/9	3/27
LF	2/9	0/9	4/6	0/3	6/27

Grey shading = "definitely abnormal".

commerce. He was described by family members as a very confident man with strong opinions, orderly and particular. His medical history included an enlarged heart that was diagnosed 16 years prior to the current event.

AP was resuscitated at the local hospital, intubated, and ventilated. An EEG performed while AP was unresponsive and ventilated showed prominent unresponsive theta activity, consistent with a diffuse cerebral incident. CT brain scan showed normal grey/white differentiation, no mass or intracranial haemorrhage, and no specific changes of early ischaemia. An MRI brain scan was degraded by movement artefact. It showed prominence of the ventricles and sulci, but no definite area of focal recent infarction. No further scans were undertaken as AP had had a dual chamber defibrillator inserted and was thought to be physically unable to undergo the associated stress.

Confabulation was noted on admission to the rehabilitation hospital. The content of the confabulations consisted of severe disorientation in time and errors concerning his age, occupation, and current illness. He was noted to act on his confabulations (e.g., he attempted to leave the hospital in the middle of the night in order to attend work). He demonstrated a severe lack of insight into his condition and was noted to become paranoid and wary of others on occasion.

Neuropsychological assessment was completed approximately 3 months postinjury. His performance indicated a reduction in intellectual functioning, working memory, and processing speed. New learning and memory were particularly impaired. A range of executive deficits were also evident, but it should be noted that his nonverbal abstract reasoning was intact. In addition, AP's ability to retrieve autobiographical information was assessed using the AMI. His performance was in the "borderline" range for childhood semantic information and in the "definitely abnormal" range for the early adult and recent life semantic categories. He was also in the "definitely abnormal" range for all age ranges on the autobiographical incidents schedule.

Patient DL

DL at the time of assessment was a 79-year-old right-handed man. Prior to his illness he was a widower who lived alone. He had completed 10 years of formal education. He had worked as an engineer for many years and was regarded as an expert in his field. He retired at 77 years of age. Work had been a major part of his life—he worked up to 7 days a week and rarely took holidays. He had an extensive history of alcohol abuse.

DL was diagnosed with meningoencephalitis of unknown cause. He was noted to confabulate frequently and to act on his confabulations. He also experienced visual hallucinations and was placed on haloperidol. This did not alleviate the hallucinations or the confabulations. CT brain scan showed periventricular low densities, enlarged ventricles, and possible communicating hydrocephalus. Small posterior right frontal haemorrhages were also noted. MRI brain scan showed extensive periventricular white matter changes with deep and peripheral white matter high signal foci in posterior right frontal, bilateral frontal, and right cerebellar hemisphere. Acute right frontal changes were also evident.

DL's awareness of his illness fluctuated. He would on one occasion claim that he was completely better and on another state that he had several problems. DL was also transiently aware that his visual hallucinations were not real. An example follows:

> DL: Something seems to be crazy about everything and I don't know what it is . . . maybe the doctor that did all the work on me . . . if he was to come and sit there it might bring something forward . . . maybe I'm hallucinating, I just don't know.
>
> Investigator: What are you hallucinating?
>
> DL: Maybe I am imagining some of this . . . I don't know . . . it doesn't seem real, for some reason none of it seems real . . . it should be real . . . because I did experience the whole thing . . . yet why doesn't it feel real?

DL's neuropsychological functioning was assessed at 2 months postinjury. Measures of intellectual functioning showed average verbal skills and low average nonverbal abilities. Memory generally fell in the borderline range.

Performance on tasks of executive functioning was variable with reductions in cognitive flexibility, problem solving, and planning, but with intact verbal generativity. His performance on the AMI was in the "borderline to acceptable" range for childhood semantic information and in the "definitely abnormal" range for the early adult and recent life semantic categories. For episodic memories, he was in the "borderline" range for childhood, the "acceptable" range for early adulthood, and the "definitely abnormal" range for his recent life on the autobiographical incidents schedule.

Patient SD

SD was a 36-year-old right-handed man who lived with his wife and three young children. He had had 15 years of formal education and was qualified as an economist/investment banker. SD was hit by a car while cycling. CT brain scans showed traumatic contusions, subarachnoid and intraventricular blood. Shallow left subdural haematoma with minimal to mild subfalcine herniation, left frontal extra-axial haemorrhage, and small contusions were seen in the right frontal lobe inferiorly and left subfrontal region. A further focal contusion was seen within the right basal ganglia. Ventricular dilatation was noted.

On admission to the rehabilitation unit, 1 month postinjury, SD was minimally conscious. Over time, SD developed a tendency to shout, swear, and act aggressively. He was placed on an antipsychotic and an antidepressant to control his aggression. His behaviour was noted to improve under these medications. He confabulated extensively about the reason for admission—for example, he claimed that he had hurt himself "while running away from birds and other animals". He also confabulated extensively about his family and his occupation and was known to act on his confabulations. Although SD mistakenly believed he would eventually make a full recovery, he had variable insight into his situation and cognitive deficits. For example:

Investigator: Do you have any memory difficulties since your accident?
SD: Only a little bit.
Investigator: Do you want to tell me what memory problems you think you've had?
SD: I can't remember things well.
Investigator: Can you give me any examples?
SD: Like my son's birthday, I'm not sure of it. My memories are not good, no good. I can't remember. It's terrible.

SD's confusion and extensive confabulation prevented neuropsychological testing until 1 year postinjury. He demonstrated a significant decline in his intellectual functioning and showed particular impairment in his speed of information processing and working memory. His new learning and memory was at floor for most tasks and he showed a range of deficits on executive tasks. His performance on the AMI was in the "probably abnormal to borderline" range for childhood semantic information and in the "definitely abnormal" range for the early adult and recent life semantic categories. For episodic memories, he was in the "acceptable" range for childhood, the "probably abnormal" range for early adulthood, and the "definitely abnormal" range for his recent life on the autobiographical incidents schedule.

Patient GM

GM was a 74-year-old right-handed man. He lived with his wife and had recently retired. He was born in Crete, moved to a Greek island, and later immigrated to Australia at 15 years of age. He never attended high school. Throughout his life he had owned and successfully run several businesses. Work had been a major part of his life. He worked long hours and up to 7 days a week. He was regarded as the patriarch of the family. GM was involved in a moped accident on a small island in Greece. Over the following month he was taken to the local hospital several times with headaches. His condition deteriorated significantly and he was flown to Athens where he underwent bilateral craniotomies. He suffered severe posterior cerebral artery vasospasms, resulting in large bilateral occipital infarctions. CT brain scans postcraniotomy showed air in front of the frontal lobes and small extraaxial collections. Bilateral posterior cerebral artery (PCA) territory infarction with swelling (subacute) was evident. MRI brain scans at this time showed a moderate left subdural haematoma and PCA infarcts with laminar necrosis and possible globus pallidus infarction (bilateral).

Following the accident GM suffered from apathy and was totally dependent on his family. His vision was severely limited and he suffered from elements of Anton's Syndrome. Damage resulting from infarction to the PCA has previously been noted to result in Anton's Syndrome (Verslegers, de Deyn, Saerens, & Marien, 1991). Confabulation was reported to occur spontaneously from shortly after his operation, but he never acted on his confabulations as his confabulations mainly revolved around past actions rather than anticipated present and future actions. GM generally denied his visual impairments and experienced anosognosia concerning his poor memory and other cognitive deficits. He was emphatic in his denial of his memory impairment; however, his awareness of his visual difficulties fluctuated. An example follows:

Investigator: Have you ever been in hospital?

GM: I think I had an operation on my eyes, because I was involved in an accident. It was OK.

Investigator: Was the operation successful?
GM: Yeah.
Investigator: After the operation could you see?
GM: Yeah.
Investigator: Can you see now?
GM: Yeah, I can see, but not 100%.
Investigator: What difficulties do you have seeing now?
GM: Old age, I think. That has happened to me after the accident. It has been very hard to see.

GM underwent formal neuropsychological testing 2 years post-TBI. Tests were limited by his vision impairment. Although English is his second language, his wife reported that he is relatively fluent and has few difficulties speaking English. Significant declines in intellectual functioning, working memory, new learning, and memory, as well as executive functioning were noted. His performance on the AMI was in the "definitely abnormal" range for all age categories for both semantic and episodic information.

Patient TW

TW was a 45-year-old right-handed man. He had had a tragic family history. Both parents passed away when TW was a child. His parents were separated when he was very young and TW and his two siblings were left in the care of his father, who later committed suicide. The siblings were then separated and adopted. Both his siblings had also deceased by the time of his injury. He was briefly married. He left home at 16 and owned a business as an electrician. He had an extensive alcohol history and was described as an alcoholic and heavy smoker by his friends. He had been diagnosed with depression and was being treated with antidepressants prior to his injury.

TW was admitted to hospital following an alleged assault. CT brain scans taken 10 days postinjury showed extensive left frontal damage, alongside large right temporal (anterior and posterior) haemorrhages with oedema. Subdural collection on the right tentorium cerebelli and in the right interhemispheric fissure anteriorly was seen as well as a small amount of left high parietal subarachnoid blood. A vertical fracture was evident in the right temporal and parietal bones. CT brain scans performed at 2 months postinjury demonstrated low density changes in the right temporoparietal and left frontotemporal regions, consistent with gliosis. The lateral ventricles were mildly to moderately enlarged, suggestive of hydrocephalus.

On admission to the rehabilitation unit, TW was extremely disorientated, confused, and agitated. He was placed on olanzapine, which was withdrawn when his agitation decreased and he was maintained on risperidone. TW confabulated extensively and was known to act on his confabulations. His most frequent confabulations concerned his tragic past. He made frequent reference to the death of his parents and siblings and related bizarre accounts of their deaths or claimed that some members of his deceased family were still alive. TW demonstrated limited insight into his situation and his cognitive deficits. He indicated that he would be soon out of the rehabilitation unit and returning to his previous place of residence and his occupation as an electrician. He showed no emotional distress when his deficits were brought to his attention and dismissed them as trivial. An example follows:

> Investigator: Why are you here?
> TW: Oh I had brain damage to my head, but I am perfect now. Yeah, great now, as fit as a fiddle, everything is perfect.

Neuropsychological functioning was conducted at 5 months postinjury. Significant declines were noted in TW's intellectual functioning, processing speed, new learning, and memory, and on measures of executive functioning. On the AMI, he was in the "definitely abnormal" range for all age categories for both semantic and episodic information. His most striking confabulation occurred during testing on Visual Reproduction. Although immediate recall contained some elements of the original figures, the delayed recall was completely unrelated to the original material (see Figure 2). The pictures depicted scenes of violence which may be reflective of his alleged assault and troubled past. Confabulation in this form has also been reported in a TBI patient studied by Demery, Hanlon, and Bauer (2001).

Patient LF

LF was a 30-year-old right-handed woman. She had 15 years of formal education and was employed as a computer graphics designer. She was described as an intelligent and outgoing woman. LF presented to the local hospital with headaches and neck stiffness. She had suffered an acute intraventricular and subarachnoid haemorrhage. CT brain scans taken one day after admission showed a tiny focus of subarachnoid blood in the right frontal lobe. LF suffered a rebleed 1 week later. An angiogram found an arterial venous malformation (AVM), which was removed via a right parietal craniotomy. She developed progressive hydrocephalus and three shunts were inserted over the following month, including a right frontal extraventricular drain and a right temporal shunt. CT brain scans following the parietal craniotomy showed extensive intraventricular haemorrhage and extensive oedema within the right parietal and occipital lobes.

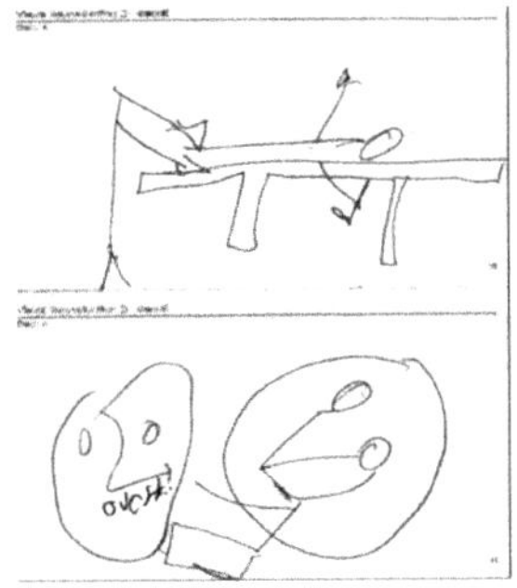

Figure 2. TW Visual Reproduction II: Example of confabulatory output.

LF was noted to become confabulatory in response to questioning about her past and her current situation. She did not spontaneously confabulate or act on any of her confabulations at the time of the current study. Her confabulations were generally constrained (i.e., not bizarre) and appeared to reflect her premorbid activities. She was placed on an antipsychotic due to her behaviour. She demonstrated variable insight into her situation and cognitive deficits. She was, on occasion, able to state that she had significant difficulty with her memory. However, her awareness into the consequences of this impairment and the likelihood of a full recovery was reduced. She would frequently become distressed when her deficits and their possible effect on her future were brought to her attention. For example:

Investigator: Do you have any memory problems?
LF: Yeah I do—lots.
Investigator: Can you give me some examples?
LF: I just can't remember a thing. I won't know what I have done in a day. I won't remember it. I won't remember whether someone was wearing purple spots. I wouldn't have a clue. It's really bad. My memory is terrible, it's like a sieve, it's f . . . ing shocking.

Neuropsychological testing at 4 months postinjury revealed relatively intact verbal intellectual abilities, a reduction in her nonverbal ability, reduced working memory and very poor processing speed. Her performance on tasks of new learning and memory was generally at floor. Impairments on tasks of executive functioning were also noted, alongside a strength in verbal inhibition. Her performance on the AMI was in the "acceptable" range for childhood semantic information and in the "borderline to acceptable" range for early adulthood, and in the "definitely impaired" range for the recent life semantic categories. For episodic memories, she was in the "acceptable" range for childhood, the "probably abnormal" range for early adulthood, and the "definitely abnormal" range for her recent life on the autobiographical incidents schedule.

METHOD

Procedure

Confabulations were gathered formally via three interviews. The first was a comprehensive interview of the patient's history. This Personal History Interview (PHI) solicited information concerning family, education, employment, medical history, drug and alcohol history, current situation, and impairments. The complete PHI consisted of 52 questions, 34 of which tapped autobiographical semantic memories (e.g., What is your date of birth?), 8 of which could be considered more episodic in nature (e.g., What is your last memory prior to your accident?), and 10 questions tapped awareness of current impairments (e.g., Do you have trouble concentrating since your accident?). Nine questions regarding orientation were also given. The second interview consisted of a modification of the Dalla Barba (1993) Confabulation Battery (MCB). This modified battery consisted of 10 "easy" questions of an episodic nature (e.g., What did you do yesterday?) matched with 10 "future" questions (e.g., What are you doing tomorrow?). Further confabulations arose as responses to the nine questions from the Autobiographical Incidents Schedule of the AMI. This resulted in a total of 90 standard questions that were given to all patients, with additional follow-up questions as appropriate.

The tasks were given to each of the five patients in a standard format with the PHI presented on the first day of testing and the other interviews within 1 week of the initial interview, with the MCB presented prior to the AMI. Answers were recorded on audiotape and later transcribed. Comprehensive interviews with family members and a close inspection of medical records were undertaken to check the accuracy of the information provided by the confabulating patients. Answers were only considered confabulatory if they could be confirmed to be untrue by family members or medical record/hospital staff. If an answer appeared to be confabulatory but this could not be confirmed it was removed from the final analysis. In the MCB, the "future" questions were only considered confabulatory if the answer could not possibly align with the patient's current circumstance. All of the confabulators were noted to confabulate outside of these specific tasks, but this additional information was not used as there was no way to standardise the circumstances under which the confabulations were elicited.

Fotopoulou et al. (2004) comment that gathering "control" confabulations from neurologically normal participants is complicated. Control participants need to consciously choose their false memories, making the task very different from that required from actual confabulators, who just need to answer questions. Detailed explanations on how to produce the confabulations would also be required, and this could lead to data that was overly prejudiced by the investigators' current aims. It was thus decided not to elicit control confabulations since these would not truly mimic the "memories" produced by the confabulators.

A list of the confabulations obtained from the tasks was presented to two naïve raters. The raters were two females (aged 32 and 35), both with 15 years of formal education. They were blind to the hypotheses of the study. Each rater was provided with the age and sex of the patients and told that the patient had suffered some form of brain damage. Several practice examples of real confabulations obtained outside the structured interviews were used to train the raters and to improve their interrater reliability. The confabulations were then presented in the order that they were elicited by the interviews. Raters were also provided with the corresponding reality of each confabulation. For example, patient LF when asked the question "Are your grandparents alive?" replied "No my grandmother is alive and my grandfather was pretty healthy, but he's dead". In fact, her grandmother had died and so this information was presented to the raters. The raters were provided with the following instructions: "Please compare the following confabulations (false memories) to their corresponding reality (true information) and answer the following question: Is the confabulation, when compared to the actual reality, more pleasant or more unpleasant than the reality? You may also select "no difference" if the confabulation is neither more pleasant nor less pleasant than the reality. An "I don't know" or an "unable to rate" category was not included. The omission of an "I don't know/unable to rate" option seems unlikely to have biased results since the two raters only differed on approximately 4% of their ratings (i.e., 5/147 responses), suggesting that it was not difficult to choose between "more pleasant", "more unpleasant", and "no difference". The five differences in ratings were for "no difference" versus "pleasant" and "no difference" versus "unpleasant". Differences were resolved by consensus discussion and the consensus results were entered in the analysis.

All participants gave written consent. Legal guardians, if appointed, also gave consent. The study was approved by the ethics committees of Macquarie University and the Royal Rehabilitation Centre, Sydney.

Examples of rated confabulations

Rated as more positive than the reality (Patient LF):

Investigator: Has anyone else in your family had a stroke?
LF: No, everyone's healthy and alive.
Reality: Her father had a stroke.

Rated as no different to the reality (Patient GM)

Investigator: When will be the next time you go on a holiday?
GM: Going away in a few months. I am going back to Australia.
Reality: His next holiday was in 1 week's time to Greece.

Rated as more negative than the reality (Patient SD)

Investigator: Have you had any previous losses of consciousness, other than the recent accident?
SD: Yes, yes I did. I got hit by a car.
Investigator: You got hit by a car once before?
SD: Yes ... and I was blacked out.
Investigator: When was this?
SD: For four weeks I was blacked out. It was about three years ago.
Investigator: Did you go back to work after this?
SD: Yes I did. It was hard at first, you know, it took a long time to recover.
Reality: He had not been involved in any prior car accidents.

RESULTS

Analysis 1a: Group analysis

In this first analysis, we compared the content of patients' confabulations to their actual situations. In line with Fotopoulou and colleagues we hypothesised that the content of confabulation will show a general positive emotional bias at a group level. The total number of confabulations produced during the interviews was 147. Of these 147, 49% were rated as more positive than the reality, 33% as neutral (i.e., not different to the reality), and 18% as more negative. For each patient, we calculated the percent of confabulations which were more positive, neutral (i.e., no difference to the reality) and more negative in order to undertake a group analysis. A one-way analysis of variance (ANOVA) revealed a significant difference, with more positively biased confabulations, $F(2,10) = 4.26$, $p = .046$. These results are summarised in Figure 3.

Analysis 1b: Individual variation in emotional bias

We then examined each patient individually to see if the positive bias was universal. For each patient, the number of positive confabulations was compared to the number of neutral and negative confabulations using chi-squared analyses. Individual patients' results can be seen in Figure 4.

AP produced 47 confabulations; 27 of these (57.4%) were rated as positive, 10 (21.3%) were neutral, and 10 (21.3%) were negative. Thus

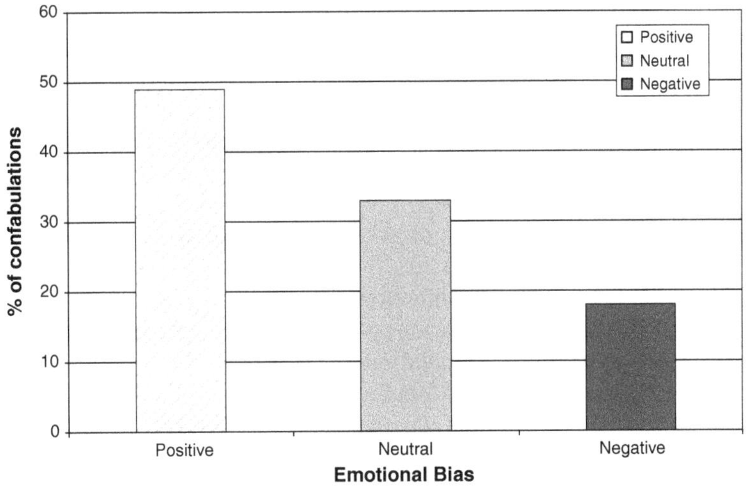

Figure 3. Overall percentages of positive, neutral, and negative confabulatory responses.

significantly more confabulations were rated as positive for AP, $\chi^2(2) = 12.30$, $p = .002$. DL produced 18 confabulations; 13 of these (72.2%) were rated as positive, 2 (11.2%) were neutral, and 3 (16.6%) was negative. Once again, significantly more confabulations were rated as positive, $\chi^2(2) = 12.33$, $p = .002$. Of the 27 confabulations produced by SD, 15 (55.6%) were rated as positive, 9 (33.3%) were neutral, and 3 (11.1%) were negative ($M = 3.43$).

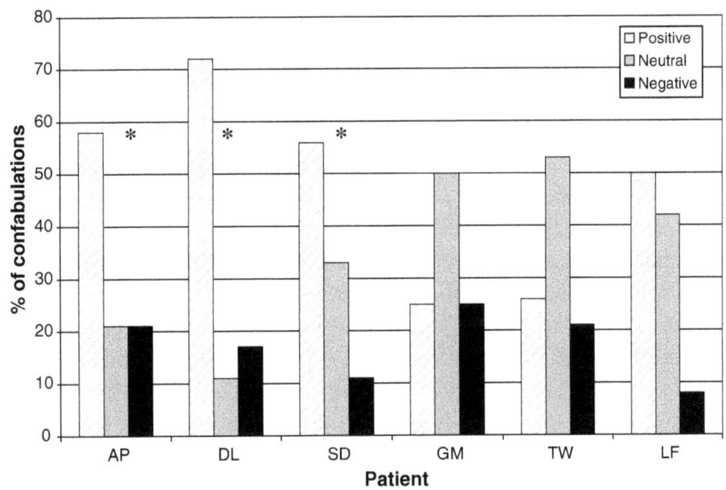

Figure 4. Percentages of positive, neutral, and negative confabulations for six individual patients. $^*p < .05$.

Here again, significantly more confabulations were rated as positive, $\chi^2(2) = 8.00$, $p = .018$. Of the 30 confabulations produced by GM, only 6 (20%) were rated as positive, 12 were neutral (40%), and 6 (20%) were negative. Thus, for GM, there was no significant evidence of a positive bias, $\chi^2(2) = 3.00$, $p = .223$. Indeed, whatever degree of bias was present was driven by a larger percent of neutral (i.e., realistic) confabulations, with much fewer and approximately equal percents of positive and negative confabulations. TW produced 19 confabulations, of which 5 (26.3%) were rated as positive, 10 (52.6%) as neutral, and 4 (21.1%) as negative. TW's pattern was thus similar to that seen in GM; while there was no significant difference, $\chi^2(1) = 2.25$, $p = .196$, more confabulations were rated as neutral and the numbers of positive and negative confabulations were lower and equal in frequency. Finally, LF produced 12 confabulations, of which 6 (50%) were rated as more positive, 5 as neutral (41.7%), and 1 (8.3%) as more negative. Although there was some indication of a positive bias, these proportions did not differ significantly, $\chi^2(1) = 2.27$, $p = .174$.

Summary of Analyses 1a and 1b

Analysis 1a revealed that the patients as a group showed a positive bias, but Analysis 1b showed that this group effect was driven primarily by three of the six confabulators (AP, DL, and SD). Of note, two patients (GM and TW) produced mostly realistic confabulations (the "no difference" category) and even when their neutral confabulations were not considered, they produced a similar number of positive and negative confabulations.

Analysis 2: Comparing current and past confabulations

Next we investigated whether the positive bias seen above was evident for all confabulations whether they regarded current postinjury or premorbid circumstances. Confabulations were therefore divided into two categories—"current" and "past". Current confabulations were defined as any confabulations that related to the patient's day-to-day life postinjury or confabulations about their injury and resulting situation. Past confabulations were defined as any confabulations that involved events from prior to the brain injury or the preinjury general life history and circumstances. The decision on whether the confabulations were current or past was predominantly based on the questions themselves. For example, all confabulatory responses to the question "What is the name of your primary school?" were regarded as past. This was the case even if a patient responded as if they were still in school (as one patient claimed). An occasional question could be regarded as past for one patient, but not another. For example, "What did you do on your last birthday?" could for one patient refer to the time period before their injury and yet be postinjury for another patient. In these cases the date of injury was taken as the decision point for deciding whether a question probed the current or the past. Therefore, the number of questions about the current or the past that a patient could respond to with a confabulatory response varied between the patients. However, the maximum difference was only four questions. Therefore, a total of 48 questions probed the current period, 38 probed the past, and four varied between patients.

Of the 147 confabulations produced throughout the interview, 96 (65.3%) were current confabulations. Of these, 66 (68.8%) were positive, 21 (21.9%) were neutral, and 9 (9.3%) were negative. An ANOVA on the percentage of each type per patient (i.e., positive, neutral, or negative) revealed a significant difference with more positively biased confabulations, $F(2, 10) = 15.46$, $p = .001$. These results are summarised in Figure 5. Of the 51(34.7%) past confabulations, 6 (11.8%) were positive, 27 (52.9%) were neutral, and 18 (35.3%) were negative. An ANOVA revealed no significant difference between the proportions of these three categories, $F(2, 10) = 2.16$, $p = .167$. These results are summarised in Figure 5. Of note, the most frequent type of past confabulation (although not significantly different in frequency than the other two types) was a neutral or a realistic confabulation (i.e., with no difference in valence between the confabulation and the reality).

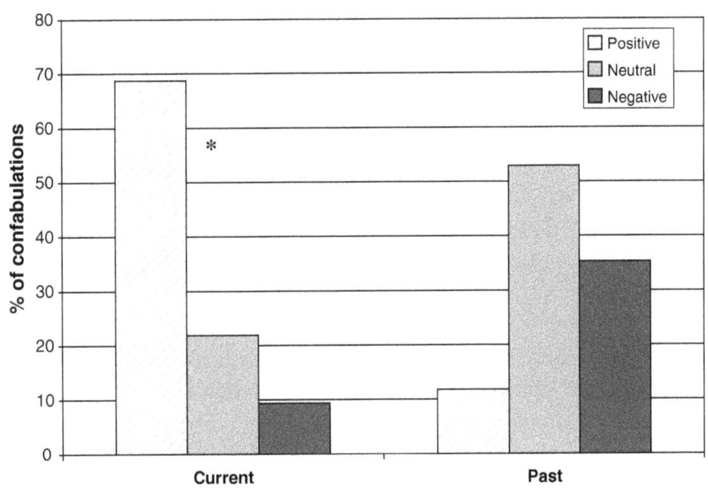

Figure 5. Overall percentages of positive, neutral, and negative confabulations for current versus past categories. $*p < .01$.

Formal analyses of each individual's current and past confabulations were not conducted due to the low incidence of ratings in some cells. However, a summary of the numbers of different types of confabulations produced by each patient is provided in Table 3. This table descriptively shows that, on an individual level, LF was the only patient to show any indication of positive bias when confabulating about past events.

In summary, positive bias was found to be a feature of current but not past confabulations and, even in the case of current confabulations, it should be noted that GM and TW were just as likely to confabulate realistically as they were to confabulate with a positive bias.

DISCUSSION

We have elsewhere proposed a cognitive neuropsychological framework for examining confabulation (Metcalf et al., 2007) in which the genesis of confabulation results from two type of damage: impairments in the retrieval of memory and in the monitoring/evaluation of memories and/or beliefs. Within this framework, personal biases play a role in nuancing the retrieval system to preferentially search for and retrieve information which is particularly salient to an individual and which is consistent with that individual's self concept. An alternate view from Fotopoulou et al. (2004) accepts the role of the premorbid self-concept in shaping confabulatory content but suggests that these biases are also self-enhancing—that is, that they play a positive emotional role.

Following on from the work of Fotopoulou et al. (2004), we investigated the role of emotional biases in six confabulating patients. Our patients were not selected according to aetiology as we focused on phenomenology, as advocated by Dalla Barba and Boissé (2010 this issue). Four patients confabulated spontaneously and were known to act on their confabulations (AP, DL, SD, and TW); one patient confabulated spontaneously but was not known to have acted on his confabulations (GM); and one other patient produced provoked confabulations in conversation about current and past activities, but was not noted to confabulate spontaneously (LF).

When confabulations, in general, were subjected to a group analysis, results revealed that our confabulators produced a significantly higher number of confabulations that were rated as more positive than the reality (compared to more negative or no difference). However, when considered case by case, three of the six patients (AP, DL, and SD) showed a significant positive bias in their confabulations, and a fourth (LF) produced roughly equal numbers of positive and neutral confabulations, as well as less negative confabulations. Two patients (GM and TW) showed no

TABLE 3
Summary of current versus past confabulations for individual patients

	Current confabulations (percentages)				*Past confabulations (percentages)*			
Subject	*Positive*	*Neutral*	*Negative*	*Total*	*Positive*	*Neutral*	*Negative*	*Total*
AP	26 (81%)	2 (6%)	4 (12%)	32	1 (7%)	8 (53%)	6 (40%)	15
DL	13 (76%)	2 (12.5%)	2 (11.5%)	17	0 (0%)	0 (0%)	1 (100%)	1
SD	14 (67%)	6 (28%)	1 (5%)	21	1 (17%)	3 (50%)	2 (33%)	6
GM	6 (50%)	5 (42%)	1 (8%)	12	0 (0%)	7 (58%)	5 (42%)	12
TW	4 (44%)	5 (56%)	0 (0%)	9	1 (10%)	5 (50%)	4 (40%)	10
LF	3 (60%)	1 (20%)	1 (20%)	5	3 (43%)	4 (57%)	0 (0%)	7
Total	66	21	9	96	6	27	18	51

indication of a positive bias, being more realistic overall, and producing roughly equal numbers of confabulations that were more positive and more negative than the reality. The results for these two patients suggested that, although the positive emotional bias may be a general characteristic of confabulation, it is not universal, at least not when confabulation is established phenomenologically—that is, with no constraints on aetiology. It thus remains possible, however, that the positive emotional bias is present in all patients with a more specific neuropathology—perhaps ventromedial frontal damage.

It has been suggested that the positive emotional bias in confabulation is caused by a dysregulated affective control system (Fotopoulou, 2010 this issue). If this is so, one might expect that such dysregulation would affect confabulations whether these are about the current or the past. To explore this possibility, we distinguished between confabulations which concerned the patients' *current* injury-related life circumstances and confabulations which concerned their *past* circumstances prior to injury. Group analysis demonstrated that it was the confabulations concerning current brain-injury circumstances that showed an overwhelming positive bias. Moreover, on a descriptive level, all of the patients individually produced more positive than negative confabulations for current events and four out of the six patients produced more positive than neutral confabulations. AP and DL demonstrated the strongest positive bias in their current confabulations, and GM and TW showed the least positive bias, generating roughly equal numbers of positive and neutral (or realistic) confabulations. In contrast, positive bias was not evident in confabulations to questions about the past (i.e., concerning the time from prior to injury and general life-circumstances). Thus, at first sight, our findings concerning past compared to current confabulations do not appear to be consistent with a dysregulated affective control system which equally affects all confabulations.

However, Fotopoulou (2010 this issue) has suggested that the degree of exaggerated self-enhancing bias in confabulation is determined by the degree of damage to systems that normally control and regulate monitoring processes. In other words, the motivational forces are more likely to take over the more that the normal retrieval processes fail, thus causing "rewarding" representations to be preferentially selected from the disordered system. In support of this view Fotopoulou, Conway, Birchall, et al. (2007) described a patient whose confabulations appeared to exaggerate premorbid values of self-esteem and positive character traits, with these themes also present in his actual memories, albeit to a lesser degree. In regards to the neuropsychological impairments of our patients, they all demonstrated evidence of memory impairment to varying degrees, which might have determined their degree of positive bias. Taken as a group, autobiographical memory impairment was particularly evident when retrieving semantic autobiographical information from the postinjury period and just prior to the injury (where retrograde amnesia may have been present). Impairments were less striking when semantic autobiographical material was retrieved about their childhood and early adulthood (e.g., location of school, first occupation). This differentially greater impairment in retrieval of information about more recent compared to more distant time periods together with our finding of a circumscribed positive bias for *current* confabulations is thus generally consistent with Fotopoulou's suggestion.

Moreover, previous PhD research (Metcalf, 2006) conducted with four of the patients in the present study—DL, SD, TW, and LF—has reported emotional bias in their accurate autobiographical memories. The study examined whether there was preferential retrieval of accurate pleasant memories compared to unpleasant memories. In these four patients, SD and LF did not demonstrate a self-enhancing bias, whereas TW and DL demonstrated more of a bias to recall unpleasant events in their accurate autobiographical memories. Thus, it would seem that the positive biases for *current* confabulations found in the present study are not the result of a general positive emotional bias, but arise only when memory retrieval fails.

However, when we consider GM and TW, it seems that it is not a universal rule that the degree of positive emotional bias is determined by the degree of damage to normal memory retrieval. On the AMI, GM and TW were in the "definitely abnormal" range for all age categories for both semantic and episodic information and yet it was GM and TW who showed least evidence of a positive bias, whether for their current or their past confabulations. In the following section we consider other patient characteristics that might influence the valence of confabulatory content, before considering the role of more general personal, and not necessarily wishful, biases in nuancing confabulatory content.

Patient characteristics that might influence positively biased confabulations

Several authors offer an interesting perspective in suggesting a combination of motivational processes and neuropsychological impairments to explain the production of an emotional bias in confabulation (e.g., Bisiach, Vallar, Perani, Papagno, & Berti, 1986; Giacino & Cicerone, 1998; Ownsworth, McFarland, & Young, 2002; Venneri & Shanks, 2004). It has been suggested that the deficits underlying confabulators who act on their confabulations may be mediated by different mechanisms to those seen in patients who do not act on their confabulations (Schnider, 2003; Schnider et al., 1996). Thus, it is possible that the mechanisms responsible for the more severe forms of spontaneous confabulation in some of our patients may have lead to the retrieval of more positive confabulations. In support of this notion three of our four spontaneous confabulators (AP, DL, and SD) drove the positive bias found in our initial group analysis. However, our other spontaneous confabulator—TW—who confabulated floridly in his daily life did not produce more positively biased confabulations. His performance suggests that the severity of the confabulations does not *necessarily* affect the strength of a positive bias.

Another individual variation that may influence the strength of the positive bias is time duration since injury. Five of the six patients were seen in the rehabilitation hospital setting, which is a negative setting for all of us. GM, on the other hand, was seen 2 years postinjury in his own home. He was settled into his life as a retired man and was managed very closely by a large and supportive family. GM's positive bias was less evident than other patients (excluding TW). The duration since his injury meant that he had been on holidays, visited his friends, and lives in his own home, and his confabulations often reflected misplacements of these events. Therefore, his confabulations, although pleasant in themselves, were no less or more pleasant than his actual corresponding situation. The implication here is that duration since injury and the current circumstances of the patient might need to be considered on a case by case basis when evaluating the role of emotional biases in confabulation.

However, there is another possibility with GM. He also showed the symptoms of Anton's Syndrome in that he generally denied his visual impairments and experienced anosognosia concerning his memory and his other cognitive deficits. He was most emphatic in his denial of his memory impairment; however, his awareness of his visual difficulties fluctuated. Fotopoulou (2010 this issue) cites research from her PhD demonstrating that patients with anosognosia for hemiplegia following right perisylvian lesions have an overall negative, rather than a positive, bias when they confabulate. Therefore, the weaker positive bias in GM may have been associated with his anosognosia. Anton's Syndrome is known to result from bilateral damage to the occipital cortex (Goldenberg, Mullbacher, & Nowak 1995), which was seen in GM's brain scans. Therefore, it is possible that the GM's weaker positive bias was the result of a lack of specific damage to the ventromedial frontal cortex—the area specifically involved in affective regulation. It would be interesting for future research to focus on the role that posterior lesion sites might play in determining the presence of less positive emotional biases in confabulation.

Although we have taken a predominantly cognitive neuropsychological approach, the above case reiterates that neuropathological difference also need consideration when looking for factors that might predispose an individual to producing positively biased confabulation. For example, damage to the ventromedial prefrontal cortex has been frequently reported in those who confabulate (Gilboa & Moscovitch, 2002; Schnider & Ptak, 1999; Schnider et al., 1996) and this region has also been associated with the retrieval of positive rather than negative emotional content (Maratos, Dolan, Morris, Henson, & Rugg, 2001; Piefke, Weiss, Zilles, Markowitsch, & Fink, 2003). Unfortunately, a fine-grained approach to looking at lesion data was not possible in the current group of patients, however, due to poor or limited scanning of some of our patients.

Another factor that might influence the production of a positive bias is the patient's current (or indeed premorbid) mood (e.g., the more depressed the patient, perhaps the greater the drive to a positive bias, or vice versa). Current mood was assessed in the current study by opinion of treating psychologist, medical professionals, and mood questionnaire where available. Of the patients who demonstrated the strongest positive bias in their *current* confabulations, none had been treated premorbidly for depression. Two of these patients (AP and DL) showed no evidence of current low mood and were not on antidepressant medication. The third (SD) did show evidence of low mood and was on antidepressant medication. In regards to the patients with *less* evidence of a positive bias, two (TW and LF) showed current evidence of low mood and were being treated with antidepressant medication. Moreover, TW had a premorbid diagnosis of depression, which had been treated for a number of years. However, GM, the third patient showing a limited positive bias, had no signs of current or past depression. Thus, if mood does contribute to the production of a positive bias, its effects are very subtle and were not readily apparent in the current study. We turn now to consider the role of personal bias in confabulation, in a more general sense.

Personal bias and confabulation

First, we note that quite a number of neutral (or realistic) confabulations were generated by our patients: 22% of current confabulations and 53% of past confabulations. We do not think that this was due to the lack of an "I don't know" response for our raters, who reported that the neutral rating was not difficult to make and that they did not use this as a default for difficult decisions. The confabulatory responses that were rated as neutral were heavily dominated by simple misplacements of events that had occurred at another time or to another related person. For example, AP stated that the last place he went on holiday was Coffs Harbour, when he really went to Forster (both pleasant beach towns). Also, GM said he had visited a good friend the day before, when in fact his brother and sister had been to visit him. In line with our own observations, Dalla Barba and Boissé (2010 this issue) have shown that the most frequent themes in confabulation involve misplacements of general memories and habits from the past. Themes of work, for example, were particularly prevalent across the confabulations of a number of our patients, particularly AP and DL. As with childhood memory, these memories of repeated daily events are likely to be well encoded and consolidated personal semantic information. In other words, the content of confabulation might primarily reflect the tendency to retrieve generic memories (Burgess & McNeil, 1999; Dalla Barba, Cappelletti, Signorini, & Denes, 1997), which are then nuanced by personal biases. Included in these personal biases will be positive emotional biases that are exaggerated, in many cases (but perhaps not all), to the degree that the patient's memory is impaired.

In general, we think that the degree and the direction of any bias in our patients' confabulations can be understood by focusing primarily on the habitual memories that best conform with a patient's premorbid concept of self. Most of the time, but not always, these premorbid self-concepts will show a positive bias. As an example, one of our patients—DL—was a strong-willed individual, who for most of his life was focused on his work and consequent success, even to the detriment of his family. These features in his personality may have enhanced the likelihood of DL retrieving material that maintained his need for stature, particularly in regards to his work. His current confabulations often revolved around the mistaken belief that he was imminently returning to work upon his discharge. In his working life he was highly regarded by his colleagues and these themes remained, and were perhaps enhanced, in his confabulations as the following conversation demonstrates:

Investigator: Will you return to work when you are discharged?
DL: Three people have offered me work already.
Investigator: What will you be doing?
DL: Hydraulic work.
Investigator: Will the work be close to here? Will it be easy to get to?
DL: It will be all around Australia.
Investigator: Are you worried about travelling?
DL: No.

Investigator: Do you want to retire and rest?
DL: No . . . I am still the best hydraulic engineer in the country.

Of course, DL's confabulations were also self-serving and so he might have been biased to generate such positive confabulations, not only because they conformed to his premorbid self-concept, but also because he was motivated to defend against confronting his current grim circumstances (whether consciously or unconsciously). Any such self-enhancing motivation to deny the current grim reality seems not to apply, however, to our patient TW, who, like GM, was more realistic (perhaps depressingly realistic) in his confabulations. TW had been diagnosed with depression premorbidly. As we have outlined in his case report, TW had also had a very sad life with numerous negative events. It is thus understandable that his retrieval of memories and confabulations might have reflected his negative, rather than his positive, sense of self. The content of his confabulations differed markedly from the other confabulating patients reported here. TW's confabulations frequently contained very dark material concerning relatives' deaths that was as morbid as the true narrative. For example, when TW was asked if his parent's were still alive, the following conversation occurred:

TW: . . . one is and one isn't. One died a week ago. Killed in a car crash, wiped his head clear off his shoulders.
Investigator: Was this your father?
TW: Yes.
Investigator: Your mother is still alive?
TW: Yeah, she just died. She just died a couple of days ago.
Investigator: How did your mother die?
TW: She died from eh . . . what do they call it . . . ah . . . you get . . . cancer.
Investigator: You said that your dad died in a car crash?
TW: Dad? We don't know nothing because we haven't seen each other since she left me?
Investigator: Who left you?
TW: My mum, she died in a car crash I think. Apparently the car wiped her head clear off her shoulder.

Negative confabulations of this type have also been described in patient JL, who had a similar sad history (Demery et al., 2001). In accord with our own views, Demery and colleagues suggested that JL's provoked confabulations reflect preferential retrieval from long-term memory of familiar negative material.

CONCLUSION

In summary, the current study has focused on the role of personal bias in explaining the content of confabulation. We adopted a cognitive neuropsychological approach to focus on phenomenology—that is, the symptom of confabulation, regardless of aetiology, and so examined a mixed group of six confabulating patients with diverse aetiologies. Consistent with previous research, we found a general positive bias in confabulations, when the patients were considered as a group. Further analyses revealed that it was the confabulations regarding the patients' *current* injury-related circumstances that were primarily responsible for this positive bias, whereas confabulations about the *past* showed no such bias. This relatively circumscribed positive bias cooccurred with generally poorer retrieval of semantic autobiographical material from the recent past and postmorbid period compared to better retrieval of semantic information from earlier life periods. Thus our group findings are consistent with Fotopoulou's (2010 this issue) suggestion that motivational mechanisms which drive a positive emotional bias take over, in degree, to the extent that normal memory retrieval fails. However, some of our confabulators did show poorer retrieval of information from the more distant past (e.g., GM and TW) and yet this poorer retrieval was not associated with more of a positive bias in these patients' past confabulations. Indeed, it was GM and TW who showed least evidence of a positive bias. We do acknowledge here, however, that a more constrained subset of confabulators (e.g., with more specific neuropathology) may all show the proposed relationship between degree of positive emotional bias and degree of memory impairment. In the case of our own confabulating patients, however, it was notable that the content of some reported confabulations seemed most consistent with a negative, rather than a positive, self-concept (in particular, for TW). We therefore concur with other researchers who suggest that the content of confabulation primarily reflects the ease with which generic memories and premorbid routines and activities are retrieved from a dysfunctional memory system coupled with a personal bias to accept memories that concur with (or inflate) past self-representations (whether positive or negative), thus serving the purpose of maintaining a consistent self-concept in the face of changing reality.

REFERENCES

Berlyne, N. (1972). Confabulation. *British Journal of Psychiatry, 120*, 31–39.

Bisiach, E., Vallar, G., Perani, D., Papagno, C., & Berti, A. (1986). Unawareness of disease following lesions of the right hemisphere: Anosognosia for hemiplegia and anosognosia for hemianopia. *Neuropsychologia, 24*, 471–482.

Bonhoeffer, K. (1904). Der korsakowsche Symptomenkomplex in seinen Beziehungen zu den verschieden Krankheitsformen. *Allgemeine Zeitschrift für Psychiatrie und Psychisch-Geritliche Medecin, 61*, 744–752.

Burgess, P. W., & McNeil, J. E. (1999). Content-specific confabulation. *Cortex, 35*, 163–182.
Burgess, P. W., & Shallice, T. (1996). Confabulation and the control of recollection. *Memory, 4*, 359–411.
Ciaramelli, E., & Ghetti, S. (2007). What are confabulators' memories made of? A study of subjective and objective measures of recollection in confabulation. *Neuropsychologia, 45*, 1489–1500.
Ciaramelli, E., Ghetti, S., Frattarelli, M., & Ladavas, E. (2006). When true memory availability promotes false memory: Evidence from confabulating patients. *Neuropsychologia, 44*, 1866–1877.
Coltheart, M. (2007). Cognitive neuropsychiatry and delusional belief. *Quarterly Journal of Experimental Psychology, 60*, 1041–1062.
Coltheart, M., Langdon, R., & McKay, R. (2007). Schizophrenia and monothematic delusions. *Schizophrenia Bulletin, 33*, 642–647.
Conway, M. A. (1996). Autobiographical knowledge and autobiographical memories. In D. C. Rubin (Ed.), *Remembering our past: Studies in autobiographical memory* (pp. 67–93). Cambridge, UK: Cambridge University Press.
Conway, M. A. (2005). Memory and the self. *Journal of Memory and Language, 53*, 594–628.
Conway, M. A., Collins, A. F., Gathercole, S. E., & Anderson, S. J. (1996). Recollections of true and false autobiographical memories. *Journal of Experimental Psychology: General, 125*, 69–95.
Conway, M. A., & Fthenaki, A. (2000). Disruption and loss of autobiographical memory. In L. S. Cermak (Ed.), *Memory and its disorders* (2nd ed., Vol. 2, pp. 281–313). Amsterdam: Elsevier.
Conway, M. A., & Pleydell-Pearce, C. W. (2000). The construction of autobiographical memories in the self-memory system. *Psychological Review, 107*, 261–288.
Conway, M. A., & Rubin, D. C. (1993). The structure of autobiographical memory. In A. F. Collins, S. E. Gathercole, M. A. Conway, & P. E. Morris (Eds.), *Theories of memory* (pp. 103–137). Hove, UK: Lawrence Erlbaum Associates Ltd.
Conway, M. A., Singer, J. A., & Tagini, A. (2004). The self and autobiographical memory: Correspondence and coherence. *Social Cognition, 22*, 491–529.
Conway, M. A., & Tacchi, P. C. (1996). Motivated confabulation. *Neurocase, 2*, 325–339.
Dalla Barba, G. (1993). Confabulation: Knowledge and recollective experience. *Cognitive Neuropsychology, 10*, 1–20.
Dalla Barba, G., & Boissé, M.-F. (2010). Temporal consciousness and confabulation: Is the medial temporal lobe "temporal"? *Cognitive Neuropsychiatry, 15*(1/2/3), 95–117.
Dalla Barba, G., Cappelletti, J. Y., Signorini, M., & Denes, G. (1997). Confabulation: Remembering "another" past, planning "another" future. *Neurocase, 3*, 425–436.
Davies, M., Coltheart, M., Langdon, R., & Breen, N. (2001). Monothematic delusions: Towards a two-factor account. Philopsophy. *Psychiatry and Psychology, 8*, 133–158.
Delis, D. C., Kaplan, E., & Kramer, J. H. (2001). *Delis Kaplan executive function system*. San Antonio, TX: Psychological Corporation.
Demery, J. A., Hanlon, R. E., & Bauer, R. M. (2001). Profound amnesia and confabulation following traumatic brain injury. *Neurocase, 7*, 295–301.
Fotopoulou, A. (2010). The affective neuropsychology of confabulation and delusion. *Cognitive Neuropsychiatry, 15*(1/2/3), 38–63.
Fotopoulou, A., Conway, M. A., Birchall, D., Griffiths, P., & Tyer, S. (2007). Confabulation: Revising the motivational hypothesis. *Neurocase, 13*, 6–15.
Foropoulou, A., Conway, M. A., & Solms, M. (2007). Confabulation: Motivated reality monitoring. *Neuropsychologia, 45*, 2180–2190.
Fotopoulou, A., Conway, M. A., Solms, M., Tyer, S., & Kopelman, M. (2008). Self-serving confabulation in prose recall. *Neuropsychologia, 26*, 1429–1441.
Fotopoulou, A., Conway, M. A., Tyer, S., Birchall, D., Griffiths, P., & Solms, M. (2008). Positive emotional biases in confabulation: An experimental study. *Cortex, 44*, 764–772.

Fotopoulou, A., Solms, M., & Turnbull, O. (2004). Wishful reality distortions in confabulation: A case report. *Neuropsychologia, 42*, 727–744.

Giacino, J. T., & Cicerone, K. D. (1998). Varieties of deficit unawareness after brain injury. *Journal of Head Trauma Rehabilitation, 13*, 1–15.

Gilboa, A., Alain, C., Stuss, D. T., Melo, B., Miller, S., & Moscovitch, M. (2006). Mechanisms of spontaneous confabulations: A strategic retrieval account. *Brain, 129*, 1339–1414.

Gilboa, A., & Moscovitch, M. (2002). The cognitive neuroscience of confabulation: A review and a model. In A. Baddeley, M. D. Kopelman, & B. Wilson (Eds.), *The handbook of memory disorders* (2nd ed., pp. 315–340). Chichester, UK: Wiley.

Goldenberg, G., Mullbacher, W., & Nowak, A. (1995). Imagery without perception: A case study of anosognosia for cortical blindness. *Neuropsychologia, 33*, 1373–1382.

Kennedy, Q., Mather, M., & Carstensen, L. L. (2004). The role of motivation in the age-related positivity effect in autobiographical memory. *Psychological Science, 15*, 208–213.

Kopelman, M. D. (1987). Two types of confabulation. *Journal of Neurology. Neurosurgery and Psychiatry, 50*, 1482–1487.

Kopelman, M. D. (1999). Varieties of false memory. *Cognitive Neuropsychology, 16*, 197–214.

Kopelman, M. D. (2010). Varieties of confabulation and delusion. *Cognitive Neuropsychiatry, 15*(1/2/3), 14–37.

Kopelman, M. D., Wilson, B., & Baddeley, A. (1990). *The Autobiographical Memory Interview (AMI)*. Bury St. Edmunds, UK: Thames Valley Test Company.

Langdon, R., & Coltheart, M. (2000a). The cognitive neuropsychology of delusions. *Mind and Language, 15*, 184–218.

Langdon, R., & Coltheart, M. (2000b). The cognitive neuropsychology of delusions. In M. Coltheart & M. Davies (Eds.), *Pathologies of belief* (pp. 183–216). Oxford, UK: Blackwell Publishers.

Langdon, R., McKay, R., & Coltheart, M. (2008). The cognitive neuropsychological understanding of persecutory delusions. In D. Freeman, R. Bentall, & P. Garety (Eds.), *Persecutory delusions: Assessment, theory and treatment* (pp. 221–236). Oxford, UK: Oxford University Press.

Maratos, E. J., Dolan, R. J., Morris, J. S., Henson, R. N. A., & Rugg, M. D. (2001). Neural activity associated with episodic memory for emotional context. *Neuropsychologia, 39*, 910–920.

Mather, M., & Carstensen, L. L. (2005). Aging and motivated cognition: The positivity effect in attention and memory. *Trends in Cognitive Science, 9*, 496–502.

Metcalf, K. (2006). *The origin and nature of confabulation: A cognitive neuropsychological perspective.* Unpublished PhD thesis, Macquarie University, Sydney, Australia.

Metcalf, K., Langdon, R., & Coltheart, M. (2007). Models of confabulation: A critical review and a new framework. *Cognitive Neuropsychology, 24*, 23–47.

Moscovitch, M. (1989). Confabulation and the frontal systems: Strategic versus associated retrieval in neuropsychological theories of memory. In H. L. Roediger III & F. I. M. Craik (Eds.), *Varieties of memory and consciousness: Essays in honour of Endel Tulving* (pp. 133–160). Hillsdale, NJ: Lawrence Erlbaum Associates, Inc.

Moscovitch, M. (1995). Confabulation. In D. L. Schacter (Ed.), *Memory distortions: How minds, brains and societies reconstruct the past* (pp. 226–251). Cambridge, MA: Harvard University Press.

Nedjam, Z., Devouche, E., & Dalla Barba, G. (2004). Confabulation, but not executive dysfunction discriminate AD from frontotemporal dementia. *European Journal of Neurology, 11*, 728–733.

Ownsworth, T. L., McFarland, K., & Young, R. M. (2002). The investigation of factors underlying deficits in self-awareness and self-regulation. *Brain Injury, 16*, 291–307.

Piefke, M., Weiss, P. H., Zilles, K., Markowitsch, H. J., & Fink, G. R. (2003). Differential remoteness and emotional tone modulate the neural correlated of autobiographical memory. *Brain, 126*, 650–668.

Schnider, A. (2003). Spontaneous confabulation and the adaptation of thought to ongoing reality. *National Review of Neuroscience, 4*, 662–671.

Schnider, A., & Ptak, R. (1999). Spontaneous confabulators fail to suppress currently irrelevant memory traces. *Nature Neuroscience, 2*, 677–681.

Schnider, A., von Daniken, C., & Gutbrod, K. (1996). The mechanisms of spontaneous and provoked confabulations. *Brain, 119*, 1365–1375.

Senior, G. (1999). *Rey Auditory Verbal Learning Test—Australian Normative Data,* 2003. Retrieved from http://www.usq.edu.au/users/senior/

Shallice, T., & Evans, M. E. (1978). The involvement of the frontal lobes in cognitive estimation. *Cortex, 14*, 294–303.

Shimamura, A. P. (2002). Memory retrieval and executive control processes. In D. T. Stuss & R. T. Knight (Eds.), *Principles of frontal lobe function* (pp. 210–220). Oxford, UK: Oxford University Press.

Talland, G. A. (1965). *Deranged Memory.* San Diego, CA: Academic Press.

Turnbull, O. H., Berry, H., & Evans, C. E. Y. (2004). A positive emotional bias in confabulatory false beliefs about place. *Brain and Cognition, 55*, 490–494.

Venneri, A., & Shanks, M. F. (2004). Belief and awareness: Reflections on a case of persistent anosognosia. *Neuropsychologia, 42*, 230–238.

Verslegers, W., de Deyn, P. P., Saerens, J., & Marien, P. (1991). Slow progressive bilateral posterior artery infarction presenting as agitated delirium, complicated with Anton's syndrome. *European Neurology, 31*, 216–219.

Wechsler, D. (1997a). *Wechsler Adult Intelligence Scale* (3rd ed.). San Antonio, TX: Psychological Corporation.

Wechsler, D. (1997b). *Wechsler Memory Scale* (3rd ed.). San Antonio, TX: Psychological Corporation.

Wechsler, D. (2001). *Wechsler Test of Adult Reading.* San Antonio, TX: Psychological Corporation.

COGNITIVE NEUROPSYCHIATRY
2010, 15 (1/2/3), 95–117

Temporal consciousness and confabulation: Is the medial temporal lobe "temporal"?

Gianfranco Dalla Barba[1,2,3,4] and Marie-Françoise Boissé[4]

[1]*INSERM Unit 610, Paris, France,* [2]*Université Pierre et Marie Curie, Paris 6, Paris, France,* [3]*Dipartimento di Psicologia, Università degli Studi di Trieste, Italy,* [4]*AP-HP, Hôpital Henri Mondor, Service de Neurologie, Créteil, France*

Since the early descriptions of this phenomenon, there is a large consensus on the distinction between two forms of confabulation. Provoked confabulations are plausible minor memory distortions in response to direct questioning, whereas spontaneous confabulations are unprovoked, often implausible, memories. However, as we show with the analysis of 284 provoked and 52 spontaneous confabulations produced by eight patients with confabulatory syndromes of different aetiologies, the provoked/spontaneous distinction fails to capture the quality of the great majority of confabulations that clearly do not fall in either of the two poles of the distinction. In this study, the majority of provoked (52%) and spontaneous (73%) confabulations consisted of what we refer to as "general memories, habits, and misplacements", i.e., either true episodes misplaced in time and place, or personal habits and routines which are considered by the patient as specific personal episodes. These observations are discussed within the framework of the Memory, Consciousness, and Temporality Theory. According to this theory, confabulation reflects an abnormal functioning of temporal consciousness (TC). The integrity of the medial temporal lobe (MTL) and related structures is crucial for the normal functioning of TC. Data from the literature show that what confabulators have in common is not a specific lesion site but rather the integrity of the MTL, which is consistent with the idea that the MTL is essential for the function of normal and confabulatory TC. In this sense the MTL is "temporal", because its integrity allows individuals to be consciously aware of a personal past, present and future. A better understanding of TC, including its neurobiological correlates, will help to better understand confabulation avoiding theoretically untenable and experimentally undemonstrated explanatory idols like memory traces and unconscious monitoring.

Keywords: Confabulation; Temporal Consciousness; Medial temporal lobe.

Correspondence should be addressed to Gianfranco Dalla Barba, INSERM, U. 610, 47, Boulevard de l'Hôpital, 75013 Paris, France. E-mail: dallabarba@chups.jussieu.fr

 DOI: 10.1080/13546800902758017

INTRODUCTION

We are all wrong. Philosophers, scientists, writers, poets, even mathematicians make huge, sometime devastating errors. We make errors in our daily life—errors of judgement, of planning, of memory, among others. Much of the time, we are not aware of our errors, we feel that we are right and we keep maintaining our position regardless of any evidence in contrast with it. In some cases, however, our mistakes in judging and remembering are so evident that we need other names to distinguish them from "normal" errors. Delusion and confabulation are the names we use to indicate "abnormal" errors in judgement and remembering.

In this paper we will focus on confabulation, providing first a tentative taxonomy of this phenomenon. We will then show how different types of confabulation can be accounted for within the framework of the Memory, Consciousness, and Temporally Theory (MCTT). Finally, we will discuss the role of the medial temporal lobe (MTL) and related structures in confabulation.

CONFABULATION: ONE, TWO, OR MANY?

Since the early descriptions of this phenomenon, clinicians and scientists have distinguished between two forms of confabulation. For example, Bleuler in his 1949 handbook of psychiatry distinguished between confabulations of embarrassment (*Verlegenheit Konfabulationen*) and productive or fantastic confabulations. The first type reflects the need to fill a memory gap when directly questioned, the second is much more context-free, unprovoked and often favoured by a euphoric mood. More recently, Kopelman (1987), following Berlyne, (1972) distinguished between provoked and spontaneous confabulations (see Kopelman, 2010 this issue). Provoked confabulations are plausible minor memory distortions in response to direct questioning or in a test situation, whereas spontaneous confabulations are unprovoked, often implausible, memories. Provoked confabulation is considered as a normal response to a faulty memory, whereas spontaneous confabulation is considered to result from the superposition of frontal/executive dysfunction to an organic amnesia. Kopelman's conceptual distinction between these two types of confabulation is certainly valuable because it underlines the qualitative difference between two extreme forms of confabulation, which may have differing underlying mechanisms. However, the line drawn between spontaneous and provoked confabulation often appears to be quite a difficult decision and in a number of cases spontaneous confabulations are plausible and provoked confabulations may be bizarre and implausible (Dalla Barba, 1993a, 1993b; Dalla Barba, Cappelletti,

Signorini, & Denes, 1997; Johnson, O'Connor, & Cantor, 1997; Nedjam, Dalla Barba, & Pillon, 2000).

We have proposed that, regardless of their modality of appearance (spontaneous vs. provoked), confabulations can be distinguished according to the semantic quality of their content. Accordingly, confabulations may be "semantically appropriate" or "semantically anomalous" according to the quality of their content. Consider the following example.

> "What did you do yesterday?" asks the doctor to patient SD
> "Yesterday I won a running race and I was awarded with a piece of meat which was put on my right knee" (Dalla Barba, 1993b)

In order to tell that SD's report is confabulatory, you don't need to know that he is a 37-year-old patient who reported a severe head trauma. In fact, SD's confabulation describes an event that not only he is unlikely to have experienced at that particular time, but which is unlikely that anybody would have or will ever experience. The content of SD's confabulation is *semantically anomalous*, in the sense that it carries meanings which are inconsistent with knowledge and information shared by the members of society. Confabulations often described as *fantastic* or *implausible* actually contain semantic anomalies (Baddeley & Wilson, 1986; Joseph, 1986; Sandson, Albert, & Alexander, 1986; Stuss, Alexander, Lieberman, & Levine, 1978; Weinstein & Lyerly, 1968). However, although semantically anomalous, these confabulations are often made of autobiographical elements put together in an inappropriate semantic structure. Consider again SD's example. SD was actually involved in running races and had spent most of his free time in this kind of activity. It was actually during a running race in the mountains that he fell reporting a severe head trauma and an open wound in his right knee. So, his confabulation about having won a running race and having been awarded with a piece of meat on his knee actually contains autobiographical elements inserted in an inappropriate semantic context.

The distinction between semantically appropriate and semantically anomalous confabulations is not an alternative to the spontaneous/provoked distinction, but is rather complementary to it in that it adds information about the content of the confabulation. However, distinctions based on the modality of appearance and on the semantic quality of content are certainly useful at a general level of description, but fail to provide an adequate description of the variety of confabulations which may reflect differing underlying cognitive and neural mechanisms. In the following sections we will show that by focusing on the content of confabulation we can identify a variety of confabulation that goes well beyond the dichotomies proposed in the literature.

VARIETIES OF CONFABULATIONS

Clinical and experimental observation shows that confabulation often consists either of true episodes misplaced in time and place or of personal habits and routines that are considered by the patient as specific personal episodes. When asked what they did today or what they will do tomorrow, confabulating patients may reply with well-established memories from their pasts, however irrelevant these memories may be to their present situation. We will refer to this as "general memories, habits, and misplacements" (GMHM).

METHOD

In order to better characterise and quantify the relative contribution of GMHM to confabulation, we analysed 284 provoked and 52 spontaneous confabulations produced by eight patients with a confabulatory syndrome. Patients' characteristics are reported in Table 1.

Provoked confabulations were collected with the Confabulation Battery, which comprises 169 questions tapping various aspects of semantic and episodic memory and also includes questions about personal future, e.g., "What are you going to do tomorrow?" and impersonal future, e.g., "What you think will be the most important medical breakthrough likely to take place in the next ten years?" (see Dalla Barba & Decaix, 2009, for a detailed description of the Confabulation Battery). Patients spontaneously confabulated in they daily life. However, the 52 spontaneous confabulations analysed in this study were collected during informal conversation, which lasted approximately 20 minutes for each patient. The examiner's participation was limited to very general cueing and specific questioning was avoided. Some patients in few occasions acted upon their confabulations, but this was not considered criteria for classifying confabulations as spontaneous.

RESULTS

The percentages of each type of confabulation (provoked and spontaneous) are reported in Table 2. The patients' number of each type of confabulation is presented in Table 3. The Wilcoxon signed-rank test was used to compare the frequency of provoked and spontaneous confabulations of each type.

GMHM accounted for 52% of provoked and 73% of spontaneous confabulations ($p > .5$). An example of confabulation consisting of GMHM is provided by patient PD.

PD is a 73 year-old woman who suffered from a rupture of anterior communicating artery aneurism which caused a left frontobasal lesion. To

TABLE 1
Patients' characteristics

Patients	*Age (years)*	*Site of lesion*	*Diagnosis*	*Digit span*	*Free and cued selective reminding test (total recall/48)*
GL	60	Bitemporal	Korsakoff's syndrome	5	15
MC	52	Diffuse cortical atrophy	Multiple Sclerosis + alcoholism	5	46
PD	73	Frontal	AACoA	6	35
AB	51	Diffuse cortical atrophy	Alcoholism	5	23
DO	48	No detectable lesion at MRI	Korsakoff's syndrome	7	17
PS	48	No detectable lesion at MRI	APCoA	5	11
VQ	78	Corpus callosum	Lymphoma	5	4
VV	43	Cerebellar angioma, frontal atrophy	Heart arrest/ anoxia	5	10

AACoA = aneurysm of the anterior communicating artery; APCoA = aneurysm of the posterior communicating artery.

the question "How did you spend last Christmas?" she answered "Last Christmas? During the day we prepared ... we opened oysters, we ate prawns, shrimps, turkey, chestnuts, some French fries, salad, cheese, fruits, a little 'bûchette'. We gave the presents to the children, we participated in the games ... we had to do something. We played dominos."

This example shows that PD, when confabulating, recalls a "general" Christmas as a specific one. Instead of recalling what she did specifically during the previous Christmas, she recalls what she has probably done on

TABLE 2
Types of confabulations

	Provoked (n = 284)	*Spontaneous (n = 52)*
General memories habits, and misplacements (GMHM)	52%	73%
Memory fabrications (MF)	18%	17%
Memory confusion (MC)	15%	5%
Autoreferential contamination (ARC)	3%	0%
Semantically inappropriate	11%	4%

TABLE 3
Number of provoked and spontaneous confabulation

	General memories, habits, and misplacements		*Memory fabrications*		*Memory confusions*		*Autoreferencial contaminations*		*Semantically inappropriate*	
Patients	*Provoked*	*Spontaneous*	*Provoked*	*Spontaneous*	*Provoked*	*Spontaneous*	*Provoked*	*Spontaneous*	*Provoked*	*Spontaneous*
GL	24	4	10	0	8	1	1	0	1	0
MC	24	1	6	2	5	2	0	0	0	0
PD	24	2	7	3	8	0	0	0	0	0
AB	22	0	5	0	0	0	0	0	1	0
DO	14	24	7	4	5	0	0	0	0	0
PS	15	6	6	0	10	0	0	0	0	0
VQ	15	0	7	0	2	0	10	0	4	0
VV	11	1	3	0	4	0	0	0	25	2
Total	149	38	51	9	42	3	11	0	31	2

many Christmas days throughout her life. This was confirmed by her husband, who also confirmed that they spent the previous Christmas alone.

Another patient, AB, who had diffuse cortical atrophy and suffered from alcoholism, reported that the previous day he went to the tomato fair. According to his wife they went many times to that fair, but certainly not on the previous day. In this case, a personal repeated event, attending an annual fair, is considered by the patient as a specific one and misplaced in time.

GMHM, though less frequently, was also observed in confabulation to semantic memory questions. For example, to the question "What happened in Nuremberg?" PD answered "There was a criminal trial against the Nazis, four years ago." In this case, a true episode and a correct memory are misplaced in time.

The second most frequent type of confabulation observed in our patients was what we called memory fabrications (MF). Fabrications are memories, episodic or semantic, without any recognisable link with personal or public events. MF accounted for 18% of provoked and 17% of spontaneous confabulations in our patients ($p > .5$). The following are examples of MF in episodic memory,

> "Why are you hospitalised?"
> PD: "Because I have lung problems [PD didn't have and never had any lung problems].

And in semantic memory, the patient PS, a 48-year-old who suffered from a rupture of the posterior communicating artery aneurism, responded to the following question:

> "Who is Delanoë (the mayor of Paris)?"
> "Delanoë? He is a war chief from ancient times."

Another type of confabulation observed in our patients is what we referred to as memory confusion (MC). MC, which accounted for 15% of provoked and 5% of spontaneous confabulations ($p > .5$), consisted of confusion with other personal or public events related to the target memory or confusion between family members. GL, for example, a 60-year-old patient with Korsakoff's syndrome, responded to the question "What happened in Waterloo?" with "Waterloo? It was like Verdun, a battle between French and Germans." The same patient answered the question "Do you have children?" with "Yes, one, Thévard, he is one year-old." Thévard was actually his grandson.

Confabulating patients when questioned about public or historical events may refer to the event in a personal context. We call this type of confabulation autoreferential contamination (ARC). In our patients ARC accounted for 3% of provoked confabulations, but were not produced spontaneously. The following are some examples of ARC.

To the question "What does the Mir station remind you of?" patient VQ, a 78-year-old with lymphoma and a lesion into the corpus callosum, answered "The Mir Station? It's very important. It is about Vietnam. We have signed something between Mir and Vietnam." VQ was the wife of a Vietnamese diplomat and she often used to talk about Vietnam and about her husband's work.

Patient GL had lost his savings in a financial scandal. To the question "What does the Dreyfus affaire remind you of?" he answered "The Dreyfus affaire? A big financial scandal." The same patient answered the question "Who was the prime minister in 1965?" with "It was Chaban [a well-known French politician]. He is my daughter's godfather."

Confabulations described in the literature as "fantastic", "semantically inappropriate", or "spontaneous", which have implausible and frankly bizarre content also occurred in our patients, but accounted for only 11% of provoked and 4% of spontaneous confabulations ($p > .5$). An example of this type of confabulation is provided by VV, a 43-year-old patient who suffered from cerebral anoxia and showed predominantly frontal cerebral atrophy. To the question "Who did you see yesterday?" he answered "I saw Régis, he does osteopathy on butterflies."

It must be noted that the boundaries between the different types of confabulation were sufficiently clear-cut, and that no particular difficulty emerged in attributing the confabulations to a particular category.

CONSCIOUSNESS AND CONFABULATION

From the analysis and characterisation of our patients' confabulations it emerges that:

1. The provoked/spontaneous distinction may be useful at a very general level of description when it refers to two extreme forms of confabulation. However, it fails to capture the quality of the great majority of confabulations that clearly do not fall in either of the two poles of the distinction.
2. Confabulations described as "fantastic", "bizarre", or semantically inappropriate are quite infrequent and are both provoked and spontaneous.
3. The great majority of confabulations, 87% in this study fall into three categories, GMHM (56%), MF (18%), and MC (13%). These confabulations have a plausible content and are more often made of

well-established memories and information that distorts or replaces all the to-be-remembered memory or information.

We have said elsewhere that patients who confabulate remember "another" past (Dalla Barba et al., 1997), in the sense that they are aware of a past but one that is different from their real past, the past they would have remembered if they didn't have had a severe amnesico-confabulatory syndrome. Most of the time this past that confabulators remember is made of recognisable elements of the patient's biography or of general semantic information. What kind of memory theory can account for this situation? Confabulation, there is no doubt, is a conscious phenomenon. Individuals who confabulate consciously remember past events and information no matter whether their remembering is inaccurate, false, or even frankly bizarre. They are not lying and they are not in bad faith. Certainly they are unaware of the fact that some malfunctioning mechanism is affecting their memory. In fact anosognosia is almost invariably associated to confabulation. But this doesn't change the fact that confabulation manifests itself as a conscious act. So, since confabulation is conscious, we need a theory that describes the type of consciousness of confabulators and its differences with the consciousness of individuals who do not confabulate, either because they are normal or because they don't remember at all, like amnesics. Some theories explain confabulation with unconscious processes. These theories emphasise the role of unconscious monitoring processes, like in the strategic retrieval hypothesis (Gilboa, 2010 this issue; Moscovitch, 1989; Turner, 2010 this issue), and in the reality monitoring hypothesis (Johnson, 1991; Schnider & Ptak, 1999). Others propose that confabulation is unconsciously motivated (Conway & Tacchi, 1996; Fotopoulou, 2010 this issue). We have extensively discussed these theories elsewhere (Dalla Barba, 2001, 2002), showing that they fall into the *fallacy of the homunculus*, that is, attributing intentionality to unconscious processes, which is unintelligible and not experimentally provable. We will not return to this subject here.

Within the framework of the Memory Consciousness and Temporality Theory (MCTT) we have argued that confabulation reflects an abnormal functioning of what we called temporal consciousness (Dalla Barba, 2002). In the following section, we will briefly describe the MCTT and show how it accounts for confabulation.

CONSCIOUSNESS: ONE OR MANY?

Intentionality is certainly the main characteristic of consciousness, the fundamental law which consciousness must obey, since it describes the necessity of consciousness to always be consciousness *of* something (Brentano, 1874/1973; Husserl, 1950; Sartre, 1943). In other words, it is impossible to separate consciousness from its object. Consciousness is not a generic and aspecific dimension that *then* becomes consciousness of its object. It is *immediately* consciousness *of* something. We would also add that consciousness is always consciousness of something *in a certain way*. This means that consciousness takes a certain point of view of its object and of the same object consciousness can take various points of view. The first consequence of this statement is that different *modes* of consciousness exist and each of these represents an original and irreducible mode of addressing the world. By "original" we mean that each mode of consciousness is different from any other. By "irreducible" we mean that the existence of each original mode of consciousness cannot be traced back to something else that precedes it in causal or ontological terms. A taxonomy of the different modes of consciousness is far beyond the aims of this work. Our aim is rather to operate certain distinctions that will allow us to see, though at a rather general level of description, the differences between two modes of consciousness, namely what we will indicate as knowing consciousness (KC) and temporal consciousness (TC).

Knowing consciousness and temporal consciousness

KC describes what is usually referred to as semantic memory. A substantial difference, however, distinguishes KC from what is presupposed in the idea of semantic memory. Unlike semantic memory, KC is not based on the idea of unconscious mental representation. KC is consciousness of the object, it is already *outside itself* and directed towards the object to be known. And it is consciousness of the object *in a certain mode*, an original mode that makes it impossible that what I know, for example, can be mistaken for what I remember or imagine. It can be argued that I could never, for example, recognise this packet of cigarettes as *red* if I had not *already* somewhere in my mind and my brain an *idea of red*. But this kind of argument is unintelligible because it presupposes the existence and the activation of unconscious representation and in so doing falls into the fallacy of the *homunculus*. If I recognise the packet of cigarettes as red it is not because I operate, unconsciously, a sort of correspondence between the packet I perceive and a mental representation that I carry in me. What one should say is that I am conscious of this packet of cigarettes as red because my present consciousness, since it is a synthesis of all my past consciousnesses, is also consciousness of red. But I can also see this packet of cigarettes as ugly, dangerous, attractive, almost finished. In short, the meanings I attribute to the packet of cigarettes are concretely infinite and depend on my being conscious here and now as synthesis of what I have been before and elsewhere. In this sense, KC is temporal since it is a synthesis of what I have been or *wesen ist was gewesen ist*, as in Hegel. But at the same time KC is also atemporal in the sense that the time of which it is made is not recognisable. KC *is* the past but it is not consciousness *of* the past, nor of the present or of the future. There is no time in the packet of cigarettes in front of me although it is thanks to time, that is of the past I am made of, that I can see the packet as red, dangerous, etc.

Consciousness *of* time, i.e., the thematisation of the object in the mode of temporality, is what we have called TC. TC, as far as it poses its object according to the structures of time, i.e., the past, the present and the future, is an organised, original and irreducible form of consciousness, for addressing the world. Unlike KC, TC transcends the mere presence of the object in order to set it in time. When I say that I remember yesterday's dinner, that now I am in my office and that later I will go out to buy some cigarettes, knowledge is presupposed, as we will see later, but it is not the aim of the temporalising act that I am making. In order to remember yesterday's dinner, to affirm that I am *now* in my office and to plan the act of buying cigarettes, I have to *know* what a dinner, an office, and cigarettes are. However, this knowledge is only the structure on which my act is founded. It is *through* knowledge that the temporalising act is realised but it is not *for* knowledge that it is realised. Although TC is an organised structure of consciousness because past, present, and future are not isolated dimensions but continuously refer to one another, consciousness of the past, of the present and of the future are nevertheless subordinate structures of TC and for the sake of clarity we will describe them separately.

Consciousness of the past is an act through which the object of consciousness is seen as absent, or as nonpresent. But, in contrast with imagining consciousness, which sees the absent object as nonexistent, for consciousness of the past the object is absent *in* the past. It is this consciousness of the past that we call remembering. But consciousness of the past is not consciousness of a generic and impersonal past. When I say that I remember that Kennedy was killed in 1963 in Dallas or that Dante wrote the *Divine Comedy*, I am not conscious of the past but of a piece of information, a notion, that joins other notions to form a certain type of knowledge. Kennedy is president of the United States *and* past, Dante is a poet, Italian, *and* past. In other words, it is about a generic and impersonal past, not *my* past. In order for consciousness of the past to exist, i.e., remembering in the mode of TC, there must be a deep link between the being I am now and a being I was before. It is to that past being of mine that consciousness of the past refers, and it is that past being that remembering represents.

In order for consciousness of the past, i.e., remembering, to exist there needs to be a present of which the past is past. It is present consciousness that is consciousness of the past. It must be emphasised here that by "present" we mean subjective or phenomenological present, which distinguishes itself from "objective", or clock-measured present. Objective present, as measured in neurophysiological experiments for example, lasts a few milliseconds and is practically instantaneous present. William James' psychological present was postulated to last a few seconds. Accordingly, present consciousness would also last a few milliseconds or a few seconds and as a consequence it would be either instantaneous or always "behind" already in the past. However, the subjective phenomenological present cannot be measured in objective time. What distinguishes subjective phenomenological present from objective neurophysiological and psychological present is its characteristic of *presence*. When I say "I am typing THESE WORDS, I am sitting at this desk writing a paper, I live in Paris, I am a neurologist, today is cloudy", I describe events and situations to which I feel myself contemporary, and which constitute my present. Some of these events and situations last a few seconds, others last some hours, others even years, but they are all constitutive of a world to which I am present. This is not to say that neurophysiological and psychological present don't exist or are wrong theoretical constructs. But they don't describe the subjectively experienced temporality, i.e., being present to a world, having a past and projecting a future.

The third subordinate structure of temporality is consciousness of the future. Consciousness of the future puts its object in the future mode. It is thematisation of my probable possible in the future mode. By probable possible we mean what is founded on knowledge of my past and present, and this radically distinguishes consciousness of the future from wishes. Tomorrow I will be in Paris and I will continue working on this paper. This is one of my probable possibles, a thematisation in the future mode of my being that founds itself and is synthesis of knowledge of my being in the world: I know I live in Paris, that I am writing this paper, and that tomorrow is not Sunday. When instead I say "I would like to be an astronaut", I don't express a probable possible, but something that transcends the knowledge of the mundane being that I am.

So TC opens the possibility of a temporal existence for the subject. A subject who is conscious of a personal past, when remembering, a personal present, in which he/she is oriented, and a personal future, in which he/she is projected. But before proceeding further and exploring the relationship between TC and confabulation, which is what interests us more, we need to know what the normal operations of TC are.

Uniqueness and multiplicity

Consciousness, we have seen, must always be consciousness *of* an object. One of the characteristics of the object of consciousness is that it represents and reveals to consciousness a uniqueness (U) and a multiplicity (M). Let's consider this point more closely. This pen on the desk is both *a pen* and *the pen*. In the first case it is an undetermined pen, something that belongs to the category of "pens", an object that I recognise and use appropriately because I recognise it. On the contrary, in the second case "the pen" is a determined object, it is exactly this pen in front of me, the pen I bought yesterday and that I will be using tomorrow. So the pen reveals a U and an M. M is reflected in its being a pen and not a different object. U manifests itself in its being this precise pen and not another. However, the U and M of the pen are not adjacent qualities, external to one another. There is a sort of hierarchy that establishes the relationship between the object as representative of an M of objects and the object as representative of itself, in being *this* object that distinguishes itself from all the other objects of the world. The U of the object, of this pen, of the room, of my feeling happy, are *this*, i.e., they manifest a U that distinguishes them from the *other* pen, room, or feeling of happiness. But their U is founded on an M, the M that acts in such a way that these objects manifest themselves to consciousness as unique but under a certain, already distinguished form, i.e., pen, room, happiness. If we consider the opposite condition, we see that for the undetermined object there is no need to represent the U. I can think of a flower, a love, a city, a world without these objects needing to be *this* flower, *this love*, etc.

But what happens when in front of me there is an object I have no experience of, that I don't know? At first sight one would say that any object that I see for the first time is unique and doesn't carry in itself that M we attributed to known objects. But in actual fact, as soon as an unknown object shows up, all the M of which it is made manifests itself instantaneously. This geometric form that I have never seen before is *already* "geometric form that I have never seen", that is it summarises and represents in the negative form what my consciousness has been before. And this can happen without my needing to notice the U of the object. So the object, be it known or unknown, is first the expression of an M and then becomes *this* object, i.e., declares its U.

However, in order for the U of the object to be revealed, it must be addressed by consciousness in the mode of TC. In other words, in order to achieve the passage from the M to the U of an object there must be an act of consciousness that selects its object as a *this*, and this can happen only if consciousness transcends the knowing mode to put itself at the level of the temporalisation of the object. One would certainly want to argue that in what we have called KC the object also appears to me as unique. The cup in front of me is in any case *this* cup, it is with this cup that I interact and not with a generic cup when I pick it up and bring it to my lips. Of course, but its U is revealed only if I consider it as a *this*, that is when I notice its presence as an object that is not my consciousness, and to which my consciousness is contemporary. When I simply use it, when I execute the appropriate sequence of gestures in order to pick it up and bring it to my lips, or when I look at it wondering whether it is full or empty, there is no U in my consciousness. I do not even need to be conscious of the cup in order to use it and when I wonder whether it is empty or full I am aware of a problem to be solved, not of the presence of *this* cup. In short, there is the continuous possibility of varying the relationship between U and M and this possibility depends on the mode in which consciousness addresses the object.

However, one could ask, where is the evidence that in TC the object manifests itself to consciousness as unique and not according to its M? I can easily, for example, remember a generic walk along the shore without being able to locate it in any specific time but only in the past in general. But this does not mean that the walk I remember is not a particular walk but instead the general idea of walking along the shore. The fact that in this memory certain details are missing, where and when, for example, does not mean that I am not remembering a specific walk. Remembering, cannot be anything other than remembering an object in its U, because the U of an object is precisely one of the elements that describe the relationship between remembering consciousness and its object.

MEMORY, CONSCIOUSNESS, AND TEMPORALITY

The ideas we have expressed so far are part of the MCTT, which we have detailed elsewhere (Dalla Barba, 2002). Aspects of the MCTT relevant to the interpretation of confabulation are summarised here and schematically represented in Figure 1.

1. Events produce atemporal and aspecific modifications in the organism and, within the organism, in the brain. These modifications, represented in Figure 1 as X, Y, and Z, are atemporal in the sense that they do not contain any information concerning time. They do not represent the past, the present or the future, nor are they organised according to the order of succession, i.e., there is nothing in Y, for example, that tells that Y comes before Z and after X. They are aspecific in the sense that they do not contain any information specifying that they are representing episodes, meanings, rules, procedures, algorithms, etc.
2. The modifications in the brain can be more or less stable and more or less vulnerable depending on a number of variables. These variables include, among others, attention at encoding, emotional value of the event, depth of encoding, rehearsal, and repeated experience of the same event, etc.

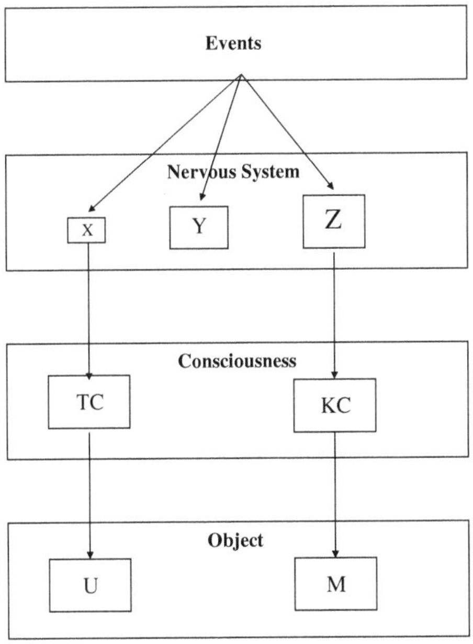

Figure 1. A hypothesis concerning the relation between memory, consciousness, and temporality. NS = nervous system; X, Y, Z = less stable (X), to more stable (Z) patterns of modification of the nervous system; TC = temporal consciousness; KC = knowing consciousness; U = uniqueness; M = multiplicity.

3. Consciousness means to be conscious *of something in a specific way*. That means that consciousness is not an aspecific dimension that passively receives and becomes aware of different types of already specified information, but rather that different types of consciousness exist, each representing an original and irreducible way of addressing the world. Different types of consciousness include, among others, TC and KC. TC means to become aware of something as part of a personal past, present or future; KC means to become aware of something as a meaning or as an element of impersonal knowledge or information.
4. The object of consciousness represents a determination and an undetermination, what we have called U(niqueness) and M(ultiplicity). TC addresses the object's U, whereas KC addresses its M.
5. Less stable and more vulnerable patterns of modifications of the brain are necessary, but not sufficient, for the interaction between TC and the object's U, whereas more stable and less vulnerable modifications of the brain are necessary, but not sufficient, for the interaction between KC and the object's M.

TEMPORAL CONSCIOUSNESS AND CONFABULATION

How do the ideas that we have described apply to the interpretation of confabulation and why is TC involved? It is known that confabulation is not limited to remembering personal past episodes, but also involves the patient's present and future (Dalla Barba, 1993a; Dalla Barba et al., 1997; Dalla Barba, Nedjam, & Dubois, 1999). Patients who confabulate not only remember "another" past but are also living "another" present and planning "another" future. In these patients the three subordinate structures of personal temporality are contaminated by confabulation, which is not a pure memory disorder but a disorder involving TC. According to the MCTT, in confabulating patients TC is still there, like in normal subjects, and addresses the object's U, just like in normal subjects. These patients can still remember their past, they are present to a world, and they can project themselves into a personal future. But in doing this they make errors, sometimes frankly bizarre errors. Actually what is happening in these patients is that TC is still there but is not interacting with less stable patterns of modification of the brain, because these modifications are abolished or inaccessible. Most frequently the result of this condition is that personal habits and routines are considered in a personal temporal framework. When asked what they have done the previous day or what they are going to do the following day, confabulating patients typically answer with memories and plans that they usually have in their daily life. Although admitted to the hospital, they will say, for example, that the previous day they went out shopping and that the following day they will be visiting some friends, acts that presumably were part of their routine life. According to the MCTT, in this condition TC interacts with more stable patterns of modification of the brain and addresses the object's M, habits, routines, repeated events, *as* U, a specific, unique past event (Figure 2).

It could be argued that patients who confabulate in episodic memory, orientation and planning tasks are not necessarily conscious of a confabulatory past, present, and future but rather they simply produce the most plausible answer without having a subjective experience of remembering, of being in that place at that time or of planning their future. If this were the case our account of confabulation in the past, present, and future would be dismissed because TC wouldn't play any role at all in confabulation. Confabulation would be just a sort of "best guess" produced as a consequence of a faulty memory. Yet there is evidence that patients who confabulate actually do become aware of their confabulatory past, present and future. For example, patient MB (Dalla Barba, 1993a) when asked to attribute a "remember" or a "know" judgement to his confabulations, he systematically gave "remember" judgements. Also, the same patient showed he was ready to carry out his confabulatory plans (see also Baddeley &

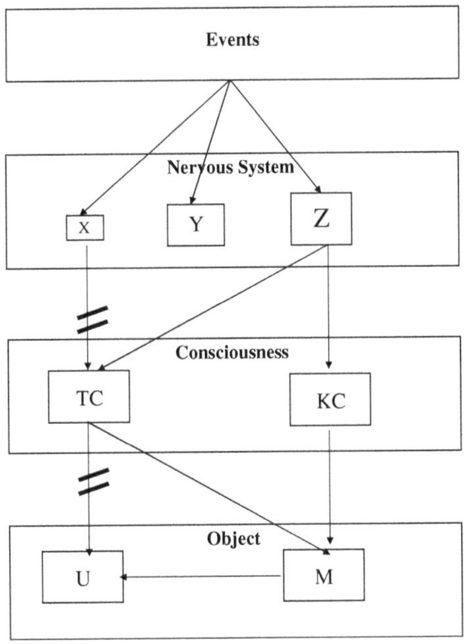

Figure 2. Confabulation: TC addresses M as U.

Wilson, 1986; Burgess & McNeil, 1999; Metcalf, Langdon, & Coltheart, 2007; Moscovitch, 1989). In addition, from a clinical point of view, confabulating patients do not look like subjects who produce their "best guess" in answering questions, but rather they seem to adhere completely to their confabulatory reports.

However, although habits, routines, and repeated events are the most frequent content of confabulation, as we have shown in this paper, confabulations are sometimes made of elements that cannot be traced back to any aspect of the patient's history, present, or future situation, like in patient PD who claimed having lung problems. Does the MCTT account for this case?

Well, it is clear that PD is immersed in a temporal existence: He *remembers* being at the hospital for lung problems. So TC is working in this case and, as it usually does, is addressing the object's U. Can we say in this case that TC interacts with more stable patterns of modification of the brain, like we said for habits, routines, and repeated events? Clearly there is no evidence in this sense. In this case confabulation appears as being created *ex nihilo*. This is difficult to understand only if we are prisoners of the idea that memories must *necessarily* be traced back memory traces. But if we consider that in PD TC is still there, the appearance of confabulation *ex nihilo* is not a problem, since we don't need to trace confabulation back to an unconscious elsewhere, memory traces, imagination whatsoever. In fact, TC cannot escape to the general law of consciousness of being consciousness *of* something. So, if TC is there, it must be consciousness of something, i.e., it must temporalise its object according to the subordinate structures of temporality, past, present, and future. There is no need to ask where the object of this temporalisation comes from because it doesn't come from any sort of unconscious world. It is not *behind* consciousness; it is down there, right in front of consciousness. If we are not in a psychoanalytic perspective, do we ask where thoughts or imagined objects come from? We don't. So why should we ask this question for TC? All we can say is that when TC temporalises its objects, in normal conditions we can recognise a *true* temporal world, a real past, present, and future, *probably* because TC interacts with less stable patterns of modification of the brain. When TC temporalises its object in confabulatory conditions, sometimes we can recognise habits, routines, and repeated events, *probably* because TC interacts with more stable patterns of modification of the brain; other times we don't recognise any meaningful element of the patient's history, present, and future situation.

So, the difference between normal memory and confabulation is that in the case of patients who confabulate we are faced with a confabulatory consciousness in which past, present, and future are somehow distorted. Distorted with respect to what? The truth, you will say; with what *actually* took place, is taking place, or will take place. But who establishes the truth? If temporality, and therefore its subordinate dimensions, are inherent to consciousness, what relationship of truth can there be between what you suppose to *actually* have taken place, to be taking place or to be going to take place and the reality of TC? And yet for a witness, the doctor or the psychologist observing the patient who confabulates, his stories about the past, his perception of the present, and his future plans are confabulatory, in that they are totally at variance with what the listener expects as an answer, so much so that they push him to consider the patient's answers as not normal, namely as confabulatory. Where does this discrepancy between what the observer expects and the answers he receives come from? In other words, what is the origin of this confabulatory temporality?

The answer to this question can only be a biological one. There is a biological difference between normal subjects and confabulators. This biological difference is represented by the brain lesion, which prevents the interaction between TC and less stable modifications of the brain.

It could be argued that we made it out with a shortcut since we have established an interaction between the biological level (patterns of modification of the brain) and the psychological level (TC). However, this is not a shortcut because TC depends on brain function and can be altered or abolished by a brain lesion. TC works normally in subjects without brain lesions, is altered in patients with brain lesions that cause confabulations, and is abolished, as we will see, in patients with brain lesions that cause amnesia. Now, the question is what are the brain structures that need to be intact for the normal functioning of TC, altered in confabulation, and damaged in amnesia? This is an experimental problem that needs more experimental work to be answered appropriately. However, the literature on amnesia and on confabulation indicate the hippocampus and the medial temporal lobe are good candidates as brain structures involved in the functioning and dysfunction of TC.

TEMPORAL CONSCIOUSNESS AND BRAIN: IS THE MEDIAL TEMPORAL LOBE "TEMPORAL"?

Patients with medial temporal lobe (MTL) lesions are known to be deeply amnesic for personal past episodes and to have relatively preserved general knowledge or semantic memory (see Kopelman, 2002, for a review). Patient HM was the first well-documented example of this condition (Milner, 1958). However, amnesic patients not only do not consciously remember their past, but neither can they imagine their personal future. These patients are lost in a *nontime*, or in a sort of instantaneous present. The patient, NN, described by Tulving (1985) is a good example of this condition. Tulving's patient had preserved semantic abilities, but was unable to retrieve any episode from his personal past or to say anything about his future.

> N.N. has no difficulties with the concept of chronological time. He knows the units of time and their relationships perfectly well, and he can accurately represent chronological time graphically. But in stark contrast to his abstract knowledge of time, his awareness of subjective time seems to be severely impaired. When asked what he did before coming to where he is now, or what he did on the previous day, he says that he does not know. When asked what he will be doing when he leaves "here", or what he will be doing "tomorrow", he says he does not know.
>
> Here is part of the transcript of the interview with me as the interviewer:
>
> E.T.: "Let's try the question again about the future. What will you be doing tomorrow?" (there is a 15-second pause.)
> N.N. smiles faintly, then says: "I don't know."
> E.T.: "Do you remember the question?"
> N.N.: "About what I'll be doing tomorrow?"
> E.T.: "Yes. How would you describe your state of mind when you try to think about it?" (A 5-second pause.)
> N.N.: "Blank. I guess."
>
> . . . When asked to compare his state of mind when he is trying to think about what he will be doing tomorrow with his state of mind when he thinks about what he did yesterday, he says it is the "*same kind of blankness.*" (Tulving, 1985, p. 4).

As emerges from the description of this patient, what characterises the core deficit of N.N. is a loss of TC. Past and future have disappeared as possible objects of his consciousness and the result is that N.N. is shut in an atemporal instantaneous present.

Further evidence of selective loss of TC in amnesia comes from patient DB described by Klein, Loftus, and Kihlstrom (2002). DB suffered severe amnesia for the personally experienced past. By contrast, his knowledge of the nonpersonal past was relatively preserved. A similar pattern was evidenced in his ability to anticipate future events. Although DB had great difficulty imagining what his experience might be like in the future, his capacity to anticipate issues and events in the public domain was comparable to that of neurologically healthy, age-matched controls. These findings show a dissociation between TC, which is impaired, and KC, which is preserved. Impairment of TC has also been documented in Alzheimer's disease (Dalla Barba et al., 1999).

So, there is increasing converging evidence that lesions which produce amnesia also produce deficits of TC. This suggests that the integrity of the MTL and related structures is crucial for the normal functioning of TC. Further evidence on the involvement of the MTL in TC comes from a recent neuroimaging study which showed that in normal subjects the hippocampus was activated both when individuals remembered their past and when they imagined their future (Addis, Wong, & Schacter, 2007).

Now, if the integrity of the MTL is crucial for the functioning of TC, what happens in confabulation, where TC is present but functioning in an abnormal way? The most plausible answer to this question is that in confabulation the MTL is intact, but lesions to other brain structures prevent its normal functioning, which is the biological counterpart of the claim that in confabulation TC is preserved but no longer interacts with less stable modifications of the brain. This seems actually to be the case. Gilboa and Moscovitch (2002) found that only 2 out of 79 patients with confabulation had lesions involving the MTL. These patients had lesions in more than 20 brain regions, although the frontal lobe was preferentially affected, but almost all these patients had preserved MTL. Twenty-eight additional confabulating patients not included in Gilboa's and Moscovitch's review also had preserved MTL (Ciaramelli & Ghetti, 2007; Ciaramelli, Ghetti, Frattarelli, & Làdavas, 2006; Dalla Barba, 1993b; Dalla Barba, Cipolotti, & Denes, 1990; Dalla Barba, Mantovan, Cappelletti, & Denes, 1998; Fotopoulou, Conway, & Solms, 2007; Fotopoulou, Solms, & Turbull, 2004). So, what these data show is that what confabulators have in common is not a specific lesion site but rather the integrity of the MTL, which is consistent with the idea that the MTL is essential for the function of normal and confabulatory TC. In this sense the MTL is "temporal", because its integrity allows individuals to be consciously aware of a personal past, present, and future.

We have shown so far that the MCTT can account for confabulation and amnesia. Can it also be applied to the interpretation of delusion? Certainly not to the interpretation of all the numerous forms of delusion. Delusional memories, however, might share similarities with the more extreme or semantically inappropriate forms of confabulation (see Kopelman, 2010 this issue). In patients with delusional memories, TC is still working, since they are aware of a personal past, but it is still unclear what are the malfunctioning mechanisms that make these memories delusional. Further experimental investigation is needed, in particular concerning the role of the MTL and possibly of its interaction with retrosplenial and prefrontal cortex in delusional memories.

There are a number of important questions that we have not addressed because they were far beyond the aims of this work. Why confabulation is often a transitory symptom? Does confabulation reflect a disconnection of the MTL? Why amnesia, i.e., loss of TC, occurs for lesions outside the MTL? Is it also a matter of disconnection of the MTL? And if this is the case, what is the difference between confabulators and nonconfabulating amnesics with preserved MTL? What is the exact role of frontal lesions in confabulation, if we reject, as we do, the possibility of unconscious monitoring? What is the exact nature of what we indicated as patterns of modification of the brain, if we reject, as we do, the notion of memory traces that would contain the past? Some of these are experimental questions that will be answered by experimental work. Others are theoretical and their discussion couldn't have been included in these pages. What we have shown in these pages is that understanding confabulation is a difficult and ambitious enterprise, an enterprise doomed to failure if based on theoretically untenable and experimentally undemonstrated explanatory idols like memory traces and unconscious monitoring. Confabulation is a conscious phenomenon, indeed a phenomenon that involves TC. A better understanding of TC, including its neurobiological correlates, is therefore demanded, legitimate, and necessary.

REFERENCES

Addis, D. R., Wong, A. T., & Schacter, D. L. (2007). Remembering the past and imaging the future: Common and distinct neural substrates during event construction and elaboration. *Neuropsychologia, 45*, 1363–1377.

Baddeley, A., & Wilson, B. (1986). Amnesia, autobiographical memory and confabulation. In D. C. Rubin (Ed.), *Autobiographical memory* (pp. 225–252). Cambridge, UK: Cambridge University Press.

Berlyne, N. (1972). Confabulation. *British Journal of Psychiatry, 120*, 31–39.

Bleuler, E. (1949). *Lehrbuch der Psychiatrie.* Berlin: Springer Verlag.

Brentano, F. (1973). *Psychology from an empirical standpoint*. London: Routledge and Kegan Paul. (Original work published 1874)

Burgess, P. W., & McNeil, J. E. (1999). Content-specific confabulation. *Cortex*, *35*, 163–182.

Ciaramelli, E., & Ghetti, S. (2007). What are confabulators' memories made of? A study of subjective and objective measures of recollection in confabulation. *Neuropsychologia*, *45*, 1489–500.

Ciaramelli, E., Ghetti, S., Frattarelli, M., & Làdavas, E. (2006). When true memory availability promotes false memory: Evidence from confabulating patients. *Neuropsychologia*, *44*, 1866–1877.

Conway, M. A., & Tacchi, P. C. (1996). Motivated confabulation. *Neurocase*, *2*, 325–339.

Dalla Barba, G. (1993a). Confabulation: Knowledge and recollective experience. *Cognitive Neuropsychology*, *10*, 1–20.

Dalla Barba, G. (1993b). Different patterns of confabulation. *Cortex*, *29*, 567–581.

Dalla Barba, G. (2001). Beyond the memory trace paradox and the fallacy of the homunculus: A hypothesis concerning the relation between memory, consciousness and temporality. *Journal of Consciousness Studies*, *8*, 51–78.

Dalla Barba, G. (2002). *Memory, consciousness and temporality*. Boston: Kluwer Academic.

Dalla Barba, G., Cappelletti, Y. J., Signorini, M., & Denes, G. (1997). Confabulation: Remembering "another" past, planning "another" future. *Neurocase*, *3*, 425–436.

Dalla Barba, G., Cipolotti, L., & Denes, G. (1990). Autobiographical memory loss and confabulation in Korsakoff's syndrome: A case report. *Cortex*, *26*, 525–534.

Dalla Barba, G., & Decaix, C. (2009). "Do you remember what you did on March 13, 1985?" A case study of confabulatory gypermnesia. *Cortex, 45,* 566–574.

Dalla Barba, G., Mantovan, M. C., Cappelletti, Y. J., & Denes, G. (1998). Temporal gradient in confabulation. *Cortex*, *34*, 417–426.

Dalla Barba, G., Nedjam, Z., & Dubois, B. (1999). Confabulation, executive functions and source memory in Alzheimer's disease. *Cognitive Neuropsychology*, *16*, 385–398.

Fotopoulou, A. (2010). The affective neuropsychology of confabulation and delusion. *Cognitive Neuropsychiatry*, *15*(1/2/3), 38–63.

Fotopoulou, A., Conway, M., & Solms, M. (2007). Confabulation: Motivated reality monitoring. *Neuropsychologia*, *45*, 2180–2190.

Fotopoulou, A., Solms, M., & Turbull, O. (2004). Wishful reality distortions in confabulation: A case report. *Neuropsychologia*, *42*, 727–744.

Gilboa, A. (2010). Strategic retrieval, confabulations and delusions: Theory and data. *Cognitive Neuropsychiatry*, *15*(1/2/3), 145–180.

Gilboa, A., & Moscovitch, M. (2002). The cognitive neuroscience of confabulation: A review and a model. In A. Baddeley, M. Kopelman, & B. Wilson (Eds.), *The handbook of memory disorders* (pp. 315–342). Chichester, UK: Wiley.

Husserl, E. (1950). *Ideen zur einen reinen Phänomenologie*. Hen Haag, The Netherlands: Martinus Nijhoff.

Johnson, M. K. (1991). Reality monitoring: Evidence from confabulation in organic brain disease patients. In G. P. Prigatano & D. L. Schacter (Eds.), *Awareness of deficit after brain injury* (pp. 176–197). New York and Oxford, UK: Oxford University Press.

Johnson, M. K., O'Connor, M., & Cantor, J. (1997). Confabulation, memory deficits, and frontal dysfunction. *Brain and Cognition*, *34*, 189–206.

Joseph, R. (1986). Confabulation and delusional denial: Frontal lobe and lateralized influences. *Journal of Clinical Psychology*, *42*, 507–520.

Klein, S. B., Loftus, J., & Kihlstrom, J. (2002). Memory and temporal experience: The effects of episodic memory loss on an amnesic patient's ability to remember the past and imagine the future. *Social Cognition*, *20*, 353–379.

Kopelman, M. D. (1987). Two types of confabulation. *Journal of Neurology, Neurosurgery and Psychiatry, 50*, 1482–1487.
Kopelman, M. D. (2002). Disorders of memory. *Brain, 125*, 2152–2190.
Kopelman, M. D. (2010). Varieties of confabulation and delusion. *Cognitive Neuropsychiatry, 15*(1/2/3), 14–37.
Metcalf, K., Langdon, R., & Coltheart, M. (2007). Models of confabulation: A critical review and a new framework. *Cognitive Neuropsychology, 24*, 23–47.
Milner, B. (1958). Psychological defects produced by temporal lobe excision. *Research Publication of the Association of Research in Nervous & Mental Diseases, 36*, 244–257.
Moscovitch, M. (1989). Confabulation and the frontal systems: Strategic versus associative retrieval in neuropsychological theories of memory. In H. L. Roedinger & F. I. M. Craik (Eds.), *Varieties of memory and consciousness: Essays in honor of Endel Tulving* (pp. 133–160). Hillsdale, NJ: Lawrence Erlbaum Associates, Inc.
Nedjam, Z., Dalla Barba, G., & Pillon, B. (2000). Confabulation in a patient with frontotemporal dementia and in a patient with Alzheimer's disease. *Cortex, 36*, 561–577.
Sandson, J., Albert, M. L., & Alexander, M. (1986). Confabulation in aphasia. *Cortex, 22*, 621–626.
Sartre, J.-P. (1943). *L'être et le néant*. Paris: Gallimard.
Schnider, A., & Ptak, R. (1999). Spontaneous confabulators fail to suppress currently irrelevant memory traces. *Nature Neuroscience, 2*, 677–681.
Stuss, D. T., Alexander, M. P., Lieberman, A., & Levine, H. (1978). An extraordinary form of confabulation. *Neurology, 28*, 1166–1172.
Tulving, E. (1985). Memory and consciousness. *Canadian Psychology, 26*, 1–12.
Turner, M., & Coltheart, M. (2010). Confabulation and delusion: A common monitoring framework. *Cognitive Neuropsychiatry, 15*(1/2/3), 346–376.
Weinstein, E., & Lyerly, O. (1968). Confabulation following brain injury. *Archives of General Psychiatry, 18*, 348–354.

COGNITIVE NEUROPSYCHIATRY
2010, 15 (1/2/3), 118–144

Novel insights into false recollection: A model of déjà vécu

Akira R. O'Connor[1], Colin Lever[2], and Chris J.A. Moulin[3]

[1] *Washington University in St. Louis, St. Louis, MO, USA,* [2] *Institute of Psychological Sciences, University of Leeds, Leeds, UK,* [3] *Leeds Memory Group, Institute of Psychological Sciences, University of Leeds, Leeds, UK*

The thesis of this paper is that déjà experiences can be separated into two forms: déjà vu, arising from the erroneous sensation of familiarity, and déjà vécu, arising from the erroneous sensation of recollection. We summarise a series of cases for whom déjà vécu is experienced frequently and for extended periods, and seek to differentiate their experiences from "healthy" déjà experiences by nonbrain-damaged participants. In reviewing our cases, we stress two novel ideas: that déjà vécu in these cases is delusion-like; and that these cases experience déjà vécu for stimuli that are especially novel or unusual. Here we present a novel cognitive neuroscientific hypothesis of déjà vécu. This hypothesis assumes that the signal of retrieval from memory is neurally dissociable from the contents of retrieval. We suggest that a region downstream of the hippocampus signals "recollection" by detecting the timing of firing in hippocampal output neurons relative to the theta oscillation. Disruptions to this "temporal coding" mechanism result in false signals of recollection which may occur without actual retrieval and which, ironically, may arise particularly during situations of contextual novelty.

Keywords: Déjà vu; Dementia; Hippocampus; Theta.

INTRODUCTION

"From the point of view of episodic memory ... each event a person experiences is always unique in the sense that in all of his previous autobiographical history there has not been another experience exactly like the present one." (Tulving, 1972, p. 399)

Correspondence should be addressed to Chris Moulin, Institute of Psychological Sciences, University of Leeds, Leeds LS2 9JT, UK. E-mail: c.j.a.moulin@leeds.ac.uk

This work stems directly from an ESRC-CNRS collaborative workshops programme awarded to Moulin (Recollection, Remembering and the Complex Nature of the Self RES-170-25-0008). We are very grateful for the contribution and cooperation of our patients and carers, without whom this work would not be possible. Finally, we are grateful for Art Funkhouser's steady mentoring of the field and ongoing questioning.

DOI: 10.1080/13546800903113071

Following an influential review on the topic (Brown, 2003), there has recently been an increase in interest amongst cognitive psychologists in the déjà vu phenomenon and associated states. Researchers have converged on a definition of déjà vu that emphasises the (erroneous) sensation of familiarity, and the subjective nature of the state. In healthy people, it is hypothesised that the state arises temporarily as a result of an erroneous sensation of familiarity. Indeed, using a fairly standard paradigm for inducing familiarity (the mere exposure paradigm) it has been possible to induce déjà vu-like sensations in the laboratory amongst undergraduates (see Brown & Marsh, 2008).

However, a major theoretical viewpoint within contemporary memory research is that memory retrieval can be based on two distinct processes or states: remembering and knowing (Tulving, 1985). In brief, these two states map on to two distinct processes. Remembering is an effortful recollective process associated with retrieval from episodic memory (corresponding to autonoetic consciousness) and knowing, or familiarity, is a more automatic process, associated with retrieval from semantic memory (corresponding to noetic consciousness; see also Gardiner, Ramponi, & Richardson-Klavehn, 1998).

Remembering and knowing have been found to be associated with distinct and dissociable neural correlates (e.g., Henson, Rugg, Shallice, Josephs, & Dolan, 1999, and see later). According to an emergent view (see Conway, 2005), memory is accompanied by experiential states that help the memory-user to infer the quality and veracity of the retrieved information—retrieval from episodic memory can be interpreted as such due to the sensation of remembering (this may be particularly important in differentiating remembering from imagining, see Addis, Wong, & Shacter, 2007), whereas a feeling of familiarity can be interpreted as resulting from a previous encounter in the absence of such evocative recall. In short, our view is that two distinct processes are also involved in abnormal memory experiences; as well as erroneous sensations of familiarity, there will be erroneous sensations of remembering.

We also propose that all sensations associated with retrieval can become dissociated from the act of retrieval itself. In these situations, there is a clash between the sensation of retrieval and the actual contents of retrieval itself. Thus, the déjà vu experient momentarily feels like she has previously visited a never-visited location in the absence of being able to retrieve memories of any such visit (and even whilst bringing to mind the knowledge that she has never been to the location). We argue that it is likewise possible to have erroneous sensations of remembering. Our argument is chiefly based on a series of cases. Moulin and colleagues (Moulin, Conway, Thompson, James, & Jones, 2005; Moulin et al., 2006) describe patients with dementia who experience erroneous sensations of *remembering*. These patients (described in detail later) report that events have happened before, even though they are experiencing them for the first time. These cases also show *recollective secondary confabulation*—the patients confabulate contextual and circumstantial material to justify their overwhelming sensations of events having happened before. We describe this recollective memory error as déjà vécu in order to differentiate it from disorders of familiarity, which can also involve clear memory deficits, and presentations just as striking as those displayed by our patients. Indeed, although erroneous familiarity is often experienced in the healthy population, it can also manifest in ways that warrant clinical attention. For instance, Ward et al. (1999) describe a set of patients who feel, on the basis of familiarity, that everyone they meet is "famous".

Therefore, in this paper we aim to extend our theory of déjà vécu as a disorder of remembering, which is qualitatively different to, rather than quantitatively different to (in terms of degree or the requirement for clinical intervention) disorders of familiarity. In doing so, we posit a possible mechanism for its formation, attempt to differentiate it from other manifestations of the déjà vu experience, and offer a more specific means by which to identify such cases: inappropriate sensations of remembering for *novel stimuli*.

DÉJÀ VU AND DÉJÀ VÉCU

The consequence of reporting these clinical cases of déjà vécu (and in particular their coverage in the mainstream media), is that the term has come to be described merely as a clinical manifestation of the déjà vu experience. This confusion is further compounded by the fact that clinicians and carers frequently and spontaneously describe their cases and family members as having déjà vu, even though there are marked differences between the clinical presentation of déjà vécu and "healthy" instances of déjà vu. We suggest that healthy people do experience a nonpathological form of déjà vécu. (For descriptions of déjà vu- and déjà vécu-like sensations induced in healthy participants see O'Connor, Barnier, & Cox, 2008.) This is possible in the same way that we may experience déjà vu for a fleeting instant when meeting a stranger in a supermarket but not have a full-blown neuropsychological deficit whereby we believe everyone to be famous (Ward et al., 1999). However, the prevalence of nonpathological déjà vécu in the healthy population is unknown.

In using the term déjà vécu, we deliberately borrowed from Funkhouser's (1996) fractionation of déjà vu into three separate experiences: déjà vécu, déjà senti, and déjà visité. Funkhouser's definition of the déjà vu states is drawn from both scientific works and literature. Notably, to describe déjà vécu he uses an oft-cited passage from Dickens' *David Copperfield*:

> "We have all some experience of a feeling, that comes over us occasionally, of what we are saying and doing having been said and done before, in a remote time—of our

> having been surrounded, dim ages ago, by the same faces, objects, and circumstances—of our knowing perfectly what will be said next, as if we suddenly *remember* it!" (Dickens, 1850, p. 236, emphasis added)

This description stresses contextual details and associated feelings and thoughts. As such, it parallels recollection, where in remembering an event we are able to draw up contextual information, and the specifics of a previously experienced event (e.g., Conway, 2005). In contrast, Funkhouser (1996) describes déjà senti as a more nebulous sensation, and differentiates it from déjà vécu thus as being "primarily or even exclusively a mental happening" with no precognitive aspects. To illustrate this sensation he draws on Hughlings Jackson's account of temporal lobe epilepsy:

> "[W]hat is occupying the attention is what has occupied it before, and indeed has been *familiar*, but has been for a time forgotten, and now is recovered with a slight sense of satisfaction as if it had been sought for." (Hughlings Jackson, 1888, p. 202, emphasis added)

This passage describes a mental event which, unlike recollection, is incomplete, with an absence of recollective detail, and the "reliving" of a situation. Funkhouser's final subdivision is déjà visité. This is a classification of déjà vu based on it occurring in particular locations—"an experience in which a person visits a new locality and nevertheless feels it to be familiar" (Funkhouser, 1996). We do not see this as a separate experiential state but a description of a déjà experience triggered by a particular cue or event. We actually have accounts of both déjà vu and déjà vécu cued by location, so suggest that this subdivision does little to help us understand the underlying memory processes at fault in the experience, although it may be important in classifying the experience in other ways not attempted here.

We emphasise the difference between the first two categories, although we chose not to use the term "déjà senti", even though it appears to resonate with our characterisation of false recognition on the basis of familiarity. This is largely because, despite Funkhouser's (1996) observant classification of the varieties of déjà vu, the literature has converged on a description of déjà vu that emphasises the experience of *familiarity*—". . . any subjectively inappropriate impression of familiarity of a present experience with an undefined past" (Neppe, 1983, p. 3). Neppe's definition of déjà vu points to another issue we see as critical. Twice in his definition, he refers to the experient's sensation of the experience. First, the experience is "subjective" and second, his definition clarifies that the experience must be combined with an "undefined" past. That is, if someone finds something familiar, and can identify why or where from, it is not déjà vu. This introduces the second area where we think the literature is lacking precision—awareness. Nonpathological déjà experiences involve self-awareness. We are not seduced by our "healthy" déjà vu experiences, no matter how strong—we will report a feeling of familiarity, but we will not be able to produce a past experience in order to justify it, and so we will acknowledge that our sense of familiarity is erroneous. Healthy individuals will not act on the basis of their experiences of déjà states, no matter how frequent or persistent.

Our patients, in contrast, are characterised by a persistent and overwhelming occurrence of déjà experiences, which they act upon and about which they mostly lack awareness. Clinical reports of persistent and debilitating forms of the déjà experience have been made of those with dementia, temporal lobe epilepsy, migraine, and schizophrenia (Kalra, Chancellor, & Zeman, 2007; Moulin et al., 2005; Neppe, 1983; Sacks, 1970), but it is not clear whether these experiences are déjà vu or déjà vécu, since the case descriptions and neuropsychological examination often provide insufficient detail to make this distinction.

A further confusion in the use of déjà vécu and déjà vu may be historical. Our interpretation of one of the early neuropsychological cases that used the then new term "déjà vu" is actually more a case of déjà vécu. Arnaud (1896) describes Louis, a 34-year-old male who had suffered anterograde and retrograde amnesia as a result of contracting cerebral malaria. Following his recovery, Louis reported recognising everything he encountered. Arnaud tested his patient's memory by exposing him to a number of events and documenting Louis' experiences of these events. One of these events was Pasteur's state funeral, a highly distinctive event attended by thousands. Arnaud reported that Louis described the funeral as an event he recognised, demonstrating that his erroneous recognition was experienced not only for mundane events, but also for highly distinctive and novel events, a theme we will pick up again later in this paper.

CASE REPORTS OF DÉJÀ VÉCU

Moulin et al. (2005) initially reported the cases of two patients, AKP and MA, who experienced déjà vécu associated with dementia. AKP was an 80-year-old man who initially presented to his family doctor with memory problems and frequent sensations, which were described as déjà vu. MA was a 70-year-old woman who presented to her doctor, convinced that things had happened before, as evidenced by her memory for them happening as they happened. AKP and MA's erroneous sensations of memory were so compelling that the patients were unwilling to engage in activities such as watching television and reading the newspaper, as they felt they had already carried them out. As mentioned previously, healthy déjà experiences do not lead to behavioural change—one is able to challenge and resist the sensation that one has encountered something before. Conversely, déjà vécu patients act on their beliefs. See Table 1 for other examples of déjà vécu patients' experiences.

TABLE 1
Accounts of déjà vécu patients' experiences as reported by correspondence with carers

Age	*Diagnosis*	*Description*
74	Memory difficulties	"Chronic déjà vu. I can't find any explanation, or correlation with any of her physical ailments ... it gets worse during stress ... but has become a chronic (multiple times a day). It is bothering to her and worrisome to me. It is triggered by both novel events and mundane, common occurrences, but much more prevalent with change of environment."
85	Early dementia	"She doesn't read or watch TV because "she's seen or read them all before". She even told me that CBC must be on strike because they are running re-runs ... we were out for a drive and were about 20 km from home. We passed a couple walking along the side of the road and mom said she had seen them earlier that morning when she was out for her walk around the block. I tried to explain that it was doubtful that it could be the same couple but she insisted that she could describe the coat the lady was wearing and proceeded to do so."
—	Stroke	"One of the most striking features of her brain injury was this newfound sense of having seen every single show on television before, years ago, when she was younger. This was, ironically I suppose, coupled with an inability to remember what had happened at the beginning of the show by the time the program ended. She also developed a tendency to make up memories from her past that had never actually happened (childhood events and the like) and recounts them very detailedly, never realising that they are in fact false."
78	Unknown	"My parents decided to not let the déjà vu's interfere with their winter vacation and went to Florida. My Dad reported that the déjà vu's were stronger and more frequent. Museums, restaurants, beaches, stores and people never visited, were all seen/felt/done before. They were worse than when at home. ... At the flower show a week back, we were standing there, looking at a display and she said 'oh I saw that before, last night on TV. I think' then, she saw a lady pass us and said, 'you've seen her, she's on TV I know I've seen her before'."
86	Unknown	"In the last two years of her life (she died at 88) I would have to say that she essentially lived in almost a constant state of déjà vécu whenever she was removed from her narrowly defined daily routine (in an assisted living residence). Whenever she spent time with me, for example, there was continual reference to 'the trees have sure grown taller,' total strangers on the road had 'gotten fat and, look, he has a new dog,' and every stranger she met was assured that she knew them already. Newspapers had been read before, she had repairmen in to find out why the television kept showing programs she had seen before, newly published books had been read years before, etc."

In order to establish the recollective nature of déjà vécu, Moulin et al. (2005) administered a recollective experience-based recognition task (Table 2) to AKP and MA. Using this task, they were able to ascertain a typical response pattern in those with déjà vécu. When they compared the déjà vécu patients' responses to those of age-matched controls, the déjà vécu patient responses were characterised by a greater number of false positives (FPs, which occurs when a new item is incorrectly identified as being seen before) and by a higher proportion of those false positive as being "remember" responses (Table 3). Thus, according to these measures of recollective experience, AKP and MA had a far greater tendency to "remember" items they had not been shown at study. Moreover, they tended to confabulate contextual details associated with items they had not previously encountered (i.e., they reported experiences and thoughts from the nonexistent study phases for nonpresented items).

In fact, this recollective secondary confabulation seems to be a critical feature of this condition. (We refer readers to Turner and Coltheart, and Langdon and Bayne, both 2010 this issue, for discussion of secondary, or post hoc, confabulations. Hereafter, we will simply use the term "recollective confabulation".) Since recollection is associated with the retrieval of

TABLE 2
The recollective experience procedure

Recollective experience memory tasks (Gardiner, Ramponi, & Richardson-Klavehn, 1998; Tulving, 1985) assess recognition memory by giving participants the opportunity to respond in the following ways to stimuli presented at test

Remember (R)	I recognise this word. I can remember aspects of my previous experience of encountering it before (e.g., what it made me think).
Familiar (F)	I recognise this word. I don't remember any aspects of previously encountering the word but I just know it was in the previous list.
Guess (G)	I think I recognise this word, but I'm guessing.
No recollection	I do not recognise this word. This is a word I didn't encounter before.

TABLE 3
Summary of results for AKP, from Experiment 2, Moulin et al. (2005)

	Hits assigned to each subjective category			*False positives assigned to each subjective category*		
Score (max. =20)	*Remember*	*Familiar*	*Guess*	*Remember*	*Familiar*	*Guess*
AKP (*z*-score)	15 (−0.78)	3 (1.93)	2 (3.34)	8 (14.55)	3 (3.73)	3 (5.67)
Controls (*SD*) (*n* =7)	17.16 (2.75)	0.84 (1.12)	0.21 (0.54)	0.21 (0.54)	0.26 (0.73)	0.16 (0.50)

contextual information and experiences at study, it is perhaps unsurprising that participants who experience high levels of déjà vécu also generate high levels of incorrect contextual information for items which they have not actually encountered before. AKP made such reports spontaneously, for instance confabulating secret early-morning trips to the newsagents to read the newspaper as it was unloaded from the lorry, whilst his wife was asleep in bed. We think that these confabulatory justifications are similar to the justifications made by anosognosic patients with hemiparesis (see Fotopoulou, 2010 this issue).

This tendency to confabulate was noted in Mr. K, reported by O'Connor (2007). Mr. K was a 92-year-old man who started experiencing memory difficulties in his 80s. Mr. K's déjà vécu became apparent to his son when they took a family holiday to France, a country Mr. K had never previously visited. His son reported an episode of recollective confabulation that is notable for the insight Mr. K had:

> "When we travelled round France, my father saw a hospital and said, "I have been here before, I visited this hospital to see my friend." He then told the story of his previous visit to confirm his memory. When he was asked how this could be possible when he had never visited France before, my father said, "I know that I have never been here when I consider my personal history seriously and logically, but I still strongly feel that I have been here before." We thought he was over-tired so we took a two-day break from sightseeing. Unfortunately, when we resumed sightseeing his memory situation had not changed." (O'Connor, 2007, p. 214)

The dissociation between Mr. K's feelings of recollection and his awareness that he could "logically" not have been to the hospital in France illustrates the conflict caused by Mr. K's déjà vécu—it was only when challenged that Mr. K would concede that his sense of recollection could be false. However, such was the strength of his memory sensation and the associated confabulation that unless he was forced to consider the consistency of his memories with what he knew about his past experience, Mr. K would believe that his memories were accurate.

Persistent déjà vécu as delusion-like

Mr. K's partial awareness of his condition is somewhat typical of our cases. We suggest that our patients are broadly speaking anosognosic, but that they do have some insight into their difficulties. Tellingly, when AKP was challenged by his wife to remember the contents of the premiere of a TV show he believed he had watched before, AKP retorted: "How should I know, I have a memory problem!" (Moulin et al., 2005, p. 1364). Similarly, a new case, Mrs. M (Moulin & Conway, 2009) reported that although it felt like everything in her life was repeating, it was often possible to just sit with her head in her hands in the kitchen, and work it all out, describing her experience as very confusing. AKP, in justifying his decision that he had previously encountered a word earlier (in fact he had not been presented with the word) reported that he was certain he had seen the word earlier, but could not remember the study phase in which he had been presented with it. His own description of his condition was that he did get confused about whether events had repeated or not, and yet, he still felt compelled to act on his memory feelings.

We suggest that it is the dimension of insight that sets apart a healthy déjà experience from a pathological one. Here we argue that the lack of insight means that our clinical cases of déjà vécu are delusion-like. During a healthy déjà experience, the experient is aware that he or she is experiencing erroneous familiarity or recollection and so does not accept or act on the sensation. During a pathological déjà experience, the experient does not seem to be aware that the sensation is erroneous, and therefore modifies his/her behaviour in accord with the sensation (e.g., withdraws from the "repeated" activity). However, not all cases are as straightforward as this. For instance, a feature of Mr. K's déjà vécu was his acknowledgment of the possibility that his sensation of recognition could be erroneous. Not only did Mr. K acknowledge that his recognition could be erroneous, but he admitted that, "logically", it probably was erroneous. When challenged, Mr. K could be made aware that his sensation of recognition was false.

Our déjà vécu patients share important features with clinical cases of delusions. The operationalisation of the DSM-IV (American Psychiatric Association, 1994) definition of delusion has been debated, but there is some consensus that delusions run counter to the beliefs of peers, are maintained despite overwhelming evidence to the contrary, and defy rational counter-argument. These same characteristics can be seen in déjà vécu. According to Langdon and Coltheart (2000), the interaction of two factors is necessary for the formation of a delusion. These are: a neuropsychological anomaly that alters perceptual or emotional processing and so disrupts the "perceived reality"; and damage to a system of belief evaluation that is responsible for the person's failure to reject the erroneous belief which stems from the first neuropsychological anomaly. In a similar vein, déjà vécu could be seen as a dysfunction of the recognition systems coincident with damage to systems responsible for evaluating and correcting the information which stems from this dysfunction. Here we develop this idea in relation to memory systems, with the notion that frontal systems should normally be able to discount erroneous sensations emanating from memory processes occurring in the temporal lobe, but that in these cases of déjà vécu, this system is deficient.

In both healthy and pathological déjà experiences, dysfunctions of recognition may result in a combination of the feeling of recognition and the awareness that this feeling is inconsistent with the knowledge and beliefs we hold about our previous experience. At this stage of the experience, healthy and pathological experiences could be said to result from similar neuropsychological anomalies. The point of divergence is in the system of belief evaluation. Whereas in healthy déjà experiences, the dysfunctional recognition is corrected in favour of the evaluation that is consistent with the rest of the experient's knowledge, in pathological déjà experiences, and particularly in our cases of déjà vécu, the dysfunction is not corrected but allowed to coexist alongside divergent knowledge and beliefs held about previous experience and the likelihood that the recognition being experienced is inappropriate. In healthy experiences, a unified experience is maintained, but in pathological déjà vécu, the absence of an appropriate evaluation of consistency results in a fragmented, inconsistent experience. The proposed evaluative dysfunction in déjà vécu can account for both recollective confabulation and the awareness that Mr. K demonstrated when asked to reconcile his recollective confabulations with his knowledge of his previous experience. He was comfortable with the use of the confabulated memory of visiting a friend in the hospital to justify his feelings of recognition in France. However, this confabulated recollection did not appear to have any consequences for the way in which Mr. K then evaluated everything else he knew about his own life, such as the fact that he had never previously visited France.

Novelty: On the triggers of déjà vécu

One of the more noteworthy features of AKP's presentation was that it seemed that it was more striking, less commonplace, distinct events that triggered more intense sensations of déjà vécu. On hearing of the death of a close friend, for instance, he claimed that he had already heard the news and he even refused to go to the funeral, claiming that he had already been. Similarly, patient MA produced déjà vécu for striking news events, such as the Bali bombing (Moulin et al., 2005), which she claimed to have already known about. In contrast, mundane and repetitive acts, such as acts of personal hygiene and eating meals, never elicited déjà vécu experiences. Table 1 shows examples of carers' reports of people with similar or identical symptoms—note how often this includes novelty, or at least the observation that this problem is magnified in new locations or nonroutine events. In our original presentation of AKP and MA, we operationalised this observation by examining false positives and recollective experience for high frequency (common) words (such as *mouse*) and low frequency (distinctive, rare) words (such as *polka*). Somewhat counterintuitively, it was the low frequency words that were more likely to elicit false positives and recollective experience. This suggested that the déjà vécu experience was not made on the basis of familiarity, or confusing the source of a highly familiar word, but due to recollective processes specifically triggered by more novel, or striking events.

We argue that demonstrating such patterns of performance is critical when investigating a state as nebulous and subjective as déjà vécu. O'Connor, Moulin, and Cohen (2007) outline a series of considerations when examining subjective states such as déjà vu. These authors emphasise the need to show that subjective evaluations and states vary predictably according to objective qualities of stimuli, that evaluations are supported by verbal justification and that the experient can spontaneously draw parallels with naturally occurring day-to-day sensations. All of these were satisfied in AKP and our other cases. Our final consideration is that neuroscientific findings should seek to support the validity of the experience and the behavioural observations. For instance, in something as subjective as the perception of Rubin's vase, markedly different patterns of brain activation have been shown according to whether the participant sees it as two faces or a vase (Andrews, Schluppeck, Homfray, Matthews, & Blakemore, 2002). We have not performed neuroimaging or electrophysiological recording on any of our cases. This should be a priority in future research. Accordingly, we proceed to outline a testable neuroscientific hypothesis on how déjà vécu, as experienced in our cases, might arise.

Importantly, the strange experiences of AKP and MA are consistent with subsequent cases. For instance, Mrs. M (Moulin & Conway, 2009) who presented to us having complained to the BBC about the high levels of repeats on television, and also as having called a television repairman to fix her television, had the same pattern of memory errors. Mrs. M was unhappy watching new television programmes, in particular, the soap opera, "Neighbours", but was happy watching old films that she had already watched before. In the case of "Neighbours", she described her experience as frustrating to the point of tears, and as waiting for the programme to stop repeating. Ironically, whilst watching DVDs of old films, she said she could happily watch them again, as she had forgotten what had happened. We operationalised such a memory error by using a "reverse" Deese-Roediger-McDermott (DRM) task. In the DRM task (Roediger & McDermott, 1995), semantically related items presented at study converge on a nonpresented lure word (e.g., *thread*, *haystack*, *cotton*, and *pin* all converge on the word *needle*). Healthy participants are likely to report that they remember the word *needle*, even though it was never presented. With Mrs. M we presented similar lists of related words but with one critical *unrelated* lure. Following presentation of related concepts such as colours (red, green, blue, black), a healthy participant is very likely to incorrectly remember a related concept such as *yellow*, whereas they are very unlikely to report remembering an unrelated, distinct item such as *Christmas*. We found that Mrs. M made the unlikely errors—even though all of the items presented at study were categorised, and she could report the title of that category, she was still liable to incorrectly recognise items that were strikingly different and not part of that category. Finally, in meeting déjà vécu cases in their own homes for the first time, it has always been our experience that they claim to have met us like this before. Interestingly, this error is not made on subsequent visits. Converging on this novelty view, several carers of patients with such déjà vécu have also reported similar situations in their e-mail correspondence (Table 1).

Deja vécu is reported with other aetiologies, for example, where a patient had received 5-hydroxytryptophan in combination with carbidopa, as treatment for palatal tremor (distressing, repetitive, and involuntary movements of the soft palate; Kalra et al., 2007). Her account also indicates that novelty is possibly a trigger:

> "I ... was a little freaked out when I watched TV as I felt I was watching repeats, although I knew I wasn't, as it was the news. I then got a phone call from my sister to tell me the kids were being sent home as there was a power cut at school. I asked her why she was telling me this again as she had told me this several days before. She asked me if I was okay and asked how she could have known that there was going to be a power cut." (Kalra et al., 2007, p. 312)

One interpretation of our novelty observation is that novel situations and events do not preferentially elicit acute instances of déjà vécu, but rather render a largely chronic déjà vécu state more noticeable. Perhaps our patients are chronically experiencing inappropriate sensations of remembering, but it is only novelty that brings these sensations to the attention of the patients (and carers). That is, when the patients are cleaning their teeth they may feel that they recollect an event, but since this event is commonplace, this sensation of remembering is not so jarring. In contrast, perhaps when Mrs. M watches a film on TV that is actually new to her, the feeling of recollection she experiences is more obviously inconsistent with her stored knowledge, which ought to support the belief that the film has not been seen before: thus the sensation of her (false) recollection is brought forcibly to the forefront of her mind. Such an account does receive some support from the literature on healthy déjà vu experience; it appears that people who travel more report more déjà vu (see Brown, 2004, for a review). Travelling may present more opportunity to experience dissociations between memory sensations and knowledge of previous events. Consider this extreme example: If you did actually attend the same places repeatedly and never travelled elsewhere, you would always have a justification for your feeling of familiarity. In the same way, patently novel events may provide time-limited windows for our patients to experience feelings of recollection that are factually unjustified.

An alternative interpretation, in line with our current thinking is that novelty does genuinely preferentially elicit acute episodes of déjà vécu in these patients. For instance, and as noted previously, we are struck by the observation that when we first meet our patients, they say they have met us before, but do not say this on the second or third time we meet them. Accordingly, we propose a specific neuroscientific mechanism underlying déjà vécu that accounts for this ironic error, and we build a case for this novel account. The account is discussed later as the encoding-experienced-as-retrieval hypothesis.

POSSIBLE MECHANISMS UNDERLYING PATHOLOGICAL DÉJÀ VÉCU

Our initial explanation of these cases is outlined in Moulin et al. (2005). We extended the recollective experience findings from AKP and MA to a tentative neuroscientific mechanism by which inappropriate recollection could be experienced as déjà vécu. According to a dual process view (Aggleton & Brown, 1999), there are different structures associated with remembering and familiarity. Aggleton and Brown (1999) proposed that the hippocampus is heavily involved in remembering, whereas the parahippocampal cortex is part of a different system responsible for familiarity. These déjà vécu patients were therefore proposed to experience déjà vécu characterised by elevated remembering for new items as a result of hippocampal dysfunction (evidenced on structural brain scans of the cases). We propose that the secondary confabulation found to be associated with justifying the sensations of remembering associated with déjà vécu was indicative of frontal decline. In short, a hippocampal dysfunction gave rise to sensations of recollection, which due to damage to the frontal lobes (evidenced in neuropsychological test scores) was not corrected, or incorrectly interpreted at a later stage. This combination of hippocampal and frontal networks in the reexperiencing and accepting of memory at retrieval received support from fMRI studies of healthy subjects making "remember" compared to "know" (or familiarity) judgements (e.g., Henson et al., 1999) and from stimulation of the hippocampal areas and associated networks by Chauvel and colleagues (e.g., Bancaud, Brunet-Bourgin, Chauvel, & Halgren, 1994; Vignal, Maillard, McGonigal, & Chauvel, 2007).

Originally, the delusion-like nature of our patients was not explored, but clearly, the role of frontal mechanisms is consistent with the second factor (causing belief evaluation failure) in Langdon and Coltheart's (2000) model of delusion. A failure in reality testing resulting from frontal decline may result in the maintenance of erroneous recollection in spite of its inconsistency with other aspects of the experient's beliefs and experiences.

In sum, déjà vécu may be a syndrome of dysfunction associated with specific problems related to both hippocampal and frontal decline.

The encoding-experienced-as-retrieval hypothesis

Our earlier account overlooks one key attribute of the déjà vécu cases: that the patients tend to experience novel or striking stimuli as having been encountered before. In fact, with these cases it is possible to identify triggers for their experiences, whereas with epilepsy, in contrast, there tends to be no external trigger at all (see Moulin & Chauvel, in press, and O'Connor & Moulin, 2008, for more about familiarity-based déjà vu not being triggered by events in the environment). Our strong impression was that whenever attention was engaged by an arousing or novel stimulus, there was an accompanying sensation of déjà vécu. We argue that the key feature of these events is that they are striking in that they are novel and that novelty detection is a key step in a process by which attention is orientated towards encoding a stimulus. As an example, when AKP was interviewed for BBC Radio 4, the journalist provocatively asked him if he felt that he had been interviewed before—he had not. AKP described how he had been interviewed before and justified his experience by noting salient perceptual features of his current situation, claiming that it was all exactly as before and using it all as justification of his memory retrieval. In such situations the memory system should be working to *encode* such features for future reference, but AKP misinterpreted such contextual and perceptual information as *retrieval* from memory. In keeping with other authors, we make the assumption that novelty is an important cue for engaging encoding mechanisms, as evidenced by the likelihood that novel events and first-time experiences are remembered for longer periods (Lisman & Grace, 2005; Tulving, Markowitsch, Craik, Habib, & Houle, 1996).

Thus, our more detailed account of the experience of déjà vécu is based on the simple principle that encoding-related activity could be misinterpreted as retrieval-related; the rest of this paper concentrates on this proposal. This proposal rests on the idea that the hippocampus supports novelty-detection as well as recollection, and that recollection normally involves a transient and distinct theta-based coupling between the hippocampus and other regions that receive information from the hippocampus. For simplicity, we shall focus our discussion on one output region within the hippocampus, CA1, and one key hippocampal efferent region, the medial prefrontal cortex, but, of course, the same principles are expected to apply to other regions. Note that other authors have suggested a similar disconnection between temporal and frontal regions and resultant confabulation (see Gilboa et al., 2006; Schnider et al., 2002). Broadly speaking, these accounts converge on the orbitofrontal prefrontal cortex as responsible for gating and monitoring outputs from temporal regions.

Our account assumes that the hippocampus is crucial for reactivating the context associated with an event, and thus for episodic recollection. It also assumes that various neocortical areas (e.g., medial parietal, visual) are involved in recreating the specific contents of the event being recollected. Another assumption is that a third region, such as the medial prefrontal cortex or retrosplenial cortex, is associated with the subjective, conscious experience that these contents evoke, resulting in recollection of one's own past. Medial prefrontal cortex and retrosplenial cortex both receive direct projections from the hippocampus, including CA1 (Amaral & Lavenex, 2007). Using these fairly standard assumptions, we outline a speculative model of how processing might proceed normally, and the consequences of it going wrong. First, we briefly discuss hippocampal involvement in recollection and novelty detection. We then summarise some data and theory on the importance of the theta oscillation in memory. Finally, we suggest a theta-based mechanism of how the encoding of novel experience could be misinterpreted by the brain as the retrieving of that information. We arrive at a specific model of how the interaction between frontal and hippocampal networks may be deficient in such a way as to produce déjà vécu. Crucially, this model explains how, in our patients, the act of encoding may be misinterpreted as the act of retrieving.

THE HIPPOCAMPUS AND NOVELTY DETECTION

There is fairly broad consensus that recollection involves the hippocampus (e.g., Duzel, Vargha-Khadem, Heinze, & Mishkin, 2001; Yonelinas, Otten, Shaw, & Rugg, 2005). A lesion study using an animal model of recollection also reached this conclusion (Fortin, Wright, & Eichenbaum, 2004). We emphasise here that several lines of evidence from different research fields demonstrate that the hippocampus also plays an important role in novelty detection (e.g., Honey, Watt, & Good, 1998; Knight, 1996; Kumaran & Maguire, 2007; Lee, Hunsaker, & Kesner, 2005; Nyberg, 2005). It seems likely that this novelty-detection function is directly related to the hippocampal role in episodic encoding of events. First, as the Tulving (1972) quotation beginning this paper implies, any event involves a unique configuration of stimuli to some extent. Second, novelty is graded—very novel, distinct events are preferentially encoded, and endure longer in memory (Lisman & Grace, 2005; Tulving et al., 1996). An episodic memory system should prioritise the recording of experience that is novel and goal-relevant (Lisman & Grace, 2005).

The precise boundaries of the novelty that the hippocampus detects are debatable. Common to most theoretical conceptualisations, however, are that the hippocampus does not detect simple stimulus novelty but rather a "higher order" novelty. In this higher order novelty, individual stimulus elements may be familiar but the stimulus configuration is novel, or there is a "mismatch" between a stimulus and its context (Honey et al., 1998; Knight, 1996; Kumaran & Maguire, 2007; Lee et al., 2005; Lever, Burton, & O'Keefe, 2006; O'Keefe & Nadel, 1978). A memorable example of potentially hippocampally mediated novelty was provided by O'Keefe and Nadel (1978, p. 241):

> "[N]ovelty typically consists of new configurations of familiar elements. ... [T]he novelty of the wife in the best friend's bed lies neither in the wife, nor the friend, nor the bed, but in the unfamiliar conjunction of the three."

Clearly, a representation can exist of a new item independent of its context, and this novelty can be detected without the hippocampus. (Such representations occur in perirhinal cortex, e.g., Aggleton & Brown, 1999). An additional novelty engendered by that item is its occurrence in an otherwise familiar, well-mapped context, as in a previously unseen neuropsychologist appearing eagerly at the front door, asking for your participation in a study investigating déjà vu. The hippocampus may well detect this item-in-context novelty (Fyhn, Molden, Hollup, Moser, & Moser, 2002; O'Keefe, 1976) and presumably participate in encoding the event.

Hippocampal novelty detection and the two input streams to CA1

Exactly how the hippocampus detects novelty is not known. Most models, however, assume that region CA1 compares current, real-world, sensory input, which it receives from the entorhinal cortex, with predictive input generated by pattern-completion based recall, which it receives from CA3 (Leutgeb, Leutgeb, Moser, & Moser, 2005; Nakazawa et al., 2002; Wills, Lever, Cacucci, Burgess, & O'Keefe, 2005). When these two input streams do not match, CA1 generates a novelty signal (Hasselmo, Wyble, & Wallenstein, 1996; Kumaran & Maguire, 2007; Lisman & Otmakhova, 2001). Importantly, these two synaptic input streams, one from the entorhinal cortex and the other from CA3, arrive in CA1 at different phases of the theta oscillation. The theta oscillation is an approximately 4–10 Hz oscillation, which is very prominent in the EEG recorded from the hippocampal formation in mammals including humans. Figure 1 shows examples of raw EEG traces recorded from rat and human hippocampus.

Novelty-responsive neuromodulation, including that generated by the hippocampus itself, can change the relative weight of the inputs from entorhinal cortex and CA3, biasing CA1 to be more responsive to its

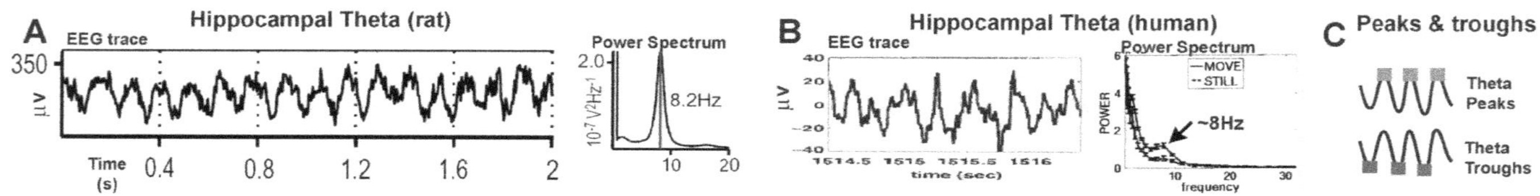

Figure 1. The theta oscillation in rats and humans. (A, B) Hippocampal EEG trace (left) and power spectrum (right) for real exploration (A, rat) and virtual-environment exploration (B, human). Rat power spectrum and human power spectrum during exploration ("MOVE") show peaks at ~8Hz. (C) Schematic theta oscillation showing peaks and troughs (used in Figure 3). (A) is adapted from Jeewajee, Lever, Burton, O'Keefe, and Burgess (2008). (B) is adapted from Ekstrom, Caplan, Ho, Shattuck, Fried, and Kahana (2005). To view this figure in colour, please visit the online version of this Journal.

entorhinal input in novelty (Hasselmo et al., 2002; Meeter, Murre, & Talamini, 2004). Since the input from entorhinal cortex and CA3 arrive at different theta phases, and novelty modulates CA1's response to this input, we might expect CA1 firing during encoding (biased towards entorhinal firing) to show a different mean theta phase from its firing during retrieval (biased towards CA3 firing). To anticipate our argument, a region downstream of CA1 capable of performing theta phase-readout of CA1 activity could underpin judgements about whether the hippocampus is encoding or retrieving.

Background to the new model: Theta, synaptic plasticity, and the separation of encoding and retrieval

Studies in humans and rats strongly indicate the importance of the theta oscillation to memory function (Buzsaki, 2006). Recently, there has been renewed interest in the human theta oscillation following demonstrations that hippocampal theta can be found in humans as well as other mammals (e.g., Kahana, Sekuler, Caplan, Kirschen, & Madsen, 1999; Tesche & Karhu, 2000). Increased theta power or theta coherence is also known to be associated with the success of both encoding and retrieval (e.g., Fell et al., 2003; Guderian & Duzel, 2005; Jacobs, Hwang, Curran, & Kahana, 2006; Klimesch, 1999; Osipova et al., 2006; Sederberg, Kahana, Howard, Donner, & Madsen, 2003). Moreover, theta synchronisation over spatially distributed networks is associated with experiential qualities of consciously remembering (Barbeau et al., 2005; Klimesch et al., 2001), and with retrieval that incorporates correct source judgements (Guderian & Duzel, 2005).

These demonstrations of the importance of theta in human memory have been inspired by work in rats showing strong associations between the temporal signal of the theta oscillation and long-term synaptic plasticity. It is well established, for instance, that long-term potentiation (LTP) in region CA1 of the hippocampus is preferentially induced when stimulation occurs at the peak of the theta oscillation in CA1 (e.g., Holscher, Anwyl, & Rowan, 1997; Huerta & Lisman, 1993). A further finding is that long-term depression (LTD), depotentation, or no change results if stimulation occurs at the opposite phase to that promoting LTP (Holscher et al., 1997; Hyman, Wyble, Goyal, Rossi, & Hasselmo, 2003). Figure 2A schematically summarises these findings.

In conclusion, a strong determinant of whether information is subsequently remembered or forgotten is the phase of theta that the information arrives at. Consistent with this idea are demonstrations that the brain can optimise memory encoding by scheduling memory-relevant sensory stimuli to arrive at the appropriate theta phase (McCartney et al., 2004; Rizzuto, Madsen, Bromfield, Schulze-Bonhage, & Kahana, 2006; Rizzuto et al., 2003).

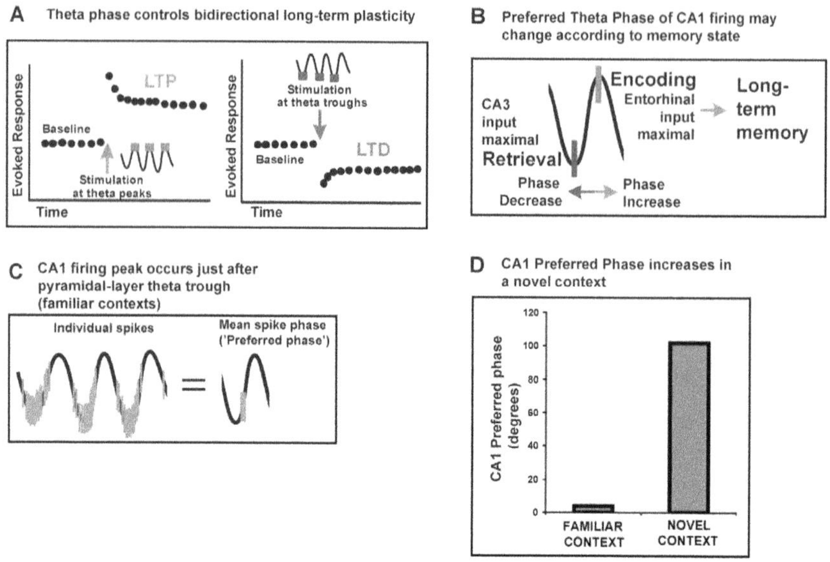

Figure 2. The relationship of theta phase to memory encoding and retrieval. (A) Theta phase controls bidirectional, long-term synaptic plasticity. The phase of theta at which stimulation occurs determines whether hippocampal synapses are subsequently strengthened (long-term potentiation, LTP), unchanged, or weakened (long-term depression, LTD). Schematic summary of data in Hyman et al. (2003) and McCartney, Johnson, Weil, and Givens (2004). (B) The model of Hasselmo, Bodelon, and Wyble (2002) proposes that encoding and retrieval in CA1 typically occur at different phases of theta. This would mean that CA1 preferred phase in novel contexts, when encoding is expected to occur, would be different to that in familiar contexts. The phase of theta when LTP can preferentially be induced in CA1 coincides with maximal entorhinal input, whereas the theta phase when LTD is preferentially induced coincides with maximal CA3 input. (C) Individual spikes of CA1 pyramidal cells occur at various phases of the theta cycle, but it is thought that the "preferred phase" (i.e., the mean phase) of CA1 pyramidal cell firing occurs just after the trough of the local pyramidal-layer theta oscillation (e.g., Csicsvari, Hirase, Czurko, Mamiya, & Buzsaki, 1999). This result was based on testing in familiar environments: Novelty variables were not studied. (D) In a novel context the preferred theta phase of firing in CA1 is increased relative to preferred phase in a familiar context. Mean all-spikes theta phase shown for one rat (two trials in familiar context, one trial in novel context).Mean theta phase is normalised such that the last trial in the familiar context is 0° (Lever et al., unpublished data). To view this figure in colour, please visit the online version of this Journal.

On the basis of such data, it has been proposed that the theta oscillation separates encoding and retrieval modes in the hippocampal memory system (Hasselmo et al., 2002; Hyman et al., 2003; Judge & Hasselmo, 2004; Kunec, Hasselmo, & Kopell, 2005). A basic prediction of these models is that the mean phase of firing across the CA1 population will differ according to whether CA1 is encoding novel information (entorhinal biased) or retrieving old information (CA3 biased). See Figure 2B for a schematic diagram of this model. Previous studies have investigated the mean phase (also called "preferred phase") of CA1 firing in rats, and found that the mean phase occurs just after the theta trough in the pyramidal layer (e.g., Csicsvari et al., 1999). See Figure 2C for a schematic summary of these findings. These studies were based on rats foraging in familiar environments. Recent work has explicitly looked at theta phase of firing during manipulations of novelty. This recent work (Lever et al., unpublished data; Manns, Zilli, Ong, Hasselmo, & Eichenbaum, 2007) supports the view that theta phase separates encoding and retrieval states. Lever et al. (unpublished data) consistently showed an *increase* in mean theta phase associated with novelty; that is, spikes of CA1 pyramidal cells tended to fire *later* in the theta cycle in a novel, unexpected environment than in an expected, familiar environment (Figure 2D).

The new model: Mean theta phase and an erroneous signal of "retrieval"

In summary, recent evidence indicates that the principal cells in CA1 (the output region of the hippocampus proper) fire at different mean phases of the theta oscillation depending on whether they are primarily encoding or primarily retrieving information. To our knowledge, in the work reviewed above Hasselmo and colleagues have not emphasised the potential consequences of the encoding versus retrieval theta phase difference for regions *downstream* of the hippocampus. If we assume that the same CA1 neurons participate in both encoding and retrieval, memory state (i.e., encoding or retrieval) cannot be inferred on the basis of which subset of CA1 neurons fire. Indeed, the more accurate the memory, the greater the overlap will be between the set of neurons that fired during the original experience and the reactivated neurons, whose firing subsequently helps to recreate, and thus subserve the remembering of that experience. What should be different about the original encoding and the subsequent retrieval is the average theta phase of CA1 spiking. Thus, it seems plausible to suggest that phase readout (e.g., Jensen, 2001) in downstream regions could play an important role in interpreting whether hippocampal output represents memory encoding or retrieval. Strength of activation per se may not be a reliable signal of hippocampal memory state.

Our proposal, then, is simply that downstream regions (e.g., medial prefrontal or retrosplenial cortex) which receive direct projections from CA1 detect this encoding versus retrieval theta phase difference. There is emerging evidence for medial prefrontal neuronal firing being phase-locked to the hippocampal theta oscillation when this is appropriate to the current behavioural task (Jones & Wilson, 2005a,b; Siapas, Lubenov, & Wilson, 2005). Interestingly, during the part of a spatial memory task when the medial prefrontal cortex most needs to read hippocampal output, theta coherence transiently increases, and the population activity of medial prefrontal neurons becomes more phase locked, indeed converging to a particular phase of the hippocampal theta rhythm that is consistent across different rats (Jones & Wilson, 2005a). The convergence to a *particular* phase of the hippocampal theta rhythm could mean that prefrontal firing at *that* particular hippocampal theta phase is associated with, and is effectively the signature of, prefrontal interpretation of hippocampal *retrieval*, thus "recollection". One might also imagine prefrontal neurons further downstream which only fire when there is sufficient input from CA1 *and* when this input arrives at the appropriate phase of theta. Interestingly, if this is the case, we would arrive at a mechanism by which a set of neurons typically only fire when there is strong theta coupling between the hippocampus and prefrontal cortex, *and* when the hippocampus is in retrieval mode. The firing of this further-downstream set of neurons would in effect signal recollection. Although these neurons in the normal situation would be under tight inhibitory control and would only fire under theta-coupling states, this coding scenario would allow for the possibility that "recollection" neurons could be activated pathologically, thus eliciting a false signal of recollection, as occurs in déjà vécu.

ENCODING STATE INTERPRETED AS RETRIEVAL STATE IN DÉJÀ VÉCU

Our account, then, assumes three states for the hypothesised downstream region (e.g., medial prefrontal cortex) with respect to hippocampal output:

1. Not receiving (no theta coupling);
2. Receiving (increased theta coupling) while hippocampus is encoding (theta encoding phase); and
3. Receiving (increased theta coupling) while hippocampus is retrieving (theta retrieval phase).

Our contention is that in pathological déjà vécu, there is a disruption to the timing of firing relative to the theta oscillation. This disruption is such that the phase of firing of prefrontal neurons is that associated with hippocampal retrieval, even though the CA1 neurons contributing to the excitation of the prefrontal neurons may actually be firing in a novelty-responsive mode supporting encoding. The precise reason why a timing disruption might occur is unclear and could result from disruption in prefrontal cortex of the integration of hippocampal synaptic input, disruption to hippocampal or prefrontal spike timings relative to a normally functioning theta oscillation, impairments in phase reset of ongoing theta, or impaired synchronisation between septohippocampal and neocortical theta. Although it is anticipated that hippocampal dysfunction plays a role in this timing disruption, what we predict is *unimpaired* in déjà vécu is the hippocampal novelty detection mechanism.

Although our hypothesis is not testable using fMRI, it can be tested using electrophysiological recordings of both EEG and single neuron firing patterns. Using electrodes implanted in the hippocampus, evidence in support of our hypothesis would include the following:

- When stimuli are presented that *elicit false recollection*, CA1 or the downstream neocortical region neurons fire with a *similar* mean theta phase of firing as that occurring during genuine recollection of past events.
- However, when stimuli are presented that *do not elicit false recollection*, the CA1 or neocortical neurons fire with a *different* mean theta phase of firing to that occurring during genuine recollection.

A complementary approach is to show that the downstream neocortical neurons, which typically fire during recollection-elicited states of high theta coupling between the hippocampus and the neocortical region in question, can also fire in abnormal circumstances (seizures, pharmacological intervention), and when they do fire, subjective sensations of "recollection" accompany such firing.

Finally, we return to the scenario of one of our déjà vécu patients making a characteristic error. Consider the act of making a false positive response, i.e., stating that an item was present at the presentation phase of the test, accompanied by the feeling of "remembering" this item. Such an error, is by definition only made for nonpresented (i.e., *novel* in that context) items. Following the first presentation of a contextually novel word, *Christmas*, hippocampal mechanisms signal that the stimulus is contextually novel. Resources are directed towards this novelty, and neuronal firing in the hippocampus attempts to encode this word and associated background features. The patient (like all of us) does not have direct conscious access to whether this hippocampal activity represents encoding or retrieving. This judgement is neocortically mediated, by a region to which the hippocampus projects, and that reads out the preferred theta phase of CA1 firing. The phase readout process is impaired such that hippocampal CA1 activity arrives at a theta phase associated with retrieval. As a result, the first presentation of a novel word, *Christmas,* results in the sensation of "recollection". The authenticity of this sensation inspires two kinds of post hoc rationalisation searching for potential causes leading to the sensation. First, stimuli in the current sensory environment are attributed the status of "having-already-been-experienced". Second, confabulations are generated, whereby actions are inserted into the narrative of the patient's past to explain just how the patient could actually have experienced the novel event.

CONCLUDING REMARKS

In this paper we have attempted to (1) outline differences between false recognition made with the sensation of recollection and familiarity, suggesting that false recognition on the basis of familiarity might be termed déjà vu and on the basis of recollection, déjà vécu, and (2) elucidate a neuroscientific mechanism by which the ironic novelty errors occur in our cases of déjà vécu. To advance our understanding of familiarity and recollection processes, we suggest that patients' false recollections be classified according to Distinction 1, in the hope that we might be able to further distinguish between the different types of memory errors that the patients make. In terms of the neuroscientific aspects of our model, we have arrived at an account that emphasises the importance of theta phase readout and theta coupling between the hippocampus and regions downstream of the hippocampus. In doing so, we have refined our original frontotemporal account of déjà vécu. Continuing to investigate similar cases with particular emphasis on responses to novelty could help to further elucidate the hypothesised, theta-mediated relationship between novelty detection and false recollection.

REFERENCES

Addis, D. R., Wong, A. T., & Schacter, D. L. (2007). Remembering the past and imagining the future: Common and distinct neural substrates during event construction and elaboration. *Neuropsychologia, 45*, 1363–1377.

Aggleton, J. P., & Brown, M. W. (1999). Episodic memory, amnesia and the hippocampal-anterior thalamic axis. *Behavioral and Brain Sciences, 22*, 425–498.

Amaral, D. G., & Lavenex, P. (2007). Hippocampal neuroanatomy. In P. Andersen, R. G. M. Morris, D. G. Amaral, T. Bliss, & J. O'Keefe (Eds.), *The hippocampus book*. New York: Oxford University Press.

American Psychiatric Association. (1994). *Diagnostic and statistical manual of mental disorders* (4th ed.; DSM-IV). Washington, DC: Author.

Andrews, T. J., Schluppeck, D., Homfray, D., Matthews, P., & Blakemore, C. (2002). Activity in the fusiform gyrus predicts perception when viewing Rubin's vase-face stimulus. *Neuroimage, 17*, 890–901.

Arnaud, F. L. (1896). Un cas d'illusion du "déjà vu" ou de "fausse mémoire". *Annales Médico-Psychologiques, 3*, 455–471.

Bancaud, J., Brunet-Bourgin, F., Chauvel, P., & Halgren, E. (1994). Anatomical origin of déjà vu and vivid "memories" in human temporal lobe epilepsy. *Brain, 117*(1), 71–90.

Barbeau, E., Wendling, F., Regis, J., Duncan, R., Poncet, M., Chauvel, P., & Bartolomei, F. (2005). Recollection of vivid memories after perirhinal region stimulations: Synchronization in the theta range of spatially distributed brain areas. *Neuropsychologia, 43*, 1329–1337.

Brown, A. S. (2003). A review of the déjà vu experience. *Psychological Bulletin, 129*(3), 394–413.

Brown, A. S. (2004). *The déjà vu experience*. New York, and Hove, UK: Psychology Press.

Brown, A. S., & Marsh, E. J. (2008). Evoking false beliefs about autobiographical experience. *Psychonomic Bulletin and Review, 15*(1), 186–190.

Buzsaki, G. (2006). *Rhythms of the brain*. New York: Oxford University Press.

Conway, M. A. (2005). Memory and the self. *Journal of Memory and Language, 53*(4), 594–628.

Csicsvari, J., Hirase, H., Czurko, A., Mamiya, A., & Buzsaki, G. (1999). Oscillatory coupling of hippocampal pyramidal cells and interneurons in the behaving rat. *Journal of Neuroscience, 19*, 274–287.

Dickens, C. (1850). *The personal history of David Copperfield*. London: Bradbury & Evans.

Duzel, E., Vargha-Khadem, F., Heinze, H. J., & Mishkin, M. (2001). Brain activity evidence for recognition without recollection after early hippocampal damage. *Proceedings of the National Academy of Sciences, 98*, 8101–8106.

Ekstrom, A. D., Caplan, J. B., Ho, E., Shattuck, K., Fried, I., & Kahana, M. J. (2005). Human hippocampal theta activity during virtual navigation. *Hippocampus, 15*, 881–889.

Fell, J., Klaver, P., Elfadil, H., Schaller, C., Elger, C. E., & Fernandez, G. (2003). Rhinal-hippocampal theta coherence during declarative memory formation: Interaction with gamma synchronization? *European Journal of Neuroscience, 17*, 1082–1088.

Fortin, N. J., Wright, S. P., & Eichenbaum, H. (2004). Recollection-like memory retrieval in rats is dependent on the hippocampus. *Nature, 431*, 188–191.

Fotopoulou, A. (2010). The affective neuropsychology of confabulation and delusion. *Cognitive Neuropsychiatry, 15*(1/2/3), 38–63.

Funkhouser, A. T. (1996). Three types of deja vu [Electronic version]. *Network, 1*. Retrieved 9 September 2008, from http://www.mentalhelp.net/poc/view_doc.php?type=doc&id=264.

Fyhn, M., Molden, S., Hollup, S., Moser, M. B., & Moser, E. (2002). Hippocampal neurons responding to first-time dislocation of a target object. *Neuron, 35*, 555–566.

Gardiner, J. M., Ramponi, C., & Richardson-Klavehn, A. (1998). Experiences of remembering, knowing and guessing. *Consciousness and Cognition, 7*, 1–26.

Gilboa, A., Alain, C., Stuss, D. T., Melo, B., Miller, S., & Moscovitch, M. (2006). Mechanisms of spontaneous confabulations: A strategic retrieval account, *Brain, 129*, 1399–1414.

Guderian, S., & Duzel, E. (2005). Induced theta oscillations mediate large-scale synchrony with mediotemporal areas during recollection in humans. *Hippocampus, 15*, 901–912.

Hasselmo, M. E., Bodelon, C., & Wyble, B. P. (2002). A proposed function for hippocampal theta rhythm: Separate phases of encoding and retrieval enhance reversal of prior learning. *Neural Computation, 14*, 793–817.

Hasselmo, M. E., Wyble, B. P., & Wallenstein, G. V. (1996). Encoding and retrieval of episodic memories: Role of cholinergic and GABAergic modulation in the hippocampus. *Hippocampus, 6*, 693–708.

Henson, R. N. A., Rugg, M. D., Shallice, T., Josephs, O., & Dolan, R. J. (1999). Recollection and familiarity in recognition memory: An event-related functional magnetic resonance imaging study. *Journal of Neuroscience, 19*, 3962–3972.

Holscher, C., Anwyl, R., & Rowan, M. J. (1997). Stimulation on the positive phase of hippocampal theta rhythm induces long-term potentiation that can be depotentiated by stimulation on the negative phase in area CA1 in vivo. *Journal of Neuroscience, 17*, 6470–6477.

Honey, R. C., Watt, A., & Good, M. (1998). Hippocampal lesions disrupt an associative mismatch process. *Journal of Neuroscience, 18*, 2226–2230.

Huerta, P. T., & Lisman, J. E. (1993). Heightened synaptic plasticity of hippocampal CA1 neurons during a cholinergically induced rhythmic state. *Nature, 364*, 723–725.

Hughlings Jackson, J. (1888). On a particular variety of epilepsy ("intellectual aura"), one case with symptoms of organic brain disease. *Brain, 11*, 179–207.

Hyman, J. M., Wyble, B. P., Goyal, V., Rossi, C. A., & Hasselmo, M. E. (2003). Stimulation in hippocampal region CA1 in behaving rats yields long-term potentiation when delivered to the peak of theta and long-term depression when delivered to the trough. *Journal of Neuroscience, 23*, 11725–11731.

Jacobs, J., Hwang, G., Curran, T., & Kahana, M. J. (2006). EEG oscillations and recognition memory: Theta correlates of memory retrieval and decision making. *Neuroimage, 32*, 978–987.

Jeewajee, A., Lever, C., Burton, S., O'Keefe, J., & Burgess, N. (2008). Environmental novelty is signaled by reduction of the hippocampal theta frequency. *Hippocampus, 18*, 340–348.

Jensen, O. (2001). Information transfer between rhythmically coupled networks: Reading the hippocampal phase code. *Neural Computation, 13*, 2743–2761.

Jones, M. W., & Wilson, M. A. (2005a). Phase precession of medial prefrontal cortical activity relative to the hippocampal theta rhythm. *Hippocampus, 15*, 867–873.

Jones, M. W., & Wilson, M. A. (2005b). Theta rhythms coordinate hippocampal-prefrontal interactions in a spatial memory task. *PLoS Biology, 3*, e402.

Judge, S. J., & Hasselmo, M. E. (2004). Theta rhythmic stimulation of stratum lacunosum-moleculare in rat hippocampus contributes to associative LTP at a phase offset in stratum radiatum. *Journal of Neurophysiology, 92*, 1615–1624.

Kahana, M. J., Sekuler, R., Caplan, J. B., Kirschen, M., & Madsen, J. R. (1999). Human theta oscillations exhibit task dependence during virtual maze navigation. *Nature, 399*, 781–784.

Kalra, S., Chancellor, A., & Zeman, A. (2007). Recurring déjà vu associated with 5-hydroxy-tryptophan. *Acta Neuropsychiatrica, 19*(5), 311–313.

Klimesch, W. (1999). EEG alpha and theta oscillations reflect cognitive and memory performance: A review and analysis. *Brain Research: Brain Research Reviews, 29*, 169–195.

Klimesch, W., Doppelmayr, M., Yonelinas, A., Kroll, N. E., Lazzara, M., Rohm, D., & Gruber, W. (2001). Theta synchronization during episodic retrieval: Neural correlates of conscious awareness. *Brain Research: Cognitive Brain Research, 12*, 33–38.

Knight, R. (1996). Contribution of human hippocampal region to novelty detection. *Nature, 383*, 256–259.

Kumaran, D., & Maguire, E. A. (2007). Which computational mechanisms operate in the hippocampus during novelty detection? *Hippocampus, 17*, 735–748.

Kunec, S., Hasselmo, M. E., & Kopell, N. (2005). Encoding and retrieval in the CA3 region of the hippocampus: A model of theta-phase separation. *Journal of Neurophysiology, 94*, 70–82.

Langdon, R., & Bayne, T. J. (2010). Delusion and confabulation: Mistakes of perceiving, remembering and believing. *Cognitive Neuropsychiatry, 15*(1/2/3), 319–345.

Langdon, R., & Coltheart, M. (2000). The cognitive neuropsychology of delusions. *Mind and Language, 15*, 184–218.

Lee, I., Hunsaker, M. R., & Kesner, R. P. (2005). The role of hippocampal subregions in detecting spatial novelty. *Behavioral Neuroscience, 119*, 145–153.

Leutgeb, S., Leutgeb, J. K., Moser, M. B., & Moser, E. I. (2005). Place cells, spatial maps and the population code for memory. *Current Opinions in Neurobiology, 15*, 738–746.

Lever, C., Burton, S., Jeewajee, A., Cacucci, F., Burgess, N., & O'Keefe, J. (unpublished data). Environmental novelty elicits a later preferred theta phase of firing in CA1 but not subiculum.

Lever, C., Burton, S., & O'Keefe, J. (2006). Rearing on hind legs, environmental novelty, and the hippocampal formation. *Reviews in the Neurosciences, 17*, 111–133.

Lisman, J. E., & Grace, A. A. (2005). The hippocampal-VTA loop: Controlling the entry of information into long-term memory. *Neuron, 46*, 703–713.

Lisman, J. E., & Otmakhova, N. A. (2001). Storage, recall, and novelty detection of sequences by the hippocampus: Elaborating on the SOCRATIC model to account for normal and aberrant effects of dopamine. *Hippocampus, 11*, 551–568.

Manns, J. R., Zilli, E. A., Ong, K. C., Hasselmo, M. E., & Eichenbaum, H. (2007). Hippocampal CA1 spiking during encoding and retrieval: Relation to theta phase. *Neurobiology of Learning and Memory, 87*, 9–20.

McCartney, H., Johnson, A. D., Weil, Z. M., & Givens, B. (2004). Theta reset produces optimal conditions for long-term potentiation. *Hippocampus, 14*, 684–687.

Meeter, M., Murre, J. M., & Talamini, L. M. (2004). Mode shifting between storage and recall based on novelty detection in oscillating hippocampal circuits. *Hippocampus, 14*, 722–741.

Moulin, C. J. A., & Chauvel, P. (in press). Déjà vu: Insights from the dreamy state and the neuropsychology of memory. In G. Davies & D. B. Wright (Eds.), *Current issues in applied memory research*. Hove, UK: Psychology Press.

Moulin, C. J. A., & Conway, M. A. (2009). The reverse DRM task and recollective confabulation. *Manuscript in preparation.*

Moulin, C. J. A., Conway, M. A., Thompson, R. G., James, N., & Jones, R. W. (2005). Disordered memory awareness: Recollective confabulation in two cases of persistent déjà vécu. *Neuropsychologia, 43*(9), 1362–1378.

Moulin, C. J. A., Turunen, M., Salter, A. J. A., O'Connor, A. R., Conway, M. A., & Jones, R. W. (2006). Recollective confabulation: Persistent déjà vécu in dementia. *Helix Review Series, 2*, 10–15.

Nakazawa, K., Quirk, M. C., Chitwood, R. A., Watanabe, M., Yeckel, M.F., Sun, L. D., et al. (2002). Requirement for hippocampal CA3 NMDA receptors in associative memory recall. *Science, 297*, 211–218.

Neppe, V. M. (1983). *The psychology of déjà vu: Have I been here before?*. Johannesburg, South Africa: Witwatersrand University Press.

Nyberg, L. (2005). Any novelty in hippocampal formation and memory? *Current Opinions in Neurology, 18*, 424–428.

O'Connor, A. R. (2007). *States of awareness and recognition: Insights from déjà vu*. Leeds, UK: University of Leeds.

O'Connor, A. R., Barnier, A. J., & Cox, R. E. (2008). Déjà vu in the laboratory: A behavioral and experiential comparison of posthypnotic amnesia and posthypnotic familiarity. *International Journal of Clinical and Experimental Hypnosis, 56*(4), 425–450.

O'Connor, A. R., & Moulin, C. J. A. (2008). The persistence of erroneous familiarity in an epileptic male: Challenging perceptual theories of déjà vu activation. *Brain and Cognition, 68*, 144–147.

O'Connor, A. R., Moulin, C. J. A., & Cohen, G. (2007). Memory and consciousness. In G. Cohen & M. A. Conway (Eds.), *Memory in the real world* (3rd ed.). Hove, UK: Psychology Press.

O'Keefe, J. (1976). Place units in the hippocampus of the freely moving rat. *Experimental Neurology, 51*, 78–109.

O'Keefe, J., & Nadel, L. (1978). *The hippocampus as a cognitive map*. Oxford, UK: Oxford University Press.

Osipova, D., Takashima, A., Oostenveld, R., Fernandez, G., Maris, E., & Jensen, O. (2006). Theta and gamma oscillations predict encoding and retrieval of declarative memory. *Journal of Neuroscience, 26*, 7523–7531.

Rizzuto, D. S., Madsen, J. R., Bromfield, E. B., Schulze-Bonhage, A., & Kahana, M. J. (2006). Human neocortical oscillations exhibit theta phase differences between encoding and retrieval. *Neuroimage, 31*, 1352–1358.

Rizzuto, D. S., Madsen, J. R., Bromfield, E. B., Schulze-Bonhage, A., Seelig, D., Schenbrenner-Scheibe, R., & Kahana, M. J. (2003). Reset of human neocortical oscillations during a working memory task. *Proceedings of the National Academy of Sciences, 100*, 7931–7936.

Roediger, H. L., & McDermott, K. B. (1995). Creating false memories: Remembering words not presented in lists. Journal of Experimental Psychology: Learning, Memory. *and Cognition, 21*, 803–814.

Sacks, O. (1970). *Migraine*. London: Faber & Faber.

Schnider, A., Valenza, N., Morand, S., et al. (2002). Early cortical distinction between memories that pertain to ongoing reality and memories that don't. *Cerebral Cortex, 12*, 54–61.

Sederberg, P. B., Kahana, M. J., Howard, M. W., Donner, E. J., & Madsen, J. R. (2003). Theta and gamma oscillations during encoding predict subsequent recall. *Journal of Neuroscience, 23*, 10809–10814.

Siapas, A. G., Lubenov, E. V., & Wilson, M. A. (2005). Prefrontal phase locking to hippocampal theta oscillations. *Neuron, 46*, 141–151.

Tesche, C. D., & Karhu, J. (2000). Theta oscillations index human hippocampal activation during a working memory task. *Proceedings of the National Academy of Sciences, 97*, 919–924.

Tulving, E. (1972). Episodic and semantic memory. In E. Tulving & W. Donaldson (Eds.), *Organization of memory* (pp. 382–402). New York: Academic Press.

Tulving, E. (1985). Memory and consciousness. *The Canadian Psychologist, 26*, 1–12.

Tulving, E., Markowitsch, H. J., Craik, F. E., Habib, R., & Houle, S. (1996). Novelty and familiarity activations in PET studies of memory encoding and retrieval. *Cerebral Cortex, 6*, 71–79.

Turner, R., & Coltheart, M. (2010). Confabulation and delusion: A common monitoring framework. *Cognitive Neuropsychiatry, 15*(1/2/3), 346–376.

Vignal, J.-P., Maillard, L., McGonigal, A., & Chauvel, P. (2007). The dreamy state: Hallucinations of autobiographic memory evoked by temporal lobe stimulations and seizures. *Brain, 130*, 88–99.

Ward, J., Parkin, A. J., Powell, G., Squires, E. J., Townshend, J., & Bradley, V. (1999). False recognition of unfamiliar people: "Seeing film stars everywhere". *Cognitive Neuropsychology, 16*, 293–315.

Wills, T. J., Lever, C., Cacucci, F., Burgess, N., & O'Keefe, J. (2005). Attractor dynamics in the hippocampal representation of the local environment. *Science, 308*, 873–876.

Yonelinas, A. P., Otten, L. J., Shaw, K. N., & Rugg, M. D. (2005). Separating the brain regions involved in recollection and familiarity in recognition memory. *Journal of Neuroscience, 25*, 3002–3008.

COGNITIVE NEUROPSYCHIATRY
2010, 15 (1/2/3), 145–180

Strategic retrieval, confabulations, and delusions: Theory and data

Asaf Gilboa

Cognitive Neurology Unit, Rambam Medical Center, Psychology Department, Haifa University, Mount Carmel, Israel

Based on Moscovitch and Winocur's "working with memory" framework, confabulation is described as a deficit in strategic retrieval processes. The present paper suggests that only a confluence of deficits on multiple memory-related processes leads to confabulation. These are divided into three categories. Core processes that are unique to confabulation and required for its evolution include: (1) an intuitive, rapid, preconscious "feeling of rightness" monitoring, (2) an elaborate conscious "editor" monitoring, and (3) control processes that mediate the decision whether to act upon a retrieved memory. The second category is deficits on constitutional processes which are required for confabulation to occur but are not unique to it. These include the formation of erroneous memory representation, (temporal) context confusion, and deficits in retrieval cue generation. Finally, associated Features of confabulations determine the content "flavour" and frequency of confabulation but are not required for their evolution. Some associated features are magnification of normal reconstructive memory processes such as reliance on generic/schematic representations, and positivity biases in memory, whereas others are abnormal such as perseveration or source memory deficits. Data on deficits in core processes in confabulation are presented. Next, the apparent correspondences between confabulation and delusion are discussed. Considering confabulation within a strategic memory framework may help elucidate both the commonalities and differences between the two symptoms. Delusions are affected by a convergence of abnormal perception and encoding of information, associated with aberrant cognitive schema structure and disordered belief monitoring. Whereas confabulation is primarily a disorder of retrieval, mnemonic aspects of delusions can be described as primarily a disorder of input and integration of information. It is suggested that delusions might share some of the associated features of confabulation but

Correspondence should be addressed to Asaf Gilboa, Cognitive Neurology Unit, Rambam Medical Center, Psychology Department, Haifa University, Mount Carmel 31905, Israel. E-mail: agilboa@psy.haifa.ac.il

I would like to thank Drs. Morre Goldsmith and Vered Galon for the use of the QAP and Sarah Adler for testing schizophrenic patients. I would also like to thank Dr. Morris Moscovitch for his inspiring mentorship. AG is supported by an EU FP06 Marie Curie IRG grant MIRG-CT-2006-046544.

DOI: 10.1080/13546800903056965

not its core and constitutional processes. Preliminary data in support of this view are presented.

Keywords: Ventromedial prefrontal cortex; Confabulation; Memory monitoring; Strategic retrieval; Working With Memory.

> Perhaps in infancy, or in a disorder of mind, things remembered may be confounded with those which are merely imagined; but in mature years, and in a sound state of mind, every man feels that he must believe what he distinctly remembers, though he can give no other reason of his belief, but that he remembers the thing distinctly; whereas, when he merely imagines a thing ever so distinctly he has no belief of it upon that account. This belief, which we have from distinct memory, we account real knowledge, no less certain than if it was grounded on demonstration; no man in his wits calls it in question, or will hear any argument against it. (Thomas Reid [1710–1796], pp. 325–326)

The earliest descriptions of confabulation have treated it as essentially a memory phenomenon. Korsakoff considered "pseudoreminiscences" a fundamental aspect of the memory disorder he observed in alcoholic patients (Victor & Yakovlev, 1955). He pointed out that the characteristic confusion of the patients he saw did not affect their current perceptions or general cognition. Rather, Korsakoff specifically attributed their confusion to representations of past events. Pseudoreminiscences reflected either inventions of complete fictions, distortions of memories, or confusing memories from different periods in the patients' lives. This conception of confabulation as belonging to the memory domain has since been eroded either directly by theorising nonmnemonic underlying mechanisms (Dalla Barba, 1993; Dalla Barba & Decaix, 2008; Schnider, 2003, 2008; Zannino, Barban, Caltagirone, & Carlesimo, 2008), or indirectly by attempting to group confabulation together with other neurocognitive disorders that appear, at least superficially, similar. Of the latter, the most influential are models that build on the commonalities between confabulations and delusions (Berrios, 1998; Gilleen & David, 2005; Joseph, 1999; Langdon & Bayne, 2010 this issue; Metcalf, Langdon, & Coltheart, 2007; Turner & Coltheart, 2010 this issue; Turner, Coltheart, Metcalf, & Langdon, 2006). These theoretical endeavours are extremely valuable in illuminating the general principles and structure governing human cognition and in particular human belief systems. However, such cross-domain analyses may also come at a cost. As is often the case with drawing analogies, such models tend to obscure important empirical differences between the disorders and consequently may fail to take into account certain constraints that should guide the construction of such universal theoretical models.

The present paper will: (1) describe a domain-specific theoretical model of confabulation, which considers it a reflection of specific impairments within the memory domain; (2) review some of the empirical evidence in support of the strategic retrieval model; and (3) present some preliminary data from patients with delusions showing that despite surface similarities, domain specific analyses of behavioural data point to important differences between the disorders, which might guide both future scientific investigations and help clinical distinctions between the disorders.

CONFABULATION: A STRATEGIC RETRIEVAL APPROACH

One influential approach to the phenomenon of confabulation is expressed by a group of theories that propose confabulation results from deficits in strategic aspects of retrieval (Burgess & Shallice, 1996; Ciaramelli & Ghetti, 2007; Gilboa & Moscovitch, 2002; Johnson, Hashtroudi, & Lindsay, 1993; Kopelman, 1999; Mercer, Wapner, Gardner, & Benson, 1977; Moscovitch, 1989, 1995b; Shapiro, Alexander, Gardner, & Mercer, 1981). The models all share the assumption that confabulation is a memory deficit, although the specifics of the disrupted memory processes differ across models. The models may also differ with regard to the extent to which other cognitive deficits (e.g., executive) contribute to confabulation.

Moscovitch (1992) and Moscovitch and Winocur (1992) have coined the term Working With Memory (WWM) as a general theoretical framework which describes the contribution of the frontal lobes to strategic memory processing, both at encoding and at retrieval. The WWM framework has been constructively and systematically applied in attempts to explain confabulation, and this application in turn has resulted in many important modifications to the theory. At the basis of these investigations is the assumption that confabulation can specifically serve as an important model of failure in retrieval processes because it often affects the time period prior to the onset of the disorder, just as much as subsequent time periods.

The WWM model: General features

The WWM model describes processes associated with different stages of memory: encoding/storage on the one hand, and retrieval on the other. The focus here will be the latter because these apply most to confabulation. It should be noted, however, that faulty encoding can contribute to confabulations associated with information learned after the onset of memory problems. The primary features of the model are described later, and represented schematically in Figure 1. Although described in a somewhat mechanistic flowchart manner, the process is obviously not conceived as

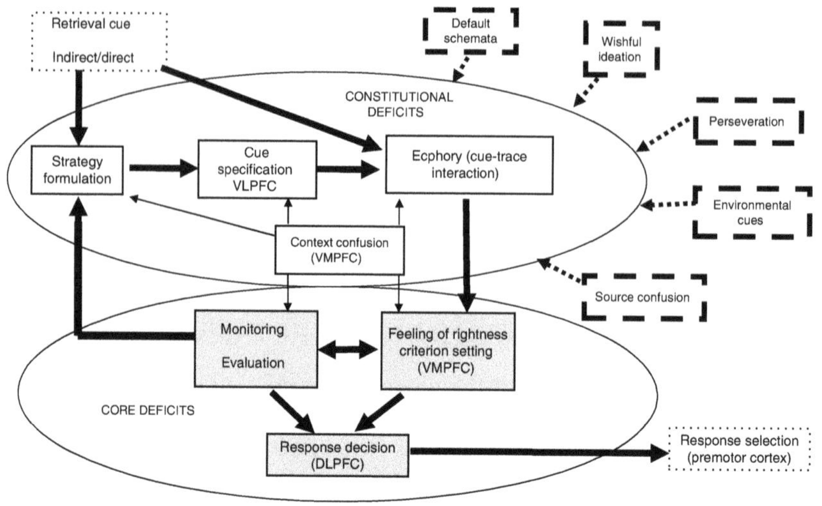

Figure 1. Working With Memory (WWM) and confabulation: Deficits in core processes (grey boxes) are critical and unique to confabulation. Deficits in constitutional processes (white boxes) are required but not unique to confabulation. Associated features (dashed boxes) may be either deficits or normal memory processes that determine the frequency and content of confabulation.

such. Information does not literally "transfer" from region to region within the PFC; rather, different regions operate on representations that are the product of complex excitatory and inhibitory processes between different PFC regions and posterior neocortical and subcortical structures, as well as intrinsic interactions among PFC regions. Thus, although different processes are assigned to different PFC structures, these should only be conceived as crucial rather than solitary regions that mediate particular functions.

Encoding and storage. According to the model (see also Hirst & Volpe, 1988), any event that is experienced consciously is automatically processed by memory-related limbic/paralimbic structures such as the hippocampus and diencephalon. Memory traces, comprising of hippocampal-neocortical ensembles, are formed to represent the conscious experience. Importantly, the hippocampal-neocortical ensembles are intrinsically devoid of any temporal order or thematic/semantic meaning. These ensembles can only represent immediate contiguity or simultaneity. During encoding, frontal lobe structures are critical for endowing information with semantic organisation (McAndrews & Milner, 1991) and temporal order (McAndrews & Milner, 1991; Milner, Petrides, & Smith, 1985; Moscovitch, 1995a; Moscovitch & Melo, 1997). The dorsolateral prefrontal cortex appears to be particularly involved in these processes. Faulty encoding due to dysfunctional limbic structures or disruption to frontally mediated WWM processes may contribute to the evolution of confabulation in that they provide retrieval processes with information that is either thematically incorrect or encoded erroneously with respect to its spatial-temporal context. However, for confabulations to arise, these erroneous details need to be produced as the end product of a retrieval process.

Retrieval. Recovery of memory traces may occur via two primary routes (Figure 1). Associative cue-dependent retrieval occurs when a retrieval cue directly activates hippocampal-neocortical ensembles that constitute the memory representation (ecphory), i.e., similar neural networks to those that were active during the original event that is being remembered, are reactivated by the cue. Erroneous direct activations may give rise to confabulatory memories or serve as potential "substrate" for confabulations, when postretrieval processes fail (see later). Associative retrieval might fail occasionally even in healthy persons (Burgess & Shallice, 1996), but of course such failures are more abundant when there is damage to memory-related limbic structures such as the hippocampus, basal forebrain, and diencephalon (Moscovitch & Melo, 1997).

The second route to retrieval involves strategic WWM processes mediated by different structures within the prefrontal cortex. Retrieval-related WWM processes involve preecphoric procedures including initiation of a search process when the associative cue is insufficient to activate a memory representation directly, organisation and maintenance of the search process, and generation of appropriate retrieval cues in accordance with the goals of the of the memory task. They also involve postecphoric evaluation, verification and response-decision processes, and postecphoric placement within a temporal or thematic contextual framework (Gilboa, Alain, et al., 2006; Gilboa & Moscovitch, 2002; Moscovitch & Winocur, 2002). Finally, postecphoric WWM processes involve the decision whether to report or withhold the product of the memory search. Different prefrontal regions are differentially involved in each of these processes.

According to the model, the dorsolateral PFC is critical for establishing a retrieval mode, which aligns the cognitive system to engage in retrieval (Lepage, Ghaffar, Nyberg, & Tulving, 2000; Rugg & Wilding, 2000) by setting the goals of the retrieval task and initiating the search process. The ventrolateral PFC plays a crucial role in specifying, describing, and generating retrieval cues that may permit access and interact with the hippocampal code to elicit the memory trace. This is a reiterative process, which continues until a specific enough cue activates a memory trace. Once a memory trace is activated, the signal is picked up by structures within the ventromedial prefrontal cortex (VMPFC), which serves in the context of memory retrieval to signal either acceptance or rejection based on an intuitive "felt rightness" quality of the recovered memory. Moscovitch and Winocur (2002) have postulated that the posterior VMPFC plays an inhibitory (rejecting) role in a dual process reciprocally complimented by the frontal pole that signals acceptance. The memory representation which was reconstructed is also monitored for compatibility with other knowledge such as the context of retrieval, other memories, semantic knowledge, etc. This slower, more deliberate "problem-solving" process is primarily mediated by the DLPFC in interaction with posterior neocortical regions and the VLPFC.

The WWM model and confabulation

Different types of confabulation including spontaneous and provoked confabulations (Kopelman, 1987) and behavioural confabulations (Schnider, von Daniken, & Gutbrod, 1996) have been interpreted within the framework of the WWM model (Ciaramelli & Ghetti, 2007; Gilboa, Alain, et al., 2006; Gilboa & Moscovitch, 2002; Moscovitch, 1995a; Moscovitch & Melo, 1997). The model can also be usefully applied to account for and to explain features of confabulation such as repetition of themes, emotional biases, and temporal context confusions (Gilboa, Alain, et al., 2006).

Moscovitch and Melo (1997; see also Moscovitch, 1989, 1995a) have suggested three basic faulty processes may underlie confabulation: (1) faulty search processes, which are reflected by confabulators' inability to initiate and maintain an orderly process of exploring the content of long-term memory; (2) faulty associations between memory cues and memory representations, which are required in order for false memories to be generated in the first place (these may arise in the context of a degraded primary memory system as in amnesia—MTL or diencephalic amnesia—but may also occur independently of any memory impairment); and (3) faulty monitoring, which was determined as the necessary and sufficient condition for confabulation to occur. Moscovitch and Winocur (2002), Gilboa and Moscovitch (2002) and later Gilboa (2004) and Gilboa, Alain, et al. (2006) have expanded on these basic principles to account for different aspects of confabulation within this strategic memory retrieval model.

The retrieval process through the indirect route begins with the formulation of a memory search strategy mediated primarily by the dorsolateral prefrontal cortex. The initiation of a search process is often deficient in confabulators leading to high rates of omissions. Alternatively patients may provide an answer without initiating a search process, relying instead on readily available retrieval cues. These may include retrieval of memories based on cues from the immediate environment or retrieval of recently activated memories, which are often referred to as perseverations (Kopelman, Ng, & van den Brouke, 1997; Mercer et al., 1977; Shapiro et al., 1981).

The launch of a retrieval process does not guarantee of course the generation of appropriate retrieval cues for the medial temporal lobe structures to operate on. Poor specification of cues by the ventrolateral prefrontal region may lead to activation of memories within the hippocampal complex that are incompatible with the memory task. In healthy persons this would normally lead to a repetition of the process (Burgess & Shallice, 1996; Moscovitch & Winocur, 2002). In confabulating patients, however, this often marks the end of the search process and an inappropriate memory is produced (Moscovitch & Melo, 1997).

Although these processes provide the occasion or substrate for confabulation to occur, Moscovitch and Melo (1997) have suggested that the necessary and sufficient condition for confabulation is the breakdown of memory monitoring processes. Faulty monitoring, by this view, leads to the indiscriminate acceptance of activated memories, and so in cases of erroneous traces, to the output of confabulation. This may also explain why in the face of contradictory evidence, confabulators continue to adhere to their original memory and instead produce secondary confabulations in an attempt to reconcile the inconsistencies. Further specification of the processes that underlie monitoring has led to the identification of at least two processes (Gilboa & Moscovitch, 2002; Moscovitch & Winocur, 2002): a preconscious intuitive "feeling of rightness" mechanism and an elaborate conscious problem-solving mechanism (see Gilboa, 2004, for discussion of other possible mechanisms).

Figure 1 and Table 1 summarise the main features of the strategic retrieval theory of confabulation. The different components of the model can be divided into core deficits, constitutional deficits, and associated features (Table 1), which will be discussed next.

Core deficits of confabulation

A dual monitoring deficit

Preconscious "feeling of rightness". One of the most apparent clinical characteristics of confabulation is the patients' absolute conviction in the truthfulness of their erroneous memories. Even when faced with the most compelling contradictory evidence, they will continue to experience a subjective sense of truthfulness of their false beliefs, and search for ways to protect the primary confabulation. This can result in quite bizarre secondary confabulations that serve to justify the contradictions when these are too obvious to ignore (Moscovitch, 1989). That is, even when conscious monitoring mechanisms (see later) appear to correctly signal an error, confabulators fail to adjust their "feeling of rightness" associated with the confabulated memory.

The conviction people have in the truthfulness of their memories is not unique to confabulators. Thomas Reid's observations quoted at the beginning of this paper specifically describe intuitive conviction as a fundamental trait of

TABLE 1
Typology of deficits leading to confabulation

Deficit types	*Contribution to confabulation*
Core deficits: • FOR monitoring • "Editor" monitoring • Control processes	Necessary for confabulation to occur. Without them, even if false memories arise, they are neither produced nor acted upon. They are unique to confabulation
Constitutional deficits: • Memory impairment • Search strategy • TCC	These occur in all or almost all confabulators. Their confluence together with core deficits may be necessary for confabulation to occur. They are not unique to confabulation.
Associated features: • Wishful ideation • Source memory deficits • Default schemata • Environmental cues • Perseveration • Familiarity	These determine the frequency of confabulations, their content and their "flavour". Some of them are normal features of memory re-construction rather than "deficits" (e.g., normal positivity biases; precedence of well-established representations).

human memory in general. Interestingly, current theories describe this trait of human memory in the same way: as an inherent characteristic of memory that is impenetrable to reason. The idea that certain memories carry with them an intrinsic sense of truthfulness has been particularly influential in theories of self-related memories. Compared with other types of information, autobiographical memories carry with them an extraordinary sense of confidence in their veracity, regardless of whether this sense is justified or not (Brewer, 1986). Moreover, one highly influential model of autobiographical memory suggests that the self (or "working self") draws on autobiographical memories as a repository of representations that help it guide behaviour to achieve current goals (Burt, Kemp, & Conway, 2001; Conway & Pleydell-Pearce, 2000). When "feeling of rightness" processes break down the result may be the acceptance of false memory traces with high confidence, and given the role of autobiographical memories in guiding behaviour could also lead to behavioural confabulations (Schnider, 2003, 2008; Schnider et al., 1996).

The physiological and neuroanatomical bases of "feeling of rightness" are poorly understood. Our data (Gilboa, Alain, et al., 2006; Gilboa & Moscovitch, 2002) as well as others' (Schnider, 2003; Turner, Cipolotti, Yousry, & Shallice, 2008) suggest that it crucially depends on networks within the ventromedial and orbitofrontal PFC. One hypothesis regarding the ventromedial PFC is that it acts to integrate cognitive processes with emotional somatic signals in order to bias decision making at a preconscious level (Bechara, Damasio, Tranel, & Damasio, 1997; Bechara, Tranel, & Damasio, 2000). It is well situated anatomically to integrate visceral cues with information from limbic and neocortical heteromodal regions, in order to allow for such biasing (Barbas, 1995). It may accomplish a similar goal in the memory domain, particularly in autobiographical memories (Gilboa, 2004) where such processes are pertinent, as memories carry emotional meaning, personal significance, and sometimes behavioural implications.

Monitoring and evaluation. Retrieved memories are constantly evaluated for their veracity by comparing them to other retrieved content, available information, and to the memory task. These processes are akin to problem-solving procedures, applied to the memory domain. They heavily rely on working memory processes for holding in mind multiple pieces of information, and performing logical operations for deciding whether various retrieved aspects are compatible with each other and with the memory task. They also heavily rely on processes such as conflict detection and conflict resolution. Burgess and Shallice (1996) call these "editing" processes and present empirical data for their involvement in retrieval in healthy controls. Breakdown of these processes can result in confabulations that not only are inaccurate in the context of retrieval but also lack internal consistency.

Interaction of monitoring systems. Early, rapid emotionally based decisions to endorse or reject an item may be followed by a more thorough, cognitive assessment of the memory's plausibility if for example the initial response is incompatible with other knowledge or memories. Faced with such contradictions, healthy individuals may reluctantly admit a failure of their memory, although the "felt rightness" phenomenology may still prevail. It appears that during the early stages of confabulation, damage to the "felt rightness" monitoring system combined with damage to the evaluation system or the interaction between them is responsible for confabulation. These are the cases where patients are aware of inconsistencies and try to make up for them with secondary confabulations, but remain convinced of the veracity of their false memory. Resolution of confabulation may be the result of one system taking over the functions of the other. It may be that some confabulators simply learn not to trust their faulty monitoring system, and learn to rely more heavily on other processes (Gilboa, Alain, et al., 2006). Long-standing confabulation, which is a rather rare occurrence, may involve significant damage to both systems. Importantly, even when both monitoring systems are dysfunctional, confabulation will not be apparent if patients decide to exercise control over their report strategy and remain silent or inactive despite having false memories.

Control processes and confabulation

Tulving (1983) makes a distinction between "ecphory", which refers to the interaction between a memory cue and a memory representation, and "conversion", which refers to the actual behavioural output of the recollective process. Our model, as well as others, has broken the latter into several stages most generally a monitoring (which as discussed earlier is itself composed of several subprocesses) and control, which we have not given much attention to. Control processes act on the products of the monitoring process to determine whether or not to volunteer the best available candidate answer (Koriat & Goldsmith, 1994, 1996; Koriat, Goldsmith, & Pansky, 2000). It is suggested that control mechanisms operate by setting a report criterion on the monitoring output on the basis of implicit or explicit payoffs. Thus, patients may be quite certain of the veracity of a particular memory; however, if the cost of acting according to that memory provided it is erroneous is too great, they might avoid action.

To test strategic regulation of memory, one needs to distinguish memory quantity (correct items as a proportion of the total input) and memory accuracy (correct items as a proportion of the total output). A critical methodological implication of this approach is that a free report condition needs to be implemented in order to allow subjects the opportunity to withhold available information so that output-bound accuracy and input-bound quantity measures can be distinguished. This contrasts with experimental tasks that have been used with confabulation in the past such as Schnider's continuous recognition task or the recognition tasks used by Gilboa, Alain, et al. (2006), which force participants to reply either through yes/no recognition or forced choice recognition. These tasks focus on input bound information and measure reliability only indirectly via input manipulations such as list membership or item plausibility. Only under free report conditions can subjects truly be held accountable for the information they produce, and their commitment to the accuracy of their memory output can be assumed. The option to withhold information is an important mechanism by which participants are able to regulate the quantity and accuracy of their memory both in real life and in the laboratory. Mercer et al. (1977) and later Dalla Barba (Dalla Barba, 1993; Dalla Barba & Decaix, 2008) as well as Schnider (Schnider et al., 1996) used this idea in what they called "I Don't Know" questions to which the normal answer for subjects is "I don't know". Numerous confabulation studies have now shown that some confabulators may have a tendency to respond with incorrect answers to such items, although this is not a universal trait. This measure, however, cannot dissociate monitoring from control processes.

To conclude, *core mechanisms* of confabulation involve deficits in three domains: FOR monitoring, "Editor" monitoring, and control mechanisms. For an overt confabulatory syndrome to occur, deficits in all three domains are required. Their cooccurrence is necessary for confabulation and unique to it.

Constitutional and associated features of confabulation

Although failure of monitoring and control systems appears to be necessary for confabulation to occur and unique to them, deficits in other process, including primary memory, search initiation, cue specification, and (temporal) context confusion, and so forth may be required for a full confabulatory syndrome to arise. I dub these processes *constitutional features* of confabulation as they appear to always be associated with confabulation, and might be necessary for a full-blown confabulatory syndrome to occur. However, they are not unique to confabulation and are not sufficient for confabulation to occur.

For example, some degree of primary memory deficits appear to always accompany confabulation, which has led some to propose the dual lesion hypothesis of confabulation (Damasio, Graff-Radford, Eslinger, Damasio, & Kassell, 1985; DeLuca, 1993; DeLuca & Diamond, 1995; Fischer, Alexander, D'Esposito, & Otto, 1995). By this view, only combined lesions to frontal executive regions and limbic memory related regions can produce confabulation. Although the dual lesion hypothesis is not well supported by neuroanatomical data (Gilboa & Moscovitch, 2002; Turner et al., 2008), cases in which spontaneous confabulations are present even with minimal anterograde memory impairment are very rare (e.g., Feinstein, Levine, & Protzner, 2000; Kapur & Coughlan, 1980; Nedjam, Dalla Barba, & Pillon, 2000; Papagno & Baddeley, 1997). Moreover, DeLuca (2000) notes that some memory impairment, especially at long delays, is always evident in those cases where such tests were conducted, and in the aforementioned case reports such testing may not have been extensive enough.

Search initiation and cue specification are two processes which are crucial for framing the memory problem, initiating search, constraining it, and guiding it towards local, proximal cues that can activate associative memory processes. Moscovitch and Melo (1997) conclude that the search component is one of the defective processes in confabulators, because prompting led to a substantial increase in both veridical and false memories in confabulators but not in nonconfabulating amnesics or normal controls (cf. Burgess & Shallice, 1996, for a similar conclusion). Faulty search and cue specification strategies cause both omissions and commissions as both veridical and misleading proximal cues are accessed, and hence are considered constitutional features of confabulation. Context confusion is another constitutional feature of confabulation by the model proposed here. Schnider and colleagues (Schnider & Ptak, 1999; Schnider, Ptak, von Daniken, & Remonda, 2000; Schnider, von Daniken, & Gutbrod, 1996) have suggested that temporal context confusion (TCC) characterises a subset of confabulating patients who act upon their confabulatory beliefs. TCC is a tendency to use information that may have been relevant in a previous context and interject it in a current context when it is no longer relevant or appropriate. They hypothesise that increased TCC emanates from an inability to suppress previously activated, but currently irrelevant, memory traces (Schnider & Ptak, 1999). Empirically, TCC has been investigated by using two runs of a continuous recognition paradigm, separated by 1 hour, to test patients' ability to differentiate currently relevant stimuli from those which were previously studied. The results normally show no difference between confabulating and nonconfabulating amnesics in the ability to store new information. However, confabulating amnesics tend to erroneously respond to targets that were relevant on the previous list, but not the current one. Schnider and colleagues argue that their performance on this task is indicative of their temporal confusion which leads to their conflating memories from widely dispersed time periods. Gilboa, Alain, et al. (2006) have devised a similar paradigm with no temporal component which yielded a similar pattern of performance, suggesting that the deficit identified by Schnider and colleagues is better characterised as a difficulty to make any sort of fine-grained distinction within memory and that the temporal hypothesis is the result of a confound in the original TCC task (cf. Schnider, Bonvallat, Emond, & Leemann, 2005, for similar evidence with another variant of their task).

Later conceptualisations of TCC indeed play down the importance to the temporal aspect of the disorder and place more emphasis on the mechanism of suppression of irrelevant stimuli (Schnider, 2008). Here the deficit is referred to as context confusion, although it may be more appropriate to simply refer to it as a suppression deficit because the word context itself is also rather ambiguous. Furthermore, our data, suggest that failure on the TCC task is uniquely associated with the posterior OFC/ VMPFC but is not unique to confabulators (Gilboa, Alain, et al., 2006). Thus, context confusion is considered a constitutional deficit of confabulation because it seems to play an important role in their evolution and is always associated with confabulation. However, since the temporal aspect appears to be incidental to the task used and because the deficit does not appear to be unique to confabulation it is not a core process.

Associated features of confabulation, such as source memory deficits, wishful ideation biases, reliance on default schemata for retrieval, persevera-tion, and so forth are commonly observed in association with confabulation. However, since there are also numerous reports of confabulation without these features, they are not considered constitutional. Associated features often determine the content of confabulation and may exacerbate their occurrence. The mechanisms of associated features are often indicative of normal reconstructive processes in memory, and may in fact represent central mechanisms that lead to erroneous memories in everyday life. Erroneous memories in everyday life, however, often take the form of distortions, omissions, misattributions, suggestibility, and so forth (Schacter, Norman, & Koutstaal, 1998; Schacter & Slotnick, 2004) and so differ greatly from the phenomenology of spontaneous confabulation, which can be quite unusual or even fantastic in nature.

A prime example of associated features of confabulation is the observation that the content of confabulation is often more positive than patients' realities, suggesting a self-serving bias is central to their evolution (Conway & Tacchi, 1996). This hypothesis has now been supported by several well-designed studies with numerous patients, showing this tendency (Fotopoulou, Conway, Griffiths, Birchall, & Tyrer, 2007; Fotopoulou, Conway, & Solms, 2007; Fotopoulou, Conway, Tyrer, et al., 2008; Fotopoulou, Solms, & Turnbull, 2004). However, even within this series of studies there are numerous examples of confabulations that are more negative in nature than current realities, suggesting motivational biases cannot be a required or even a primary mechanism of confabulation and cannot explain their formation. One way of conceiving these biases is in terms of adherence to coherent premorbid self-schema. Indeed, Metcalf (2005) suggested that her patients who tended to have extremely negative confabulations had very negative life histories and the valance of their confabulations was compatible with their self image.

The idea that powerful generic representations may determine the content of confabulation has been suggested by several authors. Most notably, Burgess and Shallice (1996) propose the existence of *description processes*, which specify the type of trace that would satisfy the demands of the retrieval task, and which we call in our model cue specification. Self-reflective comments such as "thinking now about meetings I have been to recently . . . " are thought to represent this type of process. They proposed that failure in descriptor processes would result in intrusion of generic or highly practised memories, as could be seen on some of their volunteers' protocols. Some evidence for such failures underlying confabulations was later obtained in two case reports of confabulating patients (Burgess & McNeil, 1999; Dab, Claes, Morais, & Shallice, 1999). Interestingly, the content specific confabulation of Burgess and McNeil's (1999) patient could also be considered a case of wishful ideation as it involved his previous employment which he could no longer perform. Note that both wishful ideation and reliance on generic schemata are instances of normal memory reconstructive processes which are enhanced in the context of brain pathology.

Other processes that are considered associated features of confabulation are pathological in themselves. For example several authors have noted the prominence of perseverations in the evolution of confabulation (Kopelman et al., 1997; Mercer et al., 1977; Shapiro et al., 1981). Faulty cue specification as well as initiation of search strategy may give rise to perseveration as previous mental content is used to address the memory problem faced by the patient. Perseveration which is a common symptom following frontal brain pathology determines in the context of confabulation what content will be produced when patients are attempting to recall.

Some empirical evidence for the WWM hypothesis and confabulation

Theoretical accounts of confabulation over the years have tended to be based primarily on clinical observations or qualitative analyses of the products of confabulation. Attempts at systematic investigations of confabulation have been relatively rare (e.g., Kopelman, 1987; Mercer et al., 1977; Shapiro et al., 1981). As models develop, however, they may serve as a basis for generating testable hypotheses for empirical research. Various aspects of confabulation have recently been examined using more controlled experimental paradigms (Ciaramelli & Ghetti, 2007; Dab, Morais, & Frith, 2004; Fotopoulou, Conway, Solms, Tyrer, & Kopelman, 2008; Fotopoulou, Conway, Tyrer, et al., 2008; Schnider et al., 1996, 2005; Turner et al., 2008). As strategic retrieval models evolved, aspects of their relevance to confabulation have also been experimentally tested (Burgess & Shallice, 1996; Gilboa, Alain, He, Stuss, & Moscovitch, 2009; Gilboa, Alain et al., 2006; Moscovitch & Melo, 1997).

The next section reviews some of the empirical data that support and elucidate the mechanisms of core processes of confabulation. Table 2 presents a brief overview of the theoretical constructs of core mechanisms of confabulation (FOR, editor mechanisms, and control mechanisms) as well as some of their characteristics. These theoretical characteristics can be

TABLE 2
Core processes of confabulation

Theoretical mechanisms	*Potential empirical measures*
Feeling of rightness (FOR) monitoring: • Preconscious; automatic; impenetrable • Cue memory trace correspondence • Strongest for self-related schema	Confidence/probability ratings; electrophysiology; galvanic skin conductance
"Editor" monitoring: • Problem-solving operations • Can override FOR (but not change it)	Introspective reports; challenging incompatible information
Control processes: • Quantity–accuracy tradeoff • Final decision to act/report • Reward sensitivity	Quality–accuracy profile methodology; manipulating reward contingencies

translated into operational hypotheses using empirical measures. For example, FOR may be indexed by subjects' confidence ratings or probability assessments, particularly in the autobiographical domain, although these measures are of course confounded by other more controlled mechanisms. FOR as perceived by the model is intuitive and rapid, which suggests it is intimately related to emotional systems and might be picked up by autonomic measures. It should also be reflected by electrophysiological signals that are early enough to reflect preconscious processing.

Evidence for a dual monitoring deficit

As a first attempt at dissociating monitoring mechanisms from search initiation and from cue specification components of strategic retrieval we used a recognition paradigm for details of remote personal events (Gilboa, Winocur, et al., 2006) in patients with VMPFC lesions with and without confabulations, and in healthy controls (Gilboa, Alain, et al., 2006). We assumed that recognition minimises search components of the retrieval process, and the use of autobiographical information still allows us to tap information that is likely to produce confabulation because it is normally associated with a stronger FOR. On recognition tasks, all the information is presented and one need not establish a search strategy or create retrieval cues to address the long-term memory store. To test the FOR idea, we included lures for the autobiographical recognition task, which were either plausible details or implausible ones. We hypothesised that whereas normal controls and nonconfabulating amnesics would endorse some plausible lures, only confabulators would also endorse implausible lures. The latter finding would suggest that confabulation may arise from a failure of a monitoring mechanism that is qualitatively different from the types of failures seen in controls.

As can be seen in Figure 2, Confabulators had a lower hit rate, and higher false alarm rate, suggesting their performance was not simply due to a general bias to endorse sentences. The differential false alarm rate between plausible and implausible lures also supports the idea that their performance does not reflect a simple bias. This is also inconsistent with the proposal that confabulation is associated with a general problem with response inhibition. Instead, confabulators appear to commit memory errors, and sometimes even gross ones, even when other aspects of strategic retrieval are minimised. Importantly, these errors were associated with high levels of confidence, again in contrast with controls. On this task, too, a qualitative difference between confabulators and controls was revealed. Both control groups endorsed some of the plausible lures, suggesting errors made by confabulators for these stimuli may represent exaggerated rates of otherwise normal

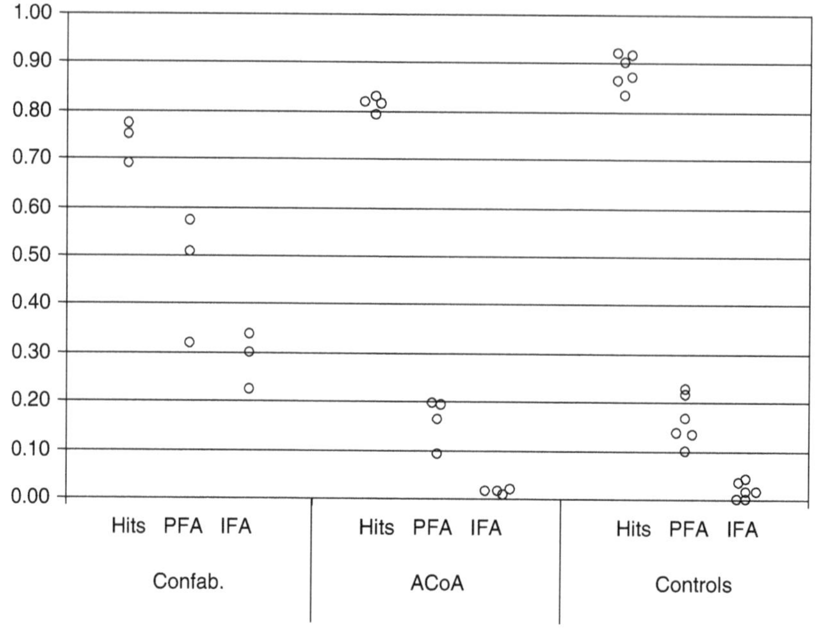

Figure 2. Proportions of hits and false alarms on autobiographical recognition. PFA = plausible false alarms; IFA = implausible false alarms.

memory failures (or disagreement between rememberers). By contrast, endorsement of implausible lures was unique to confabulators suggesting a qualitatively different mechanism may have led to these types of errors. As discussed later, we believe this represents a failure of a system that facilitates early, intuitive rejection of false memories that is particularly strongly associated with self-related memories.

Following each sentence, participants were required to indicate whether their confidence in their response was high or low. Overall, participants were quite confident in their responses. Even healthy controls had a surprisingly high percentage of high confidence for misses and false alarms (Figure 3). This may have occurred because we only provided them with two options, which may not have been sensitive enough to detect subtle differences in confidence. Nonetheless, a clear pattern emerged in which confabulators had high rates of confident responses even for implausible false alarms, although it was somewhat lower than that of hits and correct rejections. Thus, it can be seen that the breakdown of the monitoring mechanisms in confabulation is associated with an indiscriminate sense of confidence, as predicted by the model. Note, however, that we do not consider confidence ratings a direct measure of FOR. Confidence judgements depend on a multitude of cognitive and personality factors beyond the sense of self-evident

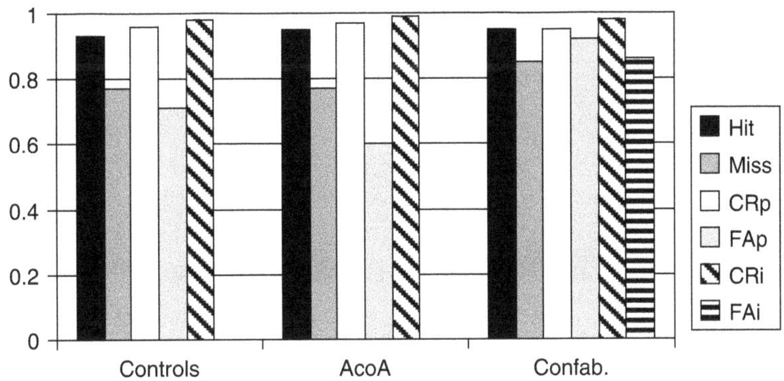

Figure 3. Proportion of high confidence ratings on autobiographical recognition. CRp =correct rejection: plausible; Cri =correct rejection: implausible; FAp =false alarms: plausible; FAi =false alarms: implausible. FAi only occurred in confabulators and so only they have a confidence score on this measure.

truthfulness that FOR produces. Confidence ratings may only be a coarse indicator of FOR, particularly at the high end of the scale, and a finer investigation of confidence and control is described later using the quantity–accuracy profile (QAP) paradigm.

The physiological basis of memory monitoring and control processes can best be examined using neuroimaging techniques with high temporal resolution. This is because an important feature of the dual monitoring hypothesis is that FOR is an early automatic preconscious process whereas "editor" monitoring is later and more elaborate. Furthermore, Gilboa (2004) proposed that FOR partially depends on a correspondence between memory cues and long-term memory representations. This correspondence would need to emerge very early in processing in order to serve as a basis for FOR. It is compatible with the idea that the VMPFC is crucial for emotion-based reinforcement processing based on a history of stimulus-stimulus associations. We examined these hypotheses by measuring event-related brain potentials (ERPs) in a group of patients with VMPFC lesions (Figure 4) following anterior communicating artery (ACoA) aneurysm rupture, and matched healthy controls during speeded decisions about remote memory representations for faces of famous, personally familiar, and unfamiliar people (Gilboa et al., 2009). Patients saw pictures of faces drawn from photos provided by their significant others. These included people they were highly familiar with as well as more remote acquaintances such as old school mates and work colleagues. They also saw faces of famous persons and unfamiliar faces and were asked to determine whether they have personally met each face (i.e., "yes" only to personal acquaintances and "no" to famous and nonfamous faces). Behaviourally, patients had a lower hit rate

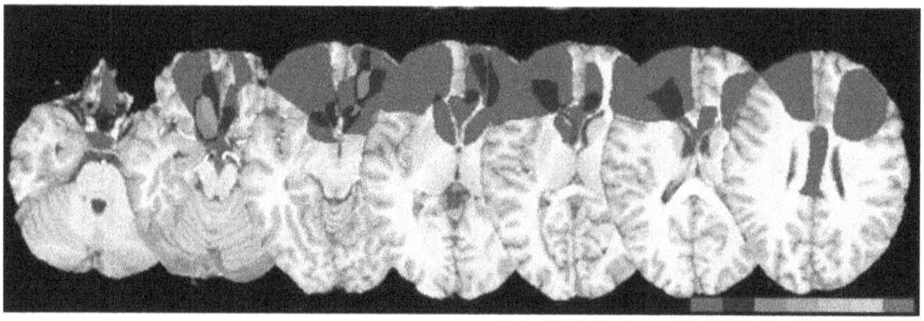

Figure 4. Lesion overlap of seven of the eight patients who participated in the ERP study.

and higher false alarm rate of both kinds (i.e., endorsing famous and nonfamous faces as personally familiar), but were far from being at floor.

As expected with an ERP study of face processing, there was a clear negative modulation larger over right inferior-posterior regions at about 170 ms poststimulus onset (N170), which was evident in both group. However, in accordance with Gilboa's (2004) hypothesis, only the controls' N170 modulation was sensitive to previous familiarity, with unfamiliar faces giving rise to a lower N170 modulation. Interestingly, even familiar faces that explicitly were erroneously judged as unfamiliar explicitly, also gave rise to a high-amplitude N170, suggesting this familiarity signature is implicit. Its absence in patients may be indicative of a lack of preconscious familiarity which could serve as a basis for FOR (Gilboa et al., 2009).

ERP waveforms over anterior sites displayed two distinct epochs where differences were noted between healthy controls and patients with VMPFC lesions (Figure 5). A very early positive modulation in controls, which peaked around 240 ms, was missing in the patients' waveform. A similar positive frontally distributed deflection, which also peaked at around 240 ms, was reported during second-run lures in an ERP study that used a variant of Schnider's task (Schnider, 2003; Schnider, Valenza, Morand, & Michel, 2002). Although no patients were tested in Schnider et al.'s (2002) ERP study, the early electrophysiological signature, associated with rapid decisions about the relevance of memory content, is very similar to the one observed in controls in our study (Gilboa et al., 2009). The neurocognitive mechanism underlying the early memory-related ERP waveforms in the two studies might be analogous. Schnider (2008) interprets this modulation as reflecting the suppression mechanism, which presumably acts by momentarily inhibiting cortical synchronisation at a preconscious stage, before explicit recognition occurs.

Also in accordance with the dual monitoring hypothesis of confabulation, there was a second anterior group difference which appeared at a later time window, beginning at 350 ms and reflecting a sustained positivity in controls

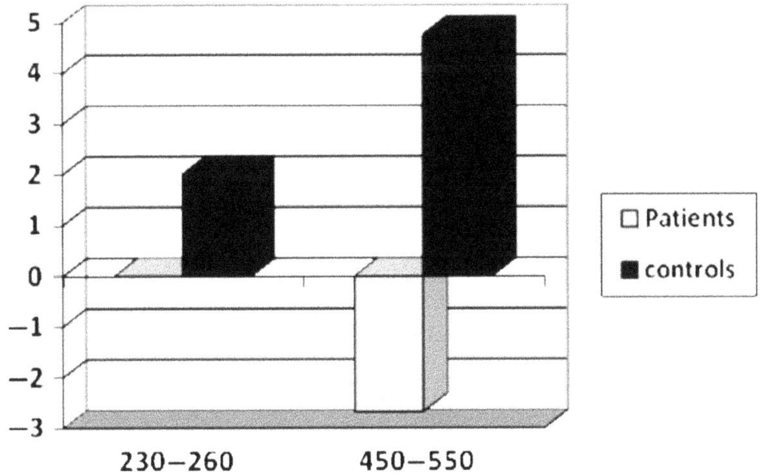

Figure 5. Mean amplitude (μV) over frontal electrodes for early (230–260 ms) and late (450–550 ms) epochs.

and sustained negativity in patients (Figure 5). These two components proved to be functionally distinct when examined against the patients' behavioural patterns. The early component was highly and negatively correlated with reaction times (Figure 6). Patients with more positive waveforms which are closer to the positive modulation observed in controls were faster on their correct memory decisions. This pattern of correlations is compatible with the idea that this positive component is associated with an immediate sense of correctness which allows for faster reaction times. The late component did not correlate with reaction times at all. By contrast, only the late component was highly and positively correlated with accuracy, such that patients with more positive waveforms which are more similar to controls' were more accurate on their responses. This pattern is compatible with the idea that the later component reflects a process that supports memory decisions and may help reduce the number of errors made during memory retrieval (Figure 6).

To conclude, there is some evidence to suggest that even when search demands are minimised, confabulators still make qualitatively different errors than healthy or patient controls, supporting the idea that a monitoring deficit is crucial and unique to confabulation. Confabulators' undifferentiated sense of confidence even for details which are highly implausible, lends some support to the hypothesis that a deficit in FOR is part of the mechanism leading to confabulation. The electrophysiological data further elucidate the nature of this mechanism, reflecting a missing early positive deflection that is associated with rapid correct endorsement or rejection of items. By contrast, later anterior differences between patients and controls appear to be associated with more elaborate accuracy-focused processing.

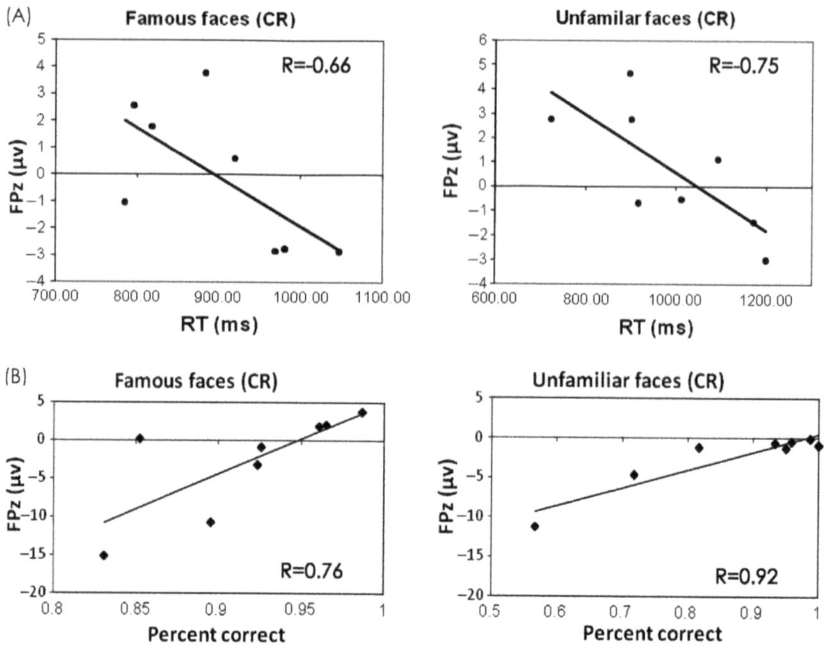

Figure 6. Correlations between RT and mean amplitude at 230–260 ms poststimulus onset (A) and correlations between accuracy and mean amplitude at 450–550 ms poststimulus onset (B).

Control processes in confabulation: The effect of free report

The third core deficit that produces confabulation by the proposed model is a deficit in control mechanism. That is, even if both monitoring mechanisms fail, patients might still refrain from reporting on their memories, depending on factors such as extent of awareness of deficit, personality factors and the interplay of environmental reinforcements available for erroneous vs. correct responses (e.g., social tolerance). We have used the QAP framework described earlier to examine the performance of a single confabulating patient. HB was a right-handed 54-year-old female at the time of testing with 16 years of education. Seventeen years earlier she had two surgeries for the removal of a suprasellar meningioma (1989/1990). She had been symptom free until May of 2005 when she again suffered from blurred vision, headaches, and went through a third surgery and a 1-month course of radiotherapy until October of 2005, about a year before we saw her. She suffered visual loss in her left eye, loss of sense of smell and taste, weight loss, frequent disorientation particularly in the morning, severe memory impairment, and confabulation. At the time of the present investigation, her husband reported that her confabulation was beginning to resolve, that she was more cautious and tended to ask whether she was making things up. In fact this question was raised many times during testing reflecting a heightened awareness of her memory problem and tendency to confabulate. Still, her husband reported confabulation occurred regularly several times a week. An MRI from August 2005 revealed extensive damage to the medial and ventromedial PFC, orbitofrontal cortex and basal forebrain and hypothalamus, as well as residual tumour (Figure 7).

The experimental task consisted of the presentation of 36 moderately related paired associates (e.g., Arrow-Apple; Error-Test). To allow for comparison of monitoring and control functions relatively independently of HB's primary memory impairment, she was presented with the encoding list twice. There were two test phases: forced and free report. During the forced report phase, participants saw the first word of each pair and the first letter of the second word as cues. They were asked to write down all of the candidate answers that came to mind and circle the one they think was the target word; they were further required to note their level of confidence in their answer, expressed as percentage probability that the answer is correct. During the second phase participants were asked to decide whether they wanted to report their candidate answer. They could win a point for every correctly reported answer and lose a point for every erroneously reported answer. They neither lost nor won points for answers they chose to withhold. This procedure allows the generation of multiple measures of memory production, memory monitoring and memory control (Koriat & Goldsmith, 1994, 1996; Koriat et al., 2000).

Memory production. As can be seen in Figure 8, HB produced an overall lower percentage of correct responses, suggesting less information was available to her than to controls, despite the fact she was exposed to the stimuli twice. Her production accuracy, on the other hand was the same as that of the controls (47% vs. 52%), which reflects a comparable level of

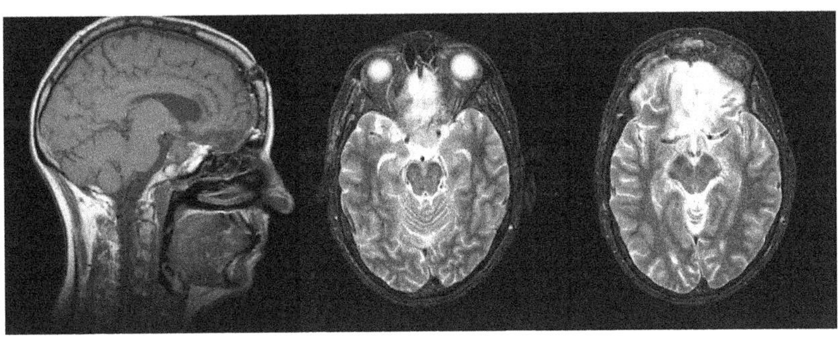

Figure 7. T1 and T2 MRIs of patient HB.

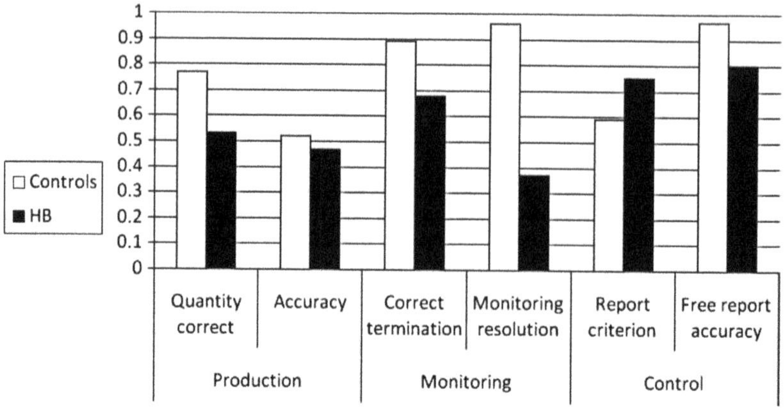

Figure 8. Primary measures of production, monitoring, and control process for HB and controls.

retrieval process accuracy, providing postretrieval processes with a similar level of challenge for filtering out wrong candidates.

Memory monitoring. Despite similar baseline of production accuracy, HB's memory QAP revealed differences both at the monitoring and at the control levels. One measure which reflects the effectiveness (and immediacy) of monitoring examines the percentage of cases in which the target item was the last item produced out of the total items in which the target item was in fact produced. In other words, this measure reflects whether the production of a target item immediately led to the termination of the search process. As can be seen in Figure 8, in about a third of the cases that HB produced the correct item, she continued to produce candidate answers suggesting she had little intuition about the correct answer. Even more apparent is HB's poor monitoring resolution reflected as the gamma correlation between the subject's assessed probability that an item is correct and the actual correctness of each best-candidate answer. Thus, whereas controls are very good at assessing the probable correctness of their answers, HB's assessment is as good as a guess despite the fact that she produced the same percentage of correct responses out of her overall production quantity. Interestingly, for HB this poor correlation reflected in fact an underconfidence in her responses, as she tended to give lower estimates of correctness (–0.23) than her actual production accuracy.

Memory control. HB's underconfidence was reflected in her control measures, which led her to adapt a rather strict report criterion (.75), meaning that on average she reported only items to which she estimated had a probability of 75% or more to be true. The corresponding criterion of controls was .56. Despite her conservatism, her free report accuracy was lower than that of controls; whereas controls' report accuracy is at ceiling, 20% of the items HB chose to report were errors. One may assume that had she been less conservative, her report accuracy would have been lower.

Thus, the most striking features of HB's QAP include very poor monitoring resolution coupled with poor report accuracy despite obvious attempts to avoid erroneous answers by adapting a conservative response criterion. This profile fits well with the clinical description of HB's growing awareness of her tendency to confabulate reflected by her constant worry that she is producing erroneous memories.

To conclude, the QAP may provide a useful instrument for quantifying monitoring and control processes in confabulation and tracking the dynamics of these processes as confabulation subsides. HB's profile may indicate that while confabulators still lack their ability to monitor the veracity of their memories, their strategic control over the memories they report may improve and lead to fewer manifestations of memory failures despite their damaged monitoring mechanisms.

NONBIZARRE DELUSIONS, CONFABULATIONS, AND MEMORY PROCESSES

Several authors (Berrios, 1998, 2000; Kopelman, 1999; Kopelman, Guinan, & Lewis, 1995; Metcalf et al., 2007; Turner et al., 2006) have noted that there are obvious resemblances between confabulation and delusions. Most prominently, both delusions and confabulations involve the production of unintentional false statements, both are resistant to contradictory evidence, and both have been shown to be influenced by motivational biases. These observed similarities have led some to propose the two disorders should be treated within the same theoretical framework, whereas others were motivated to try and better dissociate them.

Kopelman and colleagues distinguish between delusional memories and delusions in their model of the mechanisms underlying confabulatory memory disorders (Kopelman, 1999; Kopelman et al., 1995). Delusional memories, which are memories interpreted in a deluded way, or false memories that arise in the context of a psychosis share the same mechanisms with confabulation in this model, although the exact details of their evolution differ. Delusions on the other hand constitute a separate entity by Kopelman's view. The basis for the distinction is the notion discussed earlier which considers confabulation as inherently a neurological memory disorder whereas delusions are psychiatric disorders of belief formation.

By contrast, Barrios (1998, 2000) argues that since confabulations are considered by many as a form of propositional attitude (or belief) it is difficult to distinguish them from delusions. Consequently, confabulations should be considered as sharing the same conceptual space with delusions and other disorders of belief. Specifically, Barrios suggests that a more flexible concept of delusion should be employed such that confabulations can be incorporated as a subset of delusions.

Others have suggested delusions and confabulations share certain mechanisms and have proposed models designed to account for the formation of both delusions and confabulations (Langdon & Bayne, 2010 this issue; Langdon & Coltheart, 2000; Metcalf et al., 2007; Turner & Coltheart, 2010 this issue). These authors have adapted a model of delusional belief formation as a common framework to account for both delusions and confabulations. They broadly distinguish between processes that may lead to the formation of an implausible thought, and those that when disrupted lead to the acceptance of these ideas as true. The specific mechanisms that lead to confabulation by this account are very similar to those proposed by models of confabulation that emphasise its mnemonic nature (Burgess & Shallice, 1996; Conway, 2001; Conway & Fthenaki, 2000; Conway & Pleydell-Pearce, 2000; Gilboa & Moscovitch, 2002; Kopelman, 1999; Moscovitch, 1995a). Metcalf and her colleagues view their model as an overarching framework, rather than an alternative model, which is based on the links between confabulation and delusions. A similar approach was advanced by Gilleen and David (2005). These authors suggest that linking disorders of beliefs to related cognitive deficits and in particular memory disorders such as false recognition and delusions can provide an indirect link to the neurocognitive mechanisms that may underlie psychopathology.

Of course the arguments made by Berrios are very different from the ones made by Metcalf and her colleagues and by Gilleen and David. Whereas the former argues that the disorders cannot be formally distinguished, the latter are more cautious and suggest that the observed correspondences between them could serve to draw conclusion regarding common cognitive and neurocognitive mechanisms that underlie these disorders.

An important methodological and theoretical conclusion drawn by Berrios (2000) is that speculations based on clinical observations with regard to the neurocognitive mechanisms that underlie confabulations and delusions are unlikely to serve as a good heuristic to understanding the significance of these disorders. Instead, Berrios recommends an empirical experimental approach which will describe not only the occurrence of erroneous propositions in either clinical population but also in the general public.

There are very few empirical studies of confabulation in patients with delusions. A landmark study by Nathaniel-James and colleagues (Nathaniel-James, Foong, & Frith, 1996; Nathaniel-James & Frith, 1996) described what they call "a new form of confabulation" in schizophrenia. They required their patients to recall a story and identify the correct moral from it. They found a significant increase in intrusion errors and an association between error rate and performance on the Hayling test, which is an executive "frontal" test of response inhibition. Other executive test scores did not correlate with intrusion errors ("confabulation"). Nathaniel-James and colleagues argued based on their findings that schizophrenics' confabulations were qualitatively different from those of neurological patients. Schizophrenics tended to introduce irrelevant or unrelated information, thus according to these authors faults occur both at input due to disorganised encoding and at output when this disorganisation is compounded by a faulty editing process. They concluded that confabulation in schizophrenia is related to an inability to monitor and suppress inappropriate responses, and to a lesser extent to formal thought disorder. Kopelman (1999) notes, however, that the schizophrenics' intrusions might simply reflect their impaired anterograde memory compared with controls, or their preoccupying delusional beliefs. Kopelman concludes that confabulations in schizophrenia may be simply momentary intrusion errors and distortions, resulting from a faulty memory and coloured by the preoccupying delusional beliefs of these patients.

Kopelman's hypothesis was supported in later studies which again reported elevated levels of "confabulations" or intrusions in story and fable learning tests, which were the result of encoding and comprehension difficulties, whereas memory monitoring appeared to be intact (Dab et al., 2004). Furthermore, confabulatory responses during story recall are strongly associated with thought disorder symptoms in schizophrenia and are related to semantic memory impairment rather than to either episodic memory or executive functions (Lorente-Rovira, Pomarol-Clotet, McCarthy, Berrios, & McKenna, 2007). To conclude, confabulation-like phenomena in schizophrenia do not appear to be related to the mechanisms of delusions, nor are they associated with the neuropsychological profile that characterises patients with neurological confabulation.

Although it appears that memory distortions or "confabulations" are related more to the negative symptomatology than to delusions in psychosis, some evidence does link delusions and memory distortions. The incorporation of additional information during encoding is affected by the existence of a relationship between the encoded information and the content of delusions (Simpson & Done, 2002). These authors suggest this relationship reflects the existence of overused delusion-related schemas that affects the way information is encoded and incorporated into the memory system. In what follows, I will present some preliminary evidence collected from patients with confabulation, patients with delusions and healthy controls on two tasks which have been shown to be sensitive to confabulation, as well as delusional patients' profile on the QAP. If these tasks capture essential features of the underlying mechanisms of confabulations, and if delusions share essential or core features of the neurocognitive deficits that characterise confabulation, a deficit should be observed in delusional patients' performance on these tasks. Additionally, I will present some data that pertain to the hypothesis that if there is a memory component to delusions, it should be reflected more during the encoding stages than during retrieval and be affected by the activation of the delusional schema.

DO DELUSIONAL PATIENTS FAIL ON TASKS KNOWN TO BE SENSITIVE TO CONFABULATION?

One of the best studied tasks in confabulation is Armin Schnider's (Schnider, 2003; Schnider & Ptak, 1999; Schnider et al., 2002; Schnider et al., 1996) continuous recognition task. On this task participants view a series of stimuli, a subset of which is repeated several times. Participants are required to indicate for each stimulus whether it is new or whether it has already been presented within that run. One hour later, participants are again presented with the continuous recognition task, using the same set of stimuli but with different targets. The instructions emphasise that only repetition of stimuli within the current run should be reported as old, whereas all other stimuli should be responded to as new. A measure of the increase in the proportion of false alarms to hits on the second compared with the first run is calculated and patients with behaviourally spontaneous confabulation score higher on this measure than amnesic controls and healthy subjects. However, nonconfabulating patients with lesions to the VMPFC may also show increased scores on this measure (Gilboa, Alain, et al., 2006), which suggests it is sensitive to confabulation, but may not be specific to the syndrome, but rather be associated with VMPFC lesions in general (but see Schnider, 2008, for a critique of our findings).

We tested two patients with a diagnosis of Delusional Disorder on Schnider's continuous recognition task. As can be seen in Figure 9, patients with delusions had lower TCC scores than confabulating patients, and comparable to those presented by healthy controls. One of the delusional patients had a TCC score that bordered the cutoff score of 0.3 observed by Schnider and colleagues as an indication of high TCC and confabulation. The other was well below that cutoff.

We further examined the performance of these two patients on a task that more specifically examines retrieval processes using semantic narratives learned long ago (fairy tales and biblical stories). In our previous study we demonstrated that whereas confabulators did have an overall higher percentage of errors in their recounts of these semantic narratives, what

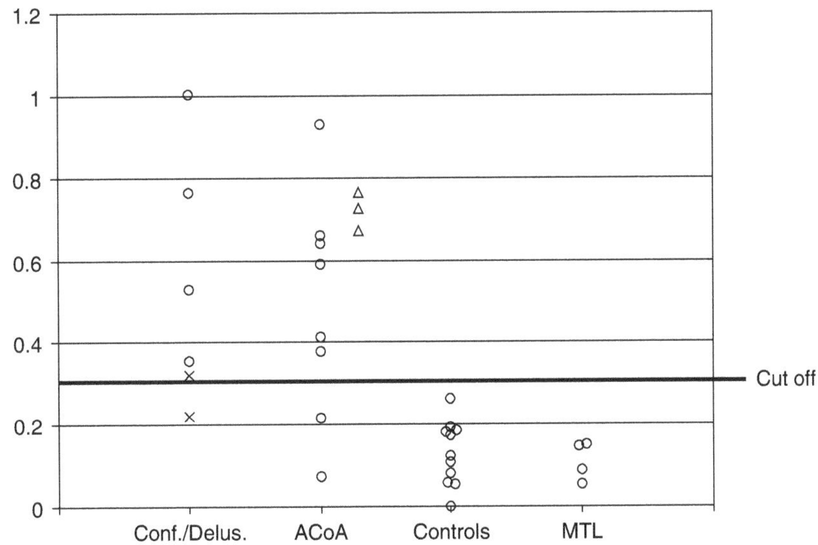

Figure 9. Temporal context confusion (TCC) scores on Schnider's task. Conf. =confabulators; ACoA =anterior communicating artery aneurysm patient controls; MTL =medial temporal lobe amnesic controls. Delusional patients are denoted by X. Three ACoA controls who were tested twice to verify their high TCC scores are denoted by triangles.

distinguished their performance from that of controls and of nonconfabulating patients was the type of errors they made. Although all participants committed errors of detail distortion, only confabulating patients had introjections of details from external sources such as other fairy tales or bible stories, and only confabulating patients had introjections of external idiosyncratic details that could not be traced to any known source. We gave the same test to the two patients with delusional disorder. As can be seen in Figure 10, their performance was equivalent to that of controls and of nonconfabulating patients in terms of overall percentage of erroneous details. Importantly, unlike confabulating patients, they did not produce a single introjections error either from other semantic narratives or from idiosyncratic sources.

Finally, patients were also tested on the verbal paired associate paradigm described eaerlier using the QAP procedure. Unlike the confabulating patient, delusional patients did not require an additional exposure to the word pairs during encoding as their performance was equivalent to that of controls following a single exposure. As can be seen in Figure 11, their performance profile differed considerably from that of patient HB. Most notably, whereas patient HB's monitoring measures were considerably lower than those displayed by controls, both delusional patients appeared to be

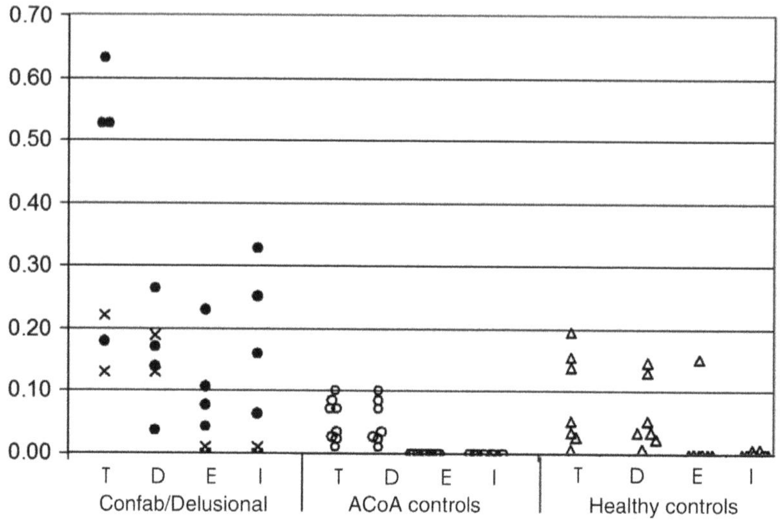

Figure 10. Error rates on free recall of semantic narratives. T = total; D = distortions of details; E = external introjections; I = idiosyncratic. Delusional patients are marked with an X.

able to terminate their search process appropriately and had intact monitoring resolution, i.e., their assessment of the probability that a particular response was true corresponded well to the actual correctness of their answers. By contrast, their control measures reflected very liberal response criteria and low report accuracy. Their production profile was not different from that of controls.

It is important to note that there is a complex relationship between monitoring effectiveness and report criterion setting. When monitoring is

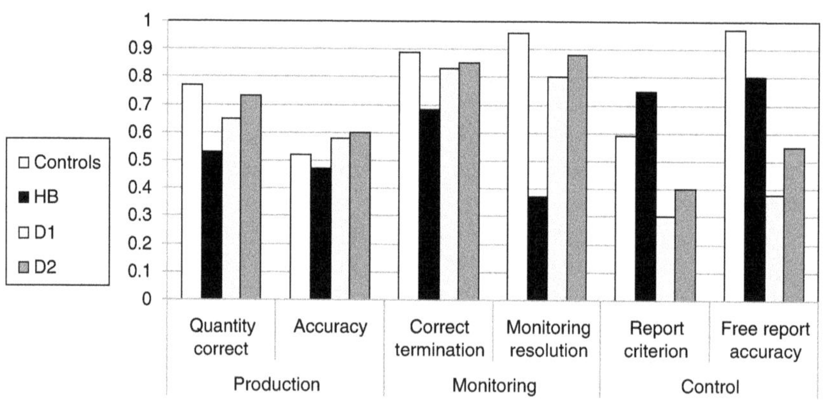

Figure 11. QAP profile for the paired associate task for controls, patient HB, and two delusional patients.

effective and a person's subjective assessment of the veracity of their answers is highly correlated with the actual probability that the answer is correct—using a conservative report criterion would result in increasing accuracy and decreasing quantity. However, when subjective probability assessments are inaccurate, conservative report criteria only result in lower quantity with little effect on quality. Thus, in confabulation where monitoring is faulty the effects of criterion setting on accuracy is reduced and primarily quantity is affected.

To conclude, the examination of the delusional patients' performance on tasks that are known to be sensitive to confabulation has yielded an overall profile that is very different from that presented by confabulators. These patients were intact on measures of neurocognitive functions that according to the strategic retrieval model of confabulation are necessary for confabulation to occur. These included both core processes (monitoring) and constitutional processes (TCC). By contrast, delusional patients did present a significant control deficit on the QAP task. Even within the control measures, however, the delusional patients differ from the confabulating patient. HB has lower control accuracy than controls (who are at ceiling for this measure); however, her report criterion in very conservative and that improves her output bound performance given her poor monitoring. By contrast, the delusional patients' poor control accuracy appears in the context of good monitoring ability but a liberal response criterion, which is typical of risk takers.

Do patients with delusions show a specific deficit in encoding rather than retrieval?

The strategic retrieval approach considers confabulation primarily a disorder of retrieval, because confabulations are just as likely to involve memories encoded long before the neurological insult occurred. That said faulty encoding can certainly play a role in the evolution of confabulation (Attali, de Anna, Dubois, & Dalla Barba, 2009) through constitutional processes and associated features. By contrast, as described previously, it has been suggested that memory processing in delusion might be affected more at the encoding stage due to the convergence of abnormal perception and encoding of information, associated with aberrant cognitive schema structure and disordered belief monitoring.

To assess this possibility we developed a task that takes advantage of the "Boundary Extension" phenomenon (Candel, Merckelbach, & Zandbergen, 2003; Intraub & Bodamer, 1993). Boundary extension describes a phenomenon in which when participants are asked to reproduce from memory a picture of an object as accurately as possible within a given boundary, they tend to draw it smaller than presented. Anecdotal reports suggest that the additional background space is sometimes completed with objects not present in the original picture even in normal controls. We hypothesised that patients with delusions would tend to have more such distortions, particularly if their aberrant cognitive schemata are activated prior to exposure, leading them to biased encoding of the picture. We further hypothesised that biasing at retrieval would have less of an effect on performance.

The study included seven male schizophrenic patients with paranoid delusions with a mean age of 40.71 ($SD = 11.07$) and an average education of 12.43 ($SD = 3.6$) as well as seven matched controls. Participants viewed 12 neutral pictures selected from the International Affective Picture System (IAPS), for 1 s each. There were two conditions: an encoding manipulation condition and a retrieval manipulation condition. On both conditions participants were told they would briefly see pictures and later be asked to reproduce them as accurately as possible with no regard to artistic ability. For the reproduction they were presented with a framed page the same size of the pictures they saw. They were told the size of the frame was the same as the picture they and asked to reproduce as accurately as possible the picture they saw within that frame.

For the encoding manipulation, three of the pictures were preceded with a sentence designed to activate delusion-related cognitive schemata (e.g., "the next picture is of an undercover agent"), whereas the other three were neutral (e.g., "the next picture is of an architect"). At retrieval participants were simply asked to draw the pictures. The retrieval manipulation was identical, except the sentences were "now draw the picture of ... that you saw before". As can be seen in Figure 12, there were overall more intrusion errors in reproduction following the encoding manipulation than following the retrieval manipulation, with no difference between the groups on the neutral sentences. However, during the biased questions, patients with delusions produced significantly more errors than controls and more errors than on neutral sentences. It is important to note that there was no difference between the groups on an overall memory score for the pictures.

These data provide preliminary evidence that distortions of memory in delusional patients ("confabulation"-like phenomena) seem to originate from the encoding or construction phase (Schacter et al., 1998) of memory rather than the retrieval or reconstruction phase. The model of confabulation espoused here would predict that if delusions and confabulations had shared core mechanisms, more distortions would occur at the retrieval or reconstruction stage, particularly when delusion-related schemata are activated. In fact one may surmise that if delusions lead to the distorted construction of memory representations, then confabulation-like phenomena are difficult to interpret in terms of faulty postretrieval mechanisms. The internal representations of previous occurrences are already formed within

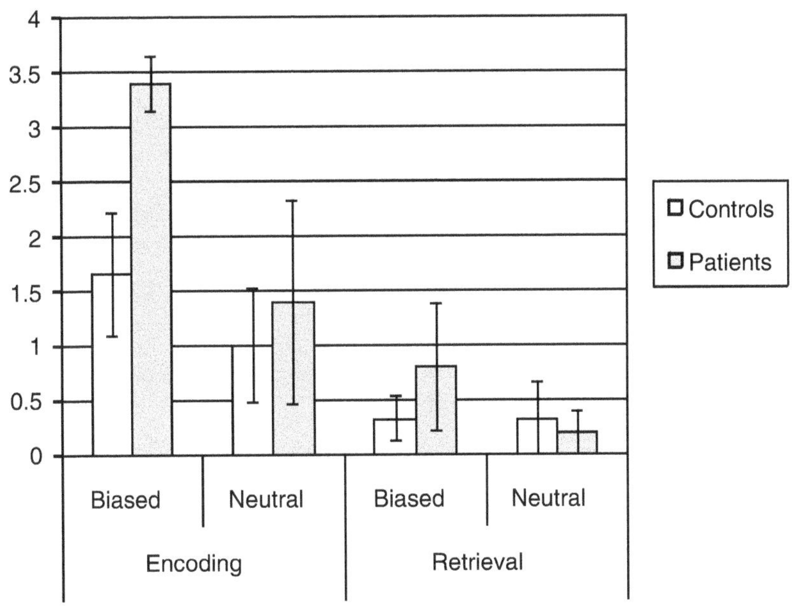

Figure 12. Mean number of errors on the boundary extension task.

the schema structure of the delusion and so postretrieval monitoring processes are hardly expected to detect inconsistencies and distortions during their reconstruction. Moreover, new information encountered that could serve to dispute the erroneous notions would also be encoded within the schema structure of the delusion. Indeed, one important difference between delusions and confabulations noted by Kopelman (1999) is that the former tend to be more systematised and all-embracing, so that information that appears odd for the outsider might fit will within the delusion schema and not require any editing.

To conclude, unlike confabulating patients, patients with delusions are not characterised by a significant memory disorder. Although some mild memory impairments can be detected, it is the result of faulty encoding, rather than retrieval and is specifically associated with the content of their delusion (Simpson & Done, 2002). These faulty encoding processes are likely influenced by perceptual and inferential biases associated with the delusion itself (Blackwood, Howard, Bentall, & Murray, 2001; Gilleen & David, 2005). Other constitutional deficits associated with confabulation, namely context confusion, also does not appear to characterise their behaviour. Of the core deficits required for confabulation to occur by our model we found no evidence that delusional patients have a monitoring deficit, although a memory control deficit was detected. The control deficit, however, was different from that seen in the confabulating patient and was characterised more by a liberal response criterion.

The obvious similarities noted above between confabulation and delusions do not seem to arise from the necessary components that lead to confabulation. One might hypothesise that the similarity is the result of common mechanisms that belong to the associated features of confabulation. Obvious candidates are wishful ideation, the use of default schemata and overdependence on environmental cues (coupled with misinterpretation of these cues in the case of delusions). These are of course hypotheses that can be empirically examined within the framework of the strategic retrieval model. It is the specificity of the framework and the emphasis on the memory domain that allows for better characterisation of differences as well as similarities between the disorders.

CONCLUSION

The present paper suggests that confabulation is best described as a confluence of deficits within the memory domain. These are divided into impairments in core processes (FOR, "editor", and control processes), whose cooccurrence is unique to confabulation and required for its evolution, impaired constitutional processes which may be required for confabulation to occur but are not unique to it, and associated features which determine the content "flavour" and frequency of confabulation but are not required for their evolution. It is argued that considering confabulation within a strategic memory framework may help elucidate both the commonalities and differences between confabulation and other symptoms such as delusions. Preliminary empirical data inspired by the model suggest that delusions share some of the associated features of confabulation, which leads to the apparent clinical overlap between them. However, the mnemonic mechanisms that contribute to the two phenomena appear to differ significantly: Whereas confabulation is primarily a disorder of retrieval, mnemonic aspects of delusions include primarily disordered input and integration of information. This is in line with models of delusions which consider them a convergence of abnormal perception and encoding of information, associated with aberrant cognitive schema structure and disordered belief monitoring.

REFERENCES

Attali, E., de Anna, F., Dubois, B., & Dalla Barba, G. (2009). Confabulation in Alzheimer's disease: Poor encoding and retrieval of over-learned information. *Brain, 113*(1), 204–214.

Barbas, H. (1995). Anatomic basis of cognitive-emotional interactions in the primate prefrontal cortex. *Neuroscience and Biobehavioral Reviews, 19*(3), 499–510.

Bechara, A., Damasio, H., Tranel, D., & Damasio, A. R. (1997). Deciding advantageously before knowing the advantageous strategy. [See comments]. *Science, 275*(5304), 1293–1295.
Bechara, A., Tranel, D., & Damasio, H. (2000). Characterization of the decision-making deficit of patients with ventromedial prefrontal cortex lesions. *Brain, 123*(11), 2189–2202.
Berrios, G. E. (1998). Confabulations: A conceptual history. *Journal of the History of the Neurosciences, 7*(3), 225–241.
Berrios, G. E. (2000). Confabulation. In G. E. Berrios & J. R. Hodges (Eds.), *Memory disorders in psychiatric practice* (pp. 348–368). Cambridge, UK: Cambridge University Press.
Blackwood, N. J., Howard, R. J., Bentall, R. P., & Murray, R. M. (2001). Cognitive neuropsychiatric models of persecutory delusions. *American Journal of Psychiatry, 158*(4), 527–539.
Brewer, W. F. (1986). What is autobiographical memory? In D. C. Rubin (Ed.), *Autobiographical memory* (pp. 25–49). New York: Cambridge University Press.
Burgess, P. W., & McNeil, J. E. (1999). Content-specific confabulation. *Cortex, 35*(2), 163–182.
Burgess, P. W., & Shallice, T. (1996). Confabulation and the control of recollection. *Memory, 4*(4), 359–411.
Burt, C. D. B., Kemp, S., & Conway, M. (2001). What happens if you retest autobiographical memory 10 years on? *Memory and Cognition, 29*(1), 127–136.
Candel, I., Merckelbach, H., & Zandbergen, M. (2003). Boundary distortions for neutral and emotional pictures. *Psychonomic Bulletin and Review, 10*(3), 691–695.
Ciaramelli, E., & Ghetti, S. (2007). What are confabulators' memories made of? A study of subjective and objective measures of recollection in confabulation. *Neuropsychologia, 45*(7), 1489–1500.
Conway, M. A. (2001). Sensory-perceptual episodic memory and its context: Autobiographical memory. *Philosophical Transactions of the Royal Society of London, Series B: Biological Sciences, 356*(1413), 1375–1384.
Conway, M. A., & Fthenaki, A. (2000). Disruption and loss of autobiographical memory. In L. S. Cermak (Ed.), *Memory and its disorders* (2nd ed., Vol. 2, pp. 281–313). Amsterdam: Elsevier.
Conway, M. A., & Pleydell-Pearce, C. W. (2000). The construction of autobiographical memories in the self-memory system. *Psychological Review, 107*(2), 261–288.
Conway, M. A., & Tacchi, P. C. (1996). Motivated confabulation. *Neurocase, 2*, 325–338.
Dab, S., Claes, T., Morais, J., & Shallice, T. (1999). Confabulation with a selective descriptor process impairment. *Cognitive Neuropsychology, 16*(3–5), 215–242.
Dab, S., Morais, J., & Frith, C. (2004). Comprehension, encoding, and monitoring in the production of confabulation in memory: A study with schizophrenic patients. *Cognitive Neuropsychiatry, 9*(3), 153–182.
Dalla Barba, G. (1993). Different patterns of confabulation. *Cortex, 29*(4), 567–581.
Dalla Barba, G., & Decaix, C. (2009). "Do you remember what you did on March 13, 1985?" A case study of confabulatory hypermnesia. *Cortex, 45*(5), 566–574.
Damasio, A. R., Graff-Radford, N. R., Eslinger, P. J., Damasio, H., & Kassell, N. (1985). Amnesia following basal forebrain lesions. *Archives of Neurology, 42*(3), 263–271.
DeLuca, J. (1993). Predicting neurobehavioral patterns following anterior communicating artery aneurysm. *Cortex, 29*(4), 639–647.
DeLuca, J. (2000). A cognitive neuroscience perspective on confabulation. *Neuro-Psychoanalysis, 2*, 119–132.
DeLuca, J., & Diamond, B. J. (1995). Aneurysm of the anterior communicating artery: A review of neuroanatomical and neuropsychological sequelae. *Journal of Clinical and Experimental Neuropsychology, 17*, 100–121.
Feinstein, A., Levine, B., & Protzner, A. (2000). Confabulation and multiple sclerosis: A rare association. *Multiple Sclerosis, 6*(3), 186–191.
Fischer, R. S., Alexander, M. P., D'Esposito, M., & Otto, R. (1995). Neuropsychological and neuroanatomical correlates of confabulation. *Journal of Clinical and Experimental Neuropsychology, 17*(1), 20–28.

Fotopoulou, A., Conway, M., Griffiths, P., Birchall, D., & Tyrer, S. (2007). Self-enhancing confabulation: Revisiting the motivational hypothesis. *Neurocase, 13*(1), 6–15.

Fotopoulou, A., Conway, M. A., & Solms, M. (2007). Confabulation: Motivated reality monitoring. *Neuropsychologia, 45*(10), 2180–2190.

Fotopoulou, A., Conway, M. A., Solms, M., Tyrer, S., & Kopelman, M. (2008). Self-serving confabulation in prose recall. *Neuropsychologia, 46*(5), 1429–1441.

Fotopoulou, A., Conway, M. A., Tyrer, S., Birchall, D., Griffiths, P., & Solms, M. (2008). Is the content of confabulation positive? An experimental study. *Cortex, 44*(7), 764–772.

Fotopoulou, A., Solms, M., & Turnbull, O. (2004). Wishful reality distortions in confabulation: A case report. *Neuropsychologia, 42*(6), 727–744.

Gilboa, A. (2004). Autobiographical and episodic memory—one and the same? Evidence from prefrontal activation in neuroimaging studies. *Neuropsychologia, 42*(10), 1336–1349.

Gilboa, A., Alain, C., He, Y., Stuss, D. T., & Moscovitch, M. (2009). Ventromedial prefrontal cortex lesions produce early functional alterations during remote memory retrieval. *Journal of Neuroscience, 29*(15), 4883–4893.

Gilboa, A., Alain, C., Stuss, D. T., Melo, B., Miller, S., & Moscovitch, M. (2006). Mechanisms of spontaneous confabulations: A strategic retrieval account. *Brain, 129*(6), 1399–1414.

Gilboa, A., & Moscovitch, M. (2002). The cognitive neuroscience of confabulation: A review and a model. In A. D. Baddeley, M. D. Kopelman, & B. A. Wilson (Eds.), *Handbook of memory disorders* (2nd ed., pp. 315–342). London: Wiley.

Gilboa, A., Winocur, G., Rosenbaum, R. S., Poreh, A., Gao, F., Black, S. E., et al. (2006). Hippocampal contributions to recollection in retrograde and anterograde amnesia. *Hippocampus, 16*(11), 966–980.

Gilleen, J., & David, A. S. (2005). The cognitive neuropsychiatry of delusions: From psychopathology to neuropsychology and back again. *Psychological Medicine, 35*(1), 5–12.

Hirst, W., & Volpe, B. T. (1988). Memory strategies with brain damage. *Brain Cognition, 8*(3), 379–408.

Intraub, H., & Bodamer, J. L. (1993). Boundary extension: Fundamental aspect of pictorial representation or encoding artifact? *Journal of Experimental Psychology: Learning, Memory, and Cognition, 19*(6), 1387–1397.

Johnson, M. K., Hashtroudi, S., & Lindsay, D. S. (1993). Source monitoring. *Psychological Bulletin, 114*(1), 3–28.

Joseph, R. (1999). Frontal lobe psychopathology: Mania, depression, confabulation, catatonia, perseveration, obsessive compulsions, and schizophrenia. *Psychiatry, 62*(2), 138–172.

Kapur, N., & Coughlan, A. K. (1980). Confabulation and frontal lobe dysfunction. *Journal of Neurology, Neurosurgery & Psychiatry, 43*(5), 461–463.

Kopelman, M. D. (1987). Two types of confabulation. *Journal of Neurology, Neurosurgery and Psychiatry, 50*(11), 1482–1487.

Kopelman, M. D. (1999). Varieties of false memory. *Cognitive Neuropsychology, 16*, 197–214.

Kopelman, M. D., Guinan, E. M., & Lewis, P. D. (1995). Delusional memory, confabulation and frontal lobe dysfunction: A case study in De Clerambault's Syndrome. *Neurocase, 1*, 71–77.

Kopelman, M. D., Ng, N., & van den Brouke, O. (1997). Confabulation extending across episodic memory, personal and general semantic memory. *Cognitive Neuropsychology, 14*, 683–712.

Koriat, A., & Goldsmith, M. (1994). Memory in naturalistic and laboratory contexts: Distinguishing the accuracy-oriented and quantity-oriented approaches to memory assessment. *Journal of Experimental Psychology: General, 123*(3), 297–315.

Koriat, A., & Goldsmith, M. (1996). Monitoring and control processes in the strategic regulation of memory accuracy. *Psychological Review, 103*(3), 490–517.

Koriat, A., Goldsmith, M., & Pansky, A. (2000). Toward a psychology of memory accuracy. *Annual Review of Psychology, 51*, 481–537.

Langdon, R., & Bayne, T. J. (2010). Delusion and confabulation: Mistakes of perceiving, remembering and believing. *Cognitive Neuropsychiatry, 15*(1/2/3), 319–345.

Langdon, R., & Coltheart, M. (2000). Cognitive neuropsychology of delusions. *Mind and Language, 15*, 183–216.

Lepage, M., Ghaffar, O., Nyberg, L., & Tulving, E. (2000). Prefrontal cortex and episodic memory retrieval mode. *Proceedings of the National Academy of Sciencess, USA, 97*(1), 506–511.

Lorente-Rovira, E., Pomarol-Clotet, E., McCarthy, R. A., Berrios, G. E., & McKenna, P. J. (2007). Confabulation in schizophrenia and its relationship to clinical and neuropsychological features of the disorder. *Psychological Medecine, 37*(10), 1403–1412.

McAndrews, M. P., & Milner, B. (1991). The frontal cortex and memory for temporal order. *Neuropsychologia, 29*(9), 849–859.

Mercer, B., Wapner, W., Gardner, H., & Benson, D. F. (1977). A study of confabulation. *Archives of Neurology, 34*(7), 429–433.

Metcalf, K. (2005). *The origin and nature of confabulation*. Unpublished doctoral dissertation. Macquarie Centre for Cognitive Science, Macquarie University, Sydney, NSW, Australia.

Metcalf, K., Langdon, R., & Coltheart, M. (2007). Models of confabulation: A critical review and a new framework. *Cognitive Neuropsychology, 24*(1), 23–47.

Milner, B., Petrides, M., & Smith, M. L. (1985). Frontal lobes and the temporal organization of memory. *Human Neurobiology, 4*(3), 137–142.

Moscovitch, M. (1989). Confabulation and the frontal systems: Strategic versus associative retrieval in neuropsychological theories of memory. In H. L. Roediger & F. I. Craik (Eds.), *Varieties of memory and consciousness: Essays in honor of Endel Tulving* (pp. 133–160). Hillsdale, NJ: Lawrence Erlbaum Associates, Inc.

Moscovitch, M. (1992). Memory and working-with-memory: A component process model based on modules and central systems. *Journal of Cognitive Neuroscience, 4*, 257–267.

Moscovitch, M. (1995a). Confabulation. In D. Schacter (Ed.), *Memory distortion* (pp. 226–251). Cambridge, MA: Harvard University Press.

Moscovitch, M. (1995b). Recovered consciousness: A hypothesis concerning modularity and episodic memory. *Journal of Clinical Experimental Neuropsychology, 17*(2), 276–290.

Moscovitch, M., & Melo, B. (1997). Strategic retrieval and the frontal lobes: Evidence from confabulation and amnesia. *Neuropsychologia, 35*(7), 1017–1034.

Moscovitch, M., & Winocur, G. (1992). The neuropsychology of memory and aging. In F. I. M. Craik & T. A. Salthouse (Eds.), *The handbook of aging and cognition* (pp. 315–372). Hillsdale, NJ: Lawrence Erlbaum Associates, Inc.

Moscovitch, M., & Winocur, G. (2002). The frontal cortex and working with memory. In D. T. Stuss & R. Knight (Eds.), *Principles of frontal lobe function* (pp. 188–209). New York: Oxford University Press.

Nathaniel-James, D. A., Foong, J., & Frith, C. D. (1996). The mechanisms of confabulation in schizophrenia. *Neurocase, 2*(6), 475–483.

Nathaniel-James, D. A., & Frith, C. D. (1996). Confabulation in schizophrenia: Evidence of a new form? *Psychological Medicine, 26*(2), 391–399.

Nedjam, Z., Dalla Barba, G., & Pillon, B. (2000). Confabulation in a patient with fronto-temporal dementia and a patient with Alzheimer's disease. *Cortex, 36*(4), 561–577.

Papagno, C., & Baddeley, A. (1997). Confabulation in a dysexecutive patient: Implication for models of retrieval. *Cortex, 33*(4), 743–752.

Reid, T. (1969). *Essays on the intellectual powers of man. III: Concerning memory*. Cambridge, MA: MIT Press.

Rugg, M. D., & Wilding, E. L. (2000). Retrieval processing and episodic memory. *Trends in Cognitive Science, 4*(3), 108–115.

Schacter, D. L., Norman, K. A., & Koutstaal, W. (1998). The cognitive neuroscience of constructive memory. *Annual Review of Psychology, 49*, 289–318.

Schacter, D. L., & Slotnick, S. D. (2004). The cognitive neuroscience of memory distortion. *Neuron*, *44*(1), 149–160.

Schnider, A. (2003). Spontaneous confabulation and the adaptation of thought to ongoing reality. *Nature Reviews Neuroscience*, *4*(8), 662–671.

Schnider, A. (2008). *The confabulating mind: How the brain creates reality*. Oxford, UK: Oxford University Press.

Schnider, A., Bonvallat, J., Emond, H., & Leemann, B. (2005). Reality confusion in spontaneous confabulation. *Neurology*, *65*(7), 1117–1119.

Schnider, A., & Ptak, R. (1999). Spontaneous confabulators fail to suppress currently irrelevant memory traces. [See comment]. *Nature Neuroscience*, *2*(7), 677–681.

Schnider, A., Ptak, R., von Daniken, C., & Remonda, L. (2000). Recovery from spontaneous confabulations parallels recovery of temporal confusion in memory. *Neurology*, *55*(1), 74–83.

Schnider, A., Valenza, N., Morand, S., & Michel, C. M. (2002). Early cortical distinction between memories that pertain to ongoing reality and memories that don't. *Cerebral Cortex*, *12*(1), 54–61.

Schnider, A., von Daniken, C., & Gutbrod, K. (1996). The mechanisms of spontaneous and provoked confabulations. *Brain*, *119*(4), 1365–1375.

Shapiro, B. E., Alexander, M. P., Gardner, H., & Mercer, B. (1981). Mechanisms of confabulation. *Neurology*, *31*(9), 1070–1076.

Simpson, J., & Done, D. J. (2002). Elasticity and confabulation in schizophrenic delusions. *Psychological Medecine*, *32*(3), 451–458.

Tulving, E. (1983). *Elements of episodic memory*. Oxford, UK: Clarendon Press.

Turner, M. S., Cipolotti, L., Yousry, T. A., & Shallice, T. (2008). Confabulation: Damage to a specific inferior medial prefrontal system. *Cortex*, *44*(6), 637–648.

Turner, M. S., & Coltheart, M. (2010). Confabulations and delusion: A common monitoring framework? *Cognitive Neuropsychiatry*, *15*(1/2/3), 346–376.

Turner, M. S., Coltheart, M., Metcalf, K., & Langdon, R. (2006). *What is the relationship between confabulation and delusion?* Paper presented at the fourth international conference on Memory, July 16–21, Sydney, Australia.

Victor, M., & Yakovlev, P. I. (1955). S. S. Korsakoff's psychic disorder in conjunction with peripheral neuritis; a translation of Korsakoff's original article with comments on the author and his contribution to clinical medicine. *Neurology*, *5*(6), 394–406.

Zannino, G. D., Barban, F., Caltagirone, C., & Carlesimo, G. A. (2008). Do confabulators really try to remember when they confabulate? A case report. *Cognitive Neuropsychology*, *25*(6), 831–852.

COGNITIVE NEUROPSYCHIATRY
2010, 15 (1/2/3), 181–201

Beauty and belief: William James and the aesthetics of delusions in schizophrenia

Vaughan J. Carr

Centre for Brain and Mental Health Research, University of Newcastle, Callaghan, and Schizophrenia Research Institute, Darlinghurst, NSW, Australia

Introduction. This paper proposes the hypothesis that aesthetics plays an important role in the construction and maintenance of delusional ideas in schizophrenia.
Method. A selective review of the literature on the cognitive science of aesthetics, beginning with the work of William James on the stream of thought, was undertaken together with a review of some of the cognitive neuroscience literature on delusion formation in schizophrenia.
Results. It is suggested that delusion formation has some similarities to to the creative process, but commences with a proto-psychotic anomalous experience in which an aberrant Jamesian fringe experience is generated. The consequence of such deviation from standard or expected conscious experience is to direct processing resources in a search for meaning, but under conditions of reduced prefrontal cortex monitoring and control mechanisms. Lowering of the usual constraints exercised by prefrontal cortex regulatory mechanisms causes the search for explanation or interpretation to be characterised by low self-reflection, temporal distortion and low volitional control, permitting relatively unfiltered ideas that do not conform to convention to emerge in consciousness. The combination of aberrant Jamesian fringe experience and reduced prefrontal regulatory mechanisms evoke idiosyncratic contextual associations and drive a hypersensitive salience assignment system in the search for meaning, out of which process nascent delusional beliefs emerge. These are accompanied by a 'sense of rightness' in the Jamesian fringe which signals the presence of a 'good fit' between the proto-psychotic anomalous experience in the centre of consciousness and the contextual associations evoked.
Conclusion. The 'sense of rightness' or 'good fit' is responsible for the aesthetic qualities of the delusion and, it is proposed, accounts for the incorrigibility of the delusions.

Keywords: Schizophrenia; Delusions; Aesthetics; Fringe.

Correspondence should be addressed to Vaughan J. Carr, School of Psychiatry, University of New South Wales at St Vincent's Hospital, 299 Forbes Street, Darlinghurst, NSW 2010, Australia. E-mail: Vaughan.Carr@hnehealth.nsw.gov.au

 DOI: 10.1080/13546800802332145

How is it that a person can be convinced that a false, even absurd, proposition is true? In spite of manifest implausibility, illogicality, absence of evidence, and even evidence to the contrary, delusional beliefs are strikingly resilient, impervious to reason or contrary evidence. Karl Jaspers (1923/1962, p. 95) stated: "delusion implies a transformation in ... total awareness of reality". In trying to understand how such a transformation comes about we need to explain two sets of phenomena; first, the creation or construction of the belief and, second, its maintenance in the face of what is real—the real, according to Jaspers, being "what resists us ... in the practice of living".

> Whatever may inhibit our bodily movements or prevent the immediate realisation of our aims and wishes is a resistance. The achievement of a goal against resistance or defeat thereby brings with it an experience of reality: all experience of reality, therefore, has a root in the practice of living. But the reality itself which we meet in practice is always an *interpretations* [sic], a meaning, the meaning of things, events or situations. When I grasp the meaning, I grasp the reality. (Jaspers, 1923/1962, p. 94)

This paper puts forward the hypothesis that aesthetics plays a key role in the construction and, especially, the maintenance of those particular forms of meaning referred to as delusions. It begins with a discussion of a phenomenology of consciousness first articulated by William James in his famous chapter on the stream of thought, particularly as elaborated upon more recently by cognitive scientists such as Bruce Mangan and Russell Epstein. The development of delusions in schizophrenia will then be examined within that framework with reference to some of the contributions of modern cognitive neuroscience to our knowledge of schizophrenia.

First, some brief, preliminary comments about aesthetics need to be made. The philosopher Immanuel Kant regarded the thinking involved in the contemplation of the beautiful as not fundamentally different from ordinary everyday cognition. Kant proposed the concept of "purposiveness" (*zweckmassigkeit*) as central to judgements of beauty, "purposiveness"—or appropriateness, suitability—implying a special sense of order, unity, and the successful accomplishment of a purpose or satisfaction of an aim. Mangan (1991), in his thesis on psycho-aesthetics, interprets "purposiveness" as a conscious experience signalling that order has been discovered by nonconscious processes conveying not pleasure but a "special feeling" of necessity, coherence, and harmony that cannot be conveyed in concrete terms; that is, a sense of meaning (i.e., meaningfulness) without conceptual representation of precisely what is meant. Mangan also applied Kant's thinking to what he terms the "alpha cluster" of aesthetic experience. The latter comprises: *ineffability*—an unstatable, incommunicable, ungraspable quality; *unity*—the integration of parts into a coherent, interconnected, unified whole or a balanced, harmonious blending of parts; the *noetic*—a form of knowledge, understanding, or recognition; and the *transcendent*—surpassing ordinary human experience, profoundness, often implying a mystical, spiritual, metaphysical, or religious interpretation of reality.

WILLIAM JAMES AND THE PHENOMENOLOGY OF CONSCIOUSNESS

> So too, we are aware that thinking consists in ordering a variety of meanings so that they move to a conclusion that all support and in which all are summed up and conserved. (Dewey, 1934/2005, p. 178)

In *The Principles of Psychology*, William James (1918/1950) proposed that consciousness is dynamic, that is, never static but constantly moving from one thought, concept, idea, sensation, feeling or perception to another. He identified two components of consciousness, a "nucleus" and a "fringe". The nucleus comprises what we might now roughly call focal attention or centre of awareness, the contents of which James referred to as "substantive" experiences—thoughts, feelings, etc.—in contrast to the "transitive" experiences occurring within the fringe. The contents of the nucleus have a number of characteristics, as summarised by Epstein (2000). First is *stability*, that is, the capacity to be "held before the mind for an indefinite time". *Memorability* refers to the fact that one is more able to remember the contents of the nucleus than the fringe. *Multimodality* reflects the notion that the substantive experiences can occur in any one of a number of modes—sensations, thoughts, images, percepts, concepts, attitudes, and so on. In addition to these three qualities, Mangan (1993) has identified a further two. *Sequentiality* indicates that one can hold only one substantive thought or experience in mind at the one time and that such experiences proceed serially from one to the next. Finally, *limited capacity* means that only a small proportion of the total amount of information being processed by the brain can be present in one substantive experience. These last two qualities call to mind the cognitive science concepts of serial information processing systems, namely, capacity-limited processing of detail within the focus of attention.

The fringe, on the other hand, comprises the vague region of experience just outside the centre of attention, on the periphery of awareness, which James referred to as transitive thoughts. The fringe primarily serves two functions. It provides a sense of *context* within which the nucleus of conscious experience is embedded and which bridges the temporal gaps between substantive thoughts. The other important function of the fringe is *retrieval*, that is, it helps to mediate the "call" for (i.e., search and extraction of) new, detailed information into consciousness (Mangan, 1993). The fringe thus provides an unobtrusive *control system that monitors and evaluates* the flow of information into consciousness.

With regard to *context*, the fringe provides what James called "feelings of relation" for the content of the nucleus, a "halo or penumbra that surrounds and escorts it", consisting of an associative memory network that provides significance, meaning, value, "inward coloring", cognitive tang, or import (Mangan, 1993) for the substantive experiences at the nucleus or centre of consciousness. In addition to the feelings of relation, the sense of context has two other components, a faint memory of preceding thoughts, and a feeling of where one's thoughts are heading or "feelings of tendency" (Epstein, 2000). With regard to *retrieval*, the feelings of relation provide a vague sense of awareness of relationships between the current thought, for example, and others that might be relevant (Epstein, 2000), and have the effect of implying that information of various kinds is available at the periphery to be called into focal attention. The fringe thus provides a target at the periphery by which the information it implies can be accessed, a transitive device by which attention may be focused on a relevant aspect of the fringe to bring it into the centre of consciousness for detailed information processing (Mangan, 1993).

According to Mangan (2001), the fringe has a number of distinguishing features. First, fringe experiences are diaphanous or translucent; that is, they have no sensory content of their own. They are of low resolution, having a "fuzzy, slurred, cloud-like character" (Mangan, 2001) as opposed to the fine-grained detail that occurs in focal attention. They are elusive, slippery, and ungraspable, eluding direct introspection, and are verified only indirectly. Fourth, they are more evident in the periphery of experience than with focused attention. Last, they are unobtrusive and, although they may vary in intensity, with some exceptions (e.g., tip-of-the-tongue, feelings of knowing, feelings of familiarity—see later) they are generally less intense than sensory experiences. Similarities are evident between the nonsensory fringe and the concept of preattentive processing described by Neisser (1967) on the basis of experimental studies and subsequently elaborated by others, including work on what has been termed "inattentive" experience (Mangan, 1993).

Some of the nonsensory experiences attributable to the operations of the fringe (see Epstein, 2000) include the feeling of *expectation* that occurs when our attention is drawn to something and we have a sense of what it might be before it is actually revealed. Others include the *feeling of knowing* when, for example, one has a word on the tip of one's tongue but is unable to recall it, the feeling of *familiarity* in the presence of well-known and recognised people or surroundings, the particular sense of *connection* contributed by words such as "but", "and", or "nevertheless" to the logical structure of thinking or sentence construction, and the feeling of *intention* when one is about to say something and has in mind a scheme of thought before articulating it. Additional examples proposed include the sense of *agency* experienced when one has intentionally executed a particular action or generated a thought and feels that one has caused the action or thought to occur, and the feeling of *ownership or mineness* when one senses an experience as one's own, belonging to oneself and no other. A further important experience attributable to the fringe, and one that is of particular importance in relation to aesthetics, is the sense of "*rightness*" or the feelings of "right and wrong relation". This refers to the sense of being on the right (or wrong) track to a conclusion, that there is a sense of harmony (vs. discord), of a right (vs. wrong) direction in the thinking and a sense of fit (vs. nonfit) between context and conclusion (i.e., between fringe and nucleus, respectively). This has also been referred to as "meaningfulness", the feeling of "making sense", a signal of tight fit, coherence, or compatibility between the nucleus and its nonconscious context provided by the fringe (Mangan, 1991).

James (1918/1950, p. 259) writes of this experience as follows: "When the sense of furtherance is there, we are 'all right;' with the sense of hindrance we are dissatisfied and perplexed, and cast about us for other thoughts." Indeed, when the feeling of rightness is present, even gibberish will make sense (Mangan, 2001), such as speaking in tongues (Mangan, 1991), and when something makes sense, even if it is objectively wrong, not rational or even incoherent, the elements will seem to "hang together" and form an integrated whole (Mangan, 2001) owing to the feeling of rightness. This is what James refers to variously as "subjective feeling of rationality", "right direction", "feeling of rational sequence", and "dynamic meaning".

A NEUROCOGNITIVE MODEL OF JAMESIAN PHENOMENOLOGY

> Oppositions of mind and body, soul and matter, spirit and flesh all have their origin, fundamentally, in fear of what life may—bring forth. They are marks of contraction and withdrawal. (Dewey, 1934/2005, p. 23)

Epstein (2000) has proposed a neurocognitive basis for the Jamesian phenomenology of consciousness just described. With regard to the nucleus he proposes that the experience of awareness within the nucleus of consciousness is a global brain process that entails the binding together of information from several cortical regions by means of synchronous firing at an EEG frequency of 40 Hz. (Synchronous EEG firing in the gamma range has been widely identified as a neural correlate of consciousness, although this is now disputed.)

According to Epstein (2000), the fringe implies the existence of two neurocognitive components, an associative memory network and a mechanism that monitors and controls the activation of this network. He identifies the medial temporal lobes, particularly the hippocampus and adjacent cortices in the parahippocampal gyrus, as the site of instantiation of the associative memory network. He proposes that this network functions as a cognitive map that mediates internal navigation through declarative memory space, just as the same anatomical structures in the laboratory rodent brain enable the animal's navigation through physical space. The medial temporal lobe structures do not contain the memory networks as such, but provide the mechanism by which a route of possible associations may be partly instantiated by neuronal connections with other cortical regions (Epstein, 2004). He argues that this view complements and is compatible with Gray's (1995) theory of the comparator functions of the hippocampus in which essentially contextual information about current perceptions and current motor programmes is used to predict change in the world 100 ms into the future by means of an efference copy in which a copy of a motor command predicts respective sensory consequences. The prediction is then compared with what actually occurs on the basis of updated information inputs. If there is congruence, that is, a match occurs between what is predicted and the updated information, then the current motor programme continues, whereas incongruence or a mismatch (e.g., novelty) causes the current motor programme to abort and the organism to orient itself towards the source of the mismatch. It has been proposed that this mechanism may operate on internal as well as external stimuli (Epstein, 2004), detecting match or mismatch between the current content of consciousness and an association, or conflict between competing associations, and on this basis provide the means by which attention may be directed to one association while suppressing others. Such outputs of the hippocampal comparison process would be a means of determining the contents of consciousness (Gray, 1995) by directing the progress of the stream of thought.

But what determines which associations will be attended to and which suppressed, associations that are assigned salience versus those that are not? How is the direction of attention governed? Is there a mechanism for distinguishing between sequences of associations, or between action sequences that are happening and those that are only imagined, between those that are remembered and those that are fantasies? The mechanism for monitoring and controlling the activation of the associative network is identified by Epstein (2000, 2004) with the frontal lobes which, he proposes, monitor for narrative consistency, including autobiographical consistency, as well as consistency with current goals. The role of the frontal cortex is to monitor the association process and to select the appropriate associations for the current context (Epstein, 2004), thereby acting as the navigator that steers through the network of potential associations offered by the hippocampus.

In summary, therefore, we have a Jamesian stream of thought in the nucleus of consciousness involving perceptual, ideational or other representations in the cerebral cortex interacting with the fringe on the periphery of consciousness through an associative network instantiated by hippocampal and related structures, and frontal lobe mechanisms that monitor and control the association process (Epstein, 2004).

SCHIZOPHRENIA

> For the mad, the insane, thing to us is that which is torn from the common context and which stands alone and isolated, as anything must which occurs in a world totally different from ours. (Dewey, 1934/2005, p. 202)

Phenomenological evidence points towards an early phase of schizophrenia marked by some kind of *protopsychotic anomalous experience.* This appears to be an altered state of consciousness whereby anomalous experiences of the world and/or the self occur, a profound and alarming, though often ineffable, change in self-experience (Parnas & Sass, 2001). Such experiences have been described as: a pervasive inability to grasp the everyday significations of the world and a correlated perplexity; an unstable sense of the groundedness, fullness, or reality of the self with a correlated feeling of alienation from the world; an experience of meaning fragmentation; an experience of one's body predominantly as an object, a sense of being detached or disconnected from one's body; a loss of automaticity of being; an experience of mental contents becoming quasi-autonomous; and a reduced ability to discriminate self from nonself (Parnas & Sass, 2001). Paraphrasing a Gestalt-influenced view of schizophrenia, these phenomena might all be regarded as instances in which individual components of consciousness become loosened from their natural or usual context with consequent alteration in the integrity or organisational coherence of consciousness so that meaning or significance is decayed or lost altogether (Uhlhaas & Mishara, 2007). Thus, the phenomenology of the protopsychotic anomalous experience can be said to entail some form of disruption in the relationship between focal attention and context, that is, between nucleus and fringe.

In fact, dysfunction in an efference copy feedforward mechanism, such as that described in relation to the comparator model of hippocampal function in the preceding section, could account for the faulty contextual binding reported to be fundamental to the cognitive deficits found in schizophrenia, leading to memories accessed with poor contextual linkage and consequent disjunction between memory content recalled and its meaning (Boyer, Phillips, Rousseau, & Ilivitsky, 2007). The initial consequence of memory retrieval without proper context would be to render the retrieved content odd or strange (Boyer et al., 2007). Indeed, Gray, Feldon, Rawlins, Hemsley, and Smith (1991) have proposed that failure to integrate actual contextual information with stored information relevant to this context may help to explain the development of delusional beliefs and the appearance of behaviours in schizophrenia that are not appropriate to the prevailing environmental context. In a slightly different vein, Hemsley (1993, p. 635) has proposed that there is a hippocampus-related "weakening of the influences of stored memories of regularities of previous input on current perception", leading to ambiguous, unstructured sensory input.

Disturbance in the fringe function of sense of agency can be related to the same hippocampal comparator-contextual model. A dysfunctional efference copy mechanism has actually been proposed by others to account for disruption in the fringe experiences of sense of agency and sense of ownership (Synofzik, Vosgerau, & Newen, 2008; David, Newen, & Vogeley, 2008). In fact, "a misbalanced integration of ... particular background beliefs, contextual cues and action intentions" has been proposed to explain agency delusions (Synofzik et al., 2008). A reduced sense of subjective control over self-initiated thoughts or actions has been described in relation to schizophrenia by Frith (1992) as a defect in the central monitoring of one's own intentions based on degradation of the efferent-copy signal. This perspective is one in which deficient self-monitoring leads to a diminished sense of control over self-initiated behaviour and gives rise to emerging discrepancy between intentions and behaviours. Mental contents and behaviours then take on a quasi-autonomous quality and motor actions lose a sense of automaticity so that habitual behaviours require conscious attention and effort (Parnas & Sass, 2001).

In schizophrenia disruptions in more than one fringe experience may occur together or over time, in contrast to typical cases of monothematic delusions where disruption in a single fringe experience appears to occur in isolation (e.g., loss of a sense of familiarity for a well known face as in Capgras syndrome) and may involve a fairly specific mechanism. In schizophrenia, on the other hand, there can be a loss of the feeling of rightness (as in the pervasive inability to grasp the meaning or significance of situations, exemplified by delusional mood/atmosphere) and loss of the sense of agency (as in delusions of control). In addition, however, in schizophrenia there may also be loss of the sense of familiarity (as in the Capgras delusion encompassing an entire family and/or community or, less specifically, in delusional mood/atmosphere), of intention (as in some forms of thought disorder) and of ownership or mineness (as in thought insertion). In other words, just as protopsychotic experiences can be understood in terms of weakening of the influence of the contextual functions of the fringe on the nucleus, some of the classic symptoms of schizophrenia and related psychoses can also be understood as being based on abnormal fringe experiences, whereas in monothematic delusional states a more circumscribed abnormality in fringe experience may be occurring.

Although the protopsychotic experience of schizophrenia appears to involve disturbances in the Jamesian fringe experiences of *context*, it is not known whether these are reflections of primary abnormalities in medial temporal or frontal lobe functioning, or both. Whether either or both are secondary to, or independent of, a further abnormality in the neurocognitive underpinnings of the nucleus of consciousness, an abnormality perhaps caused by a deficit in the feedforward mechanisms that maintain integration of consciousness and which may depend on the integrity of synchronous gamma-band (30–80 Hz) oscillations in the EEG signal, is also not known.

The genesis of delusions can thus be understood in terms of fringe alterations that are inherent in the protopsychotic experience. For example, as intimated previously, disruption in the fringe contextual feeling of rightness would be prone to generate the clinical symptom of delusional atmosphere (Jaspers, 1923/1962, p. 98) in which the person feels that something odd is going on that cannot be explained, that familiar surroundings have become strange, as if altered in some undefinable way. Jaspers described this as "some change which envelops everything with a subtle, pervasive and strangely uncertain light ... a distrustful, uncomfortable uncanny tension invades the patient" (p. 98). Disruption in the fringe contextual sense of agency would be prone to generate so-called passivity phenomena in which the person experiences their own thoughts or actions as not being self-generated but "made" by other means. Here thoughts occur that the patient does not intend, as if "made" by an external agent, or actions such as walking, speaking, and gesturing occur without the patient intending them, or automaticity may be compromised. The thoughts or actions are recognised as one's own, but they are experienced as not intentionally generated. Disruption in the sense of ownership or mineness, on the other hand, would be prone to generate failure in recognising thoughts, feelings and perceptions as one's own or belonging to the self, but rather seeming to be "not-me", foreign or alien, as if interposed from an external source, as in thought insertion.

It is suggested that protopsychotic experiences give rise, with varying degrees of urgency, to a sense of uncertainty and puzzlement, with things taking on a strange, uncanny or mysterious quality that generates perplexity and discomfort. Such a profoundly unsettling problem or puzzle, involving a state of dissonance, that is, disjunction between the centre of awareness and context, between nucleus and fringe (or repeated mismatch between the expected and the obtained to recall the model of the hippocampal comparator) produces the "angst" or drive to seek a solution, to find meaning in, interpretation of, or explanation for the new state of the world and the self—or even the human condition if the experience is taken to have universal implications. Such a state of mind, teetering on the brink of frank psychosis, has parallels with what has been described as the beginning of the creative process (Dietrich, 2004).

PARALLELS BETWEEN THE CREATIVE PROCESS AND PSYCHOSIS

> Moreover, I do not think it can be denied that an element of reverie, of approach to a state of dream, enters into the creation of a work of art. (Dewey, 1934/2005, p. 287)

Two sets of operations, in varying combinations over time, are thought to be involved in creativity. The first entails a subtle defocusing of attention which, in the Jamesian framework, might be regarded as a relaxation or loosening of the boundaries of the nucleus and an opening up to fringe experiences, or in Dewey's terms a dreamlike state of reverie. In schizophrenia, rather than normative defocusing of attention, it is proposed instead that a protopsychotic anomalous experience occurs. In creativity, momentary defocused attention is accompanied by a partial surrender of the monitoring and control functions exercised by the frontal cortex. The prefrontal cortex in schizophrenia is well known to exhibit structural and functional abnormalities and the phenomenon of hypofrontality in this disorder has been repeatedly demonstrated using a variety of neuropsychological tests and functional brain imaging techniques. Defocused attention is thought to allow the emergence into working memory of hitherto nonconscious material retrieved from the associative memory network through the fringe. "Ideas are floating, not anchored to any existence as its property, its possession of meanings. Emotions that are equally loose and floating cling to these ideas" (Dewey, 1934/2005, p. 284). This is not unlike the "intrusion into consciousness of unintended material from memory" described in the context of schizophrenia by Hemsley (1993). Under conditions of defocused attention and reduced frontal monitoring and control functions, such material is said to be comparatively more random, unfiltered, and bizarre, and is marked by such features as absent self-reflection, temporal distortions, lowered volitional control, concrete thinking, and less conformity to internalised values or belief systems (Dietrich, 2004). Comparisons with the features of dreaming have been drawn (Dietrich, 2004), and similarities to both the psychotic experience and what psychoanalysis refers to as primary process thinking are apparent.

The second set of operations proposed in the creative process involves a voluntary, deliberate, effortful search for meaning, interpretation, or explanation, to assign suitable significance to and make sense of one's experiences that arise from the defocusing of attention. This is essentially a problem-solving exercise that entails sustained attention (a function that is weakened in schizophrenia) and involves a search for salient elements of the experience by means of a more deliberate search for meaning in a structured, rational way that conforms more to internalised values and belief systems. (Its similarity to the psychoanalytic concept of secondary process thinking is also apparent.) It is in association with this process that the cognitive biases to which various individuals may be prone can begin to assert themselves. For example, confirmation bias, illusory correlation, the clustering illusion and so on are widely distributed in normal populations and can be brought to bear in the search for meaning. As another example, the clinical decision making of medical practitioners has been described to be influenced by a number of cognitive biases such as attribution error, availability error, search satisfying error (premature closure), confirmation bias, and commission bias (Groopman, 2007). Similarly, in delusional patients a variety of cognitive biases have been described such as externalising attributional style and personalised attributions (Bentall, Corcoran, Howard, Blackwood, & Kinderman, 2001), confirmation bias (Maher, 1974), jumping to conclusions (Garety & Hemsley, 1994), need for closure (Colbert, Peters, & Garety, 2006; McKay, Langdon, & Coltheart, 2006), lack of belief flexibility and extreme responding or dichotomous thinking style (Garety et al., 2005), and hindsight bias (Woodward et al., 2006).

In schizophrenia it is proposed that the protopsychotic anomalous experience, with its inherent disruptions in fringe experiences (e.g., loss of feelings of familiarity, rightness, agency, ownership, etc.), leads to an effortful, deliberate search for salience as a basis for constructing meaning or explanation for that experience, but under conditions of impaired prefrontal monitoring and control functions. As reviewed by Kapur (2003), the mesolimbic dopamine system is thought to be critical to the process of salience attribution. The mesolimbic dopamine pathway in schizophrenia is especially sensitive to stressors of various kinds (including psychostimulants such as amphetamine) and prone to phasic hyperactivity. This is possibly due to reduced cortical-subcortical NMDA receptor-mediated glutamatergic regulation of dopamine neurons in the ventral tegmentum (Laruelle, Kegeles, & Abi-Dargham, 2003), and/or perhaps down-regulation of inhibitory tegmental GABA interneurons (Lewis, Hashimoto, & Volk, 2005). Spikes of transient activity in this pathway that, according to Kapur (2003), are "stimulus-independent" are proposed to usurp the normal process of contextually driven salience attribution and lead to an aberrant assignment of salience to inappropriate external and internal stimuli. Taking this concept on a somewhat different path, I propose that under conditions of the protopsychotic anomalous experience and reduced prefrontal monitoring and control functions, unusual, random, or bizarre (primary process) relational content that is, at least initially, nonconscious is accessed through the fringe from the associative memory network, generating an *aberrant relational context* in the fringe, which drives the hypersensitive salience assignment system. I propose that the aberrant contextual elements emergent through the fringe provide the internal stimulus material for salience assignment under conditions of urgency (i.e., hunger for meaning) brought about by the protopsychotic experiences of altered sense of familiarity, agency, ownership, and so on experienced in the fringe. Meanwhile, the salience assignment system is also operating on external stimuli, in which the stimuli to which salience is attributed are selected on the basis that they imply or can be forced into some degree of harmony, consistency, or congruence with the aberrant relational items accessed through the fringe. Salience assignment would also be influenced by dispositional inclinations such as the cognitive biases mentioned previously. Particular instances of salience attribution, in turn, then evoke a fringe experience of rightness or right relations that replace the fringe feelings of loss of familiarity, agency, ownership, etc. The belief content emerging from this process thereby acquires a convincing quality of "truth" about it owing to that feeling of rightness.

On occasions, it is possible that this mechanism could account for the sudden appearance of psychotic insight in the form of an epiphany, an instantaneous revelation sometimes referred to as the "ah-ha!" phenomenon or "eureka experience". That is, a flash of intuition in which everything falls into place around a central delusional idea that suddenly crystallises and explains everything that has been going on but has hitherto been inexplicable. The fringe experience of rightness or "fit" on these occasions would be particularly intense and taken to attest particularly strongly to the "truth" of the revelation.

More usually, however, this mesolimbic, dopamine-mediated, salience assignment system transforms the patient's protopsychotic experiences less dramatically, giving them meaning, guided by feelings of rightness, on a more gradual basis. The model is readily applicable to the genesis of delusions other than those mentioned in the previous section (i.e., "passivity" phenomena, thought insertion) such as those referred to by Jaspers (1923/1962) as primary delusions. These include delusional perceptions (pp. 99–100), in which more-or-less clear meaning or significance is assigned to ordinary stimuli, and delusions of reference, in which the patient experiences external events as having an obvious and specific relation to the self.

The content of the delusions would derive from a combination of (1) the nature and intensity of the protopsychotic anomalous experience, (2) the formerly nonconscious associative material that is accessed through the fringe under conditions of reduced prefrontal monitoring and control processes, and (3) effortful, deliberate processing whereby a hypersensitive salience assignment system, influenced by certain dispositional inclinations (i.e., cognitive biases), becomes engaged in the selection of experiential elements to form the basis for the construction of meaning or explanation for the protopsychotic experience (i.e., delusions). The weakening of the monitoring and control functions of the prefrontal cortex would facilitate access to contents of the associative network implied in the fringe and thereby allow a rich array of relatively unfiltered memories, images, ideas, and feelings to become available. Such contextual material would then drive the mesolimbic, dopaminergic salience assignment system on the basis of which delusions would then be constructed. Prefrontal cortex dysfunction may have a further contributing role in failing to inhibit inappropriate salience assignment.

The intensity, duration, and recurring nature of the anomalous protopsychotic experiences provide ample ongoing or repeated learning opportunities for the reconfirmation of initial appraisals, refinement of salience assignment, and further elaboration and consolidation of belief influenced by the application of a variety of the aforementioned cognitive biases.

Although these processes in the proposed model contribute to the construction of delusions, what about the question of their maintenance in spite of implausibility, absence of objective evidence for the delusions, or compelling evidence that contradicts them? In other words, why are delusions maintained and elaborated in spite of these factors?

THE ROLE OF AESTHETICS IN DELUSION CONSTRUCTION AND MAINTENANCE

> Memories, not necessarily conscious but retentions that have been organically incorporated in the very structure of the self, feed present observation. (Dewey, 1934/2005, p. 93)

According to Epstein (2004), Marcel Proust, author of the novel *Remembrance of Things Past*, like William James, distinguished between the conscious sensory stimuli that dominate the content of individual thoughts and the accompanying network of associations that controls the transition from one thought to another. According to Proust, elements of certain current external stimuli (such as the famous madeleine) evoke memories of past sensations and, in turn, their accompanying network of associations (sensations, thoughts, emotions, desires, and other impressions) that comprise a complex remembered scene or sequence of events. In Proust's case this amounted to a vivid involuntary reinstantiation of an earlier experience as it actually occurred in which the memories are so life-like that they seem to be occurring in the present (in contrast to voluntary memory, which Proust regarded as a worked over interpretation of past events). As we saw, the Jamesian stream from one substantive thought or sensation to another, with the more salient information contained in the immediate focus or nucleus of consciousness, is accompanied by a fringe of normally *dimly* perceived contextual information that provides a vague suffusion or overtone giving the thought or sensation in focus added savour and playing a role in conveying its meaning. It is this relational information network that is recovered in the involuntary memories described by Proust and brought with unusual vividness into the foreground to make up the Proustian "true" reality about which he wrote in his novel. The moments in which this phenomenon occurred (*moments bienheureux*) were accompanied by intense emotion of a kind that Proust regarded as aesthetic and that could be explored through his art.

I propose that a similar relational information network is recovered, sometimes as a vivid involuntary reinstantiation, in the memories, images, ideas, and feelings evoked through the fringe by the protopsychotic anomalous experience in schizophrenia, under the condition of loss of the normal inhibitory influence exercised by the monitoring and control mechanisms of the prefrontal cortex.

As explained by Epstein (2004), in conveying the experience of such moments of involuntary memory, Proust reconstructed in his novel the nexus of associations making up such moments by the use of metaphor whereby the immediate salient sense impressions contained within the focus of consciousness are connected to the network of memories, impressions and sensations that make up the penumbra of associations in the fringe of awareness. The metaphor in Proust's case has high aesthetic value to both the author and the reader. That is, it conveys an ineffable sense of knowledge or recognition, an integration of parts into wholeness or unity, and the implication of something profound or transcendent.

In the deluded schizophrenia patient I propose that a similar process is operating, the salience assigned to impressions in the focus of consciousness under the influence of the protopsychotic anomalous experience and impaired prefrontal inhibitory control are likewise connected to an association network in the fringe of awareness by the use of metaphor, but an idiosyncratic metaphor in the case of schizophrenia, one that conveys no public meaning but is instead solipsistic and holds significance primarily to the self, namely a delusion. Its conveyance of ineffable knowledge, wholeness, and profundity, that is, its aesthetic qualities, are felt only by the patient, often with a particular intensity that reflects the tight fit achieved by the delusion between consciousness and context. Here the metaphor's aesthetic qualities are appreciated and felt with intensity by the author, the patient, and only very rarely by others (e.g., *folie à deux*).

Just as Proust creates a metaphor that acts as a symbol for something that cannot be directly represented in everyday cognition, namely the fringe of associations that normally only convey an overtone to conscious impressions, so does the schizophrenic patient create a symbol for something that cannot be directly represented, the fringe of associations evoked by the protopsychotic anomalous experience underlying psychosis.

William James argued that the most important of all the fringe feelings (i.e., experiences, awareness) was the feeling of harmony (i.e., rightness, being on-track) because it guides the progression of thought, and plays a role in sustaining or aborting searches, including searches of memory. He also proposed that as one's search progresses, the feeling of rightness appears each time one's latest percept is closer to one's inner goal image, which, in the case of schizophrenic psychosis, is to find meaning or explanation for the protopsychotic anomalous experiences occurring within the nucleus of consciousness, and this feeling of rightness as one's inner goal is approached in some way validates and encourages the search direction. It has further been proposed by Mangan (1993) that aesthetic feelings are particularly intense versions of this same feeling of rightness or degree of fit between features in the nucleus and the associated nonconscious knowledge structure in the fringe that gives those features meaning.

I suggest that delusions achieve this same intense feeling of rightness or degree of fit with the protopsychotic anomalous experience on the one hand and, on the other, with the associated nonconscious knowledge structure implied in and accessed through the fringe of the psychotic patient. When a protopsychotic anomalous experience occurs in the nucleus of consciousness there is a sense of dissonance generated in the fringe conveyed as a sense of wrongness or absence of rightness, a feeling that is also implicit in the feelings of loss of agency, loss of ownership, or loss of familiarity. This is discomforting. The delusion puts this right and eliminates the discord. The delusion is formed by knitting together the anomalous experience and items from among those accessible in the associative network by a hypersensitive salience assignment mechanism to construct an explanation for the changed state of the world. The delusional explanation thereby creates harmony between the contents of consciousness in the nucleus and the patient's associative network, and in so doing induces a feeling of rightness or good fit in the fringe. The rightness or goodness of fit engendered by the delusion has the potential to give it aesthetic value to the patient and the more intense the experience of rightness the greater is the aesthetic experience of the individual.

I propose that the feeling of rightness accounts for the resistance to change of delusions, their maintenance in the face of disconfirmatory evidence, and their continuation despite reasoned argument to the contrary. The rightness of the delusion signals coherence between the content of consciousness and the nonconscious context in which it is embedded, and the feeling of rightness is even able to guide conscious activity before any clear content (i.e., delusion in the case of schizophrenia) appears as an explicit evaluative criterion (Mangan, 2001). In particular, the feeling of rightness validates any entity in consciousness as if it were appropriate to its context, whatever the objective state of affairs may be.

Ludwig Wittgenstein (Barrett, 1966) spoke of the aesthetic experience as an occasion in which there is a subjective feeling that occurs when a stimulus evokes a response or reminiscence that gives rise to a sense that "it clicks", "it fits", that one is "satisfied" with the "rightness" of it, that somehow things have "fallen into place" or that there is a certain "charm" to it. In particular, Wittgenstein states: "The attraction of certain kinds of explanation is overwhelming. At a given time the attraction of a certain kind of explanation is greater than you can conceive—in particular, explanation of the kind 'This is really only this'" (Barrett, 1966, p. 24). Further, and this is of relevance to both the fact that popular notions of beauty are not central to aesthetics and that delusions often involve the grotesque and the frightening, Wittgenstein states "It may be the fact that the explanation is extremely repellent that drives you to adopt it" (p. 24).

CLINICAL ILLUSTRATION

A 40-year-old single man had a system of persecutory delusions that centred on his "feeling" (his word, he rejected the term "belief") that a microchip had been implanted in his body. This explained a large number of his experiences, including that people knew in advance what he was doing and knew generally about what was going on in his life, as well as numerous instances of alien control of his thoughts and actions, and feeling that people were reading his mind. The central idea of the microchip came to him in adulthood after a developmental history marked by traumatic family break-ups and emotional and physical cruelties of various kinds. As a child he had witnessed verbal and physical abuse in the home and his step-father had "played mind games" with him in which intimidation, humiliation, and sadistic manipulation were the hallmarks. The microchip explanation occurred to him at a time when people's behaviour and motivations no longer made sense to him, events seemed inexplicable, and he had the sense that his thoughts and actions were no longer his own or under his full control. On one occasion, in which he had an uncanny feeling of "being set up" while people were approaching him to engage in conversation in ways that did not make sense to him, someone used the word "chip". He immediately fastened upon this as conveying the message that a microchip had been inserted in his body through which he was being controlled and monitored. This explanation "clicked" and everything then fell into place, all of his current anomalous experiences now made sense to him and fitted with memories of his traumatic earlier development. There was a peculiar ineffability about this interpretation, it knitted together so many otherwise disparate and puzzling experiences into a coherent whole, it had an irresistibly captivating explanatory power, it had profound implications for the nature of his being-in-the-world, and there was a compelling "rightness" about the quality of understanding or insight it conveyed.

CONCLUDING REMARKS

The role of aesthetics in the construction and maintenance of belief is almost certainly not confined to delusions in schizophrenia or other mental disorders, but has a role in everyday belief as intimated by Kant. John Dewey wrote in the 1930s of the aesthetic dimensions of meaning construction in relation to everyday thinking and belief, stating that "an experience of thinking has its own esthetic quality ... [it] has a satisfying emotional quality because it possesses internal integration and fulfilment reached through ordered and organized movement" (see Johnson, 2007, pp. 103–105). He outlined a similar sequence to that already described in relation to the development of delusions: a problematic situation requiring interpretation or explanation and engagement in an inquiring search for generalisations in which the "unity of qualitativeness [i.e., rightness or degree of fit] regulates pertinence or relevancy and force of every distinction and relation; it guides selection and rejection and the manner of utilization of all explicit terms" (p. 78).

> Different ideas have their different "feels," their immediate qualitative aspects, just as much as anything else. One who is thinking his way through a complicated problem finds direction on his way by means of this property of ideas. Their qualities stop him when he enters the wrong path and send him ahead when he hits the right one. They are signs of an intellectual "Stop" and "Go." If a thinker had to work out the meaning of each idea discursively, he would be lost in a labyrinth that had no end and no center. Whenever an idea loses its immediate felt quality, it ceases to be an idea and becomes, like an algebraic symbol, a mere stimulus to execute an operation without the need of thinking. For this reason certain trains of ideas leading to their appropriate consummation (or conclusion) are beautiful or elegant. They have esthetic character. (Dewey, 1934/2005, pp. 124–125)

It is possible that nonrational ways of thinking and the maintenance of false beliefs among nonpsychotic individuals may be due to the aesthetics of everyday thinking and belief formation. For example, in some places AIDS deniers claim that HIV does not exist, or that if it does exist it does not cause AIDS, and they proffer alternative explanations for the widespread death and morbidity caused by this disease. Influential groups in developed countries claim that autism is caused by childhood vaccinations even though rigorous studies do not support this belief (Editorial, 2007). Members of certain eschatological religious groups prepare for the Rapture and Tribulation of the end time, which they believe is imminent, reflecting the beliefs of similar millenarian sects over hundreds of years. At a more commonplace level there are the widely held beliefs in astrology. Adherence to false or highly improbable propositions may be based on a variety of factors, such as to obtain acceptance within a particular social group and thereby achieve status of "insider" comforted by shared knowledge systems. However, the aesthetic experience arising from the sense of rightness outlined in this paper is one further factor that could play a role in the acquisition and maintenance of false beliefs among people other than those with clinical delusions, and is worth further exploration in this context.

It is also possible that the feeling of rightness could be relevant to the genesis of confabulation and the adherence to false memories. Similarly, a feeling of rightness could be generated in affective disorders by delusional ideas that "fit" with intense affective experiences. However, the present hypothesis was developed to account for the maintenance of delusions in schizophrenia and the role, if any, of the feeling of rightness in other delusional states and in confabulation constitute separate questions that may be worth pursuing.

James asserted that feelings of rightness played a role in everyday thinking and problem solving, and not just creative or artistic thinking. Yet, the roots of aesthetic experience have been proposed to derive from the feeling of rightness, and the more intense the feeling of rightness the more intense the aesthetic experience. What makes for an intense feeling of rightness in delusional and other beliefs is not clear, but the number and aptness, or fittingness, of associations evoked by the thought, conclusion, or belief in the relational memory network, by encapsulating a sense of necessity, coherence, and harmony, and thereby enriching the meaning and feeling tone (meaningfulness) of the thought or belief, may be the key to answering this question.

The defective belief evaluation system that has been proposed to account for the incorrigibility of delusions in the two-factor model of delusions (Coltheart, 2005; Davies, Coltheart, Langdon, & Been, 2001) is rendered redundant if the present rightness/aesthetic hypothesis is confirmed as the sole means of accounting for the incorrigibility of delusional beliefs. This particular two-factor position appears to assume that beliefs are generally grounded in logical reasoning and the capacity to evaluate empirical evidence, which are somehow rendered defective in psychosis. On the contrary, not only is there no evidence of a general incapacity to reason logically or critically evaluate evidence in psychosis, in everyday thinking human beings do not operate predominantly on the basis of such principles—they play no more than a minor role in real world belief formation and maintenance. Instead, I contend that the Jamesian fringe experience of meaningfulness or rightness involved in the construction of delusional interpretations or explanations for the protopsychotic anomalous experience gives the delusion, via the aesthetic experience generated, its own validity or internal "truth", just like any other belief. In other words, the aesthetics of meaning making or rightness trumps logical reasoning every time in the deluded and the artist alike—and, for that matter, in every one of us.

Confirming this hypothesis represents a formidable challenge. Case examples such as the one outlined earlier represent a useful place to start, but by themselves they are insufficient for confirmation. What is required is a reliable and valid psychometric of aesthetic experience against which to test delusions (and other beliefs for that matter). Mapping the brain networks involved in the aesthetic experience using neuroimaging techniques and applying this to deluded patients would also help to provide confirmation when such techniques have been developed and similarly tested for reliability and validity. In the meantime, perhaps the competing aesthetics of the defective belief evaluation model and the meaning-making or rightness model will appeal to the collective sensibility of the research community.

REFERENCES

Barrett, C. (Ed.).(1966). *L. Wittgenstein: Lectures and conversations on aesthetics, psychology and religious belief.* Oxford, UK: Blackwell.

Bentall, R. P., Corcoran, R., Howard, R., Blackwood, N., & Kinderman, P. (2001). Persecutory delusions: A review and theoretical integration. *Clinical Psychology Review, 21*, 1143–1192.

Boyer, P., Phillips, J. L., Rousseau, F. L., & Ilivitsky, S. (2007). Hipppocampal abnormalities and memory deficits: New evidence of a strong pathophysiological link to schizophrenia. *Brain Research Reviews, 54*, 92–112.

Colbert, S. M., Peters, E. R., & Garety, P. A. (2006). Need for closure and anxiety in delusions: A longitudinal investigation in early psychosis. *Behaviour Research and Therapy, 44*, 1385–1396.

Coltheart, M. (2005). Conscious experience and delusional belief. *Philosophy, Psychiatry and Psychology, 12*, 153–157.

David, N., Newen, A., & Vogeley, K. (2008). The "sense of agency" and its underlying cognitive and neural mechanisms. *Consciousness and Cognition, 17*, 523–534.

Davies, M., Coltheart, M., Langdon, R., & Been, N. (2001). Monothematic delusions: Towards a two-factor account. *Philosophy, Psychiatry and Psychology, 8*, 133–158.

Dewey, J. (2005). *Art as experience.* New York: Berkley Publishing Group and Perigee. (Original work published 1934)

Dietrich, A. (2004). The cognitive neuroscience of creativity. *Psychonomic Bulletin and Review, 11*, 1011–1026.

Editorial: Silencing debate over autism. (2007). *Nature Neuroscience, 10*, 531.

Epstein, R. (2000). The neural-cognitive basis of the Jamesian stream of thought. *Consciousness and Cognition, 9*, 550–575.

Epstein, R. (2004). Consciousness, art and the brain: Lessons from Marcel Proust. *Consciousness and Cognition, 13*, 213–240.

Frith, C. D. (1992). *The cognitive neuropsychology of schizophrenia*. Hove, UK: Lawrence Erlbaum Associates, Inc.

Garety, P. A., Freeman, D., Jolley, S., Dunn, G., Bebbington, P. E., Fowler, D. G., et al. (2005). Reasoning, emotions, and delusional conviction in psychosis. *Journal of Abnormal Psychology, 114*, 373–384.

Garety, P. A., & Hemsley, D. R. (1994). *Delusions: Investigations into the psychology of delusional reasoning*. New York: Oxford University Press.

Gray, J. A. (1995). The contents of consciousness: A neuropsychological conjecture. *Behavioural and Brain Sciences, 18*, 659–676.

Gray, J. A., Feldon, J., Rawlins, J. N. P., Hemsley, D. R., & Smith, A. D. (1991). The neuropsychology of schizophrenia. *Behavioural and Brain Sciences, 14*, 1–84.

Groopman, J. (2007). *How doctors think*. New York: Houghton Mifflin.

Hemsley, D. R. (1993). A simple (or simplistic?) cognitive model for schizophrenia. *Behaviour Research and Therapy, 31*, 633–645.

James, W. (1950). *The principles of psychology, Vol. 1*. New York: Dover Publications, Inc. (Original work published 1918)

Jaspers, K. (1962). *General psychopathology* (J. Hoenig & M. W. Hamilton, Trans.). Manchester, UK: Manchester University Press. (7th ed. published 1923 in German)

Johnson, M. (2007). *The meaning of the body: Aesthetics of human understanding*. Chicago: University of Chicago Press.

Kapur, S. (2003). Psychosis as a state of aberrant salience: A framework linking biology, phenomenology, and pharmacology in schizophrenia. *American Journal of Psychiatry, 160*, 13–23.

Laruelle, M., Kegeles, L. S., & Abi-Dargham, A. (2003). Glutamate, dopamine, and schizophrenia: From pathophysiology to treatment. *Annals of the New York Academy of Science, 1003*, 138–158.

Lewis, D. A., Hashimoto, T., & Volk, D. W. (2005). Cortical inhibitory neurons and schizophrenia. *Nature Reviews Neuroscience, 6*, 312–324.

Maher, B. A. (1974). Delusional thinking and perceptual disorder. *Journal of Individual Psychology, 30*, 98–113.

Mangan, B. (2001). Sensations' ghost: The non-sensory "fringe" of consciousness. *Psyche*, 7(18). Retrieved from http://psyche.cs.monash.edu.au/v7/psyche-7-18-mangan.html

Mangan, B. B. (1991). *Meaning and the structure of consciousness: An essay in psycho-aesthetics*. Unpublished PhD thesis, University of California, Berkeley, CA.

Mangan, B. B. (1993). Taking phenomenology seriously: The "fringe" and its implications for cognitive research. *Consciousness and Cognition, 2*, 89–108.

McKay, R., Langdon, R., & Coltheart, M. (2006). Need for closure, jumping to conclusions, and decisiveness in delusion-prone individuals. *Journal of Nervous and Mental Disease, 194*, 422–426.

Neisser, U. (1967). *Cognitive psychology*. New York: Appleton-Century-Crofts.

Parnas, J., & Sass, L. A. (2001). Self, solipsism and schizophrenic delusions. *Philosophy, Psychiatry and Psychology, 8*, 101–120.

Proust, M. (1981). *Remembrance of Things Past* (Vols. 1–12) (C. K. Scott-Moncrieff & Terence Kilmartin, Trans.). London: Chatto and Windus.

Synofzik, M., Vosgerau, G., & Newen, A. (2008). I move, therefore I am: A new theoretical framework to investigate agency and ownership. *Consciousness and Cognition*, *17*, 411–424.

Uhlhaas, P. J., & Mishara, A. L. (2007). Perceptual anomalies in schizophrenia: Integrating phenomenology and cognitive neuroscience. *Schizophrenia Bulletin*, *33*, 142–156.

Woodward, T. S., Moritz, S., Arnold, M. M., Cuttler, C., Whitman, J. C., & Lindsay, D. S. (2006). Increased hindsight bias in schizophrenia. *Neuropsychology*, *20*, 461–467.

COGNITIVE NEUROPSYCHIATRY
2010, 15 (1/2/3), 202–232

Hypnotic illusions and clinical delusions: Hypnosis as a research method

Rochelle E. Cox and Amanda J. Barnier

Macquarie Centre for Cognitive Science, Macquarie University, Sydney, Australia

Introduction. Hypnosis is not only intrinsically interesting, but it can be used instrumentally as a powerful tool to investigate phenomena outside its immediate domain. In focusing on instrumental hypnosis research, we first sketch the many contributions of hypnosis across a range of areas in experimental psychopathology. In particular, we summarise the historical and more recent uses of hypnosis to create and explore clinically relevant, temporary delusions.

Methods. We then describe in detail the steps that hypnosis researchers take in constructing a hypnotic paradigm to map the features and processes shared by clinical and hypnotic delusions, as well as their impact on information processing (including autobiographical memory). We illustrate with hypnotic versions of mirrored-self misidentification, somatoparaphrenia, alien control, and identity delusions.

Results. Findings indicate that hypnotic analogues can produce compelling delusions with features that are strikingly similar to their clinical counterparts. These similarities encompass phenomenological features of delusions, delusional resistance to challenge, and autobiographical memory during delusions.

Conclusion. We recognise important methodological issues and limitations of such hypnotic analogues, including: indexing response (behaviour vs. experience), alternative explanations (e.g., social compliance), the need for converging data, the need for close and continuing dialogue between the clinic and the laboratory, and generalisability of the findings.

Keywords: Hypnosis; Delusions; Confabulation; Hypnotic analogues.

Correspondence should be addressed to Amanda J. Barnier, Macquarie Centre for Cognitive Science (MACCS), Macquarie University, Sydney, NSW 2109, Australia. E-mail: abarnier@maccs.mq.edu.au

The preparation of this manuscript and the research reported in it were supported by a Macquarie University Research Fellowship to RC and by funding to AB from the Australian Research Council (Queen Elizabeth II Fellowship, Australian Research Fellowship, Discovery-Project Grant) and Macquarie University (MQRDG). We are grateful for that support. We would like to thank Lisa Bortolotti, Chris Moulin, and Martha Turner and for their comments on an earlier version of this manuscript.

 DOI: 10.1080/13546800903319884

INTRODUCTION

People can believe the most extraordinary, clearly false things. Delusional patients may mistakenly believe, for instance, that: "My wife has been replaced by an imposter" or "Whenever I look in the mirror, I see a stranger, not me" (Davies, Coltheart, Langdon, & Breen, 2002). Delusions are common, often cardinal features of a range of neuropsychological and psychiatric disorders (Coltheart, 2007). Delusions can be distressing for the patient and for their families, and can make everyday living extremely difficult. We must understand them fully to treat them effectively.

Langdon and Coltheart (2000; see also Coltheart, 2007; Metcalf, Coltheart, & Langdon, 2007) proposed that we can understand delusions by answering just two questions: (1) What generates the false proposition (belief) in the first place? (2) Once generated, why isn't it rejected as untrue? Langdon and Coltheart's two-factor theory answers these questions by identifying "breaks" in the way the healthy human mind processes information about self and the world. The first break, Factor 1, explains the content of the false belief and why it is generated (e.g., my wife has been replaced by an impostor). The second break, Factor 2, explains why the person fails to reject it as untrue. These breaks are often, but not always, neuropsychological in origin (Coltheart, 2007). According to Langdon and Coltheart (see also Johnson & Raye, 1998), there are other ways to break normal information processing.

In this paper we argue that one such way is with hypnosis. Hypnotic suggestions can break normal cognitive processing, both to generate false beliefs (akin to Factor 1) and to disrupt their normal evaluation (akin to Factor 2), turning these effects on and off with no lasting consequences (Johnson & Raye, 1998; Kihlstrom & Hoyt, 1988; Oakley & Halligan, 2009). Thus, hypnosis offers a way to recreate clinical delusions in the laboratory. This is potentially of great value since there is currently no proven way to experimentally study pathological forms of false belief. With reliable and valid analogues of clinical delusions, we can explore the influence of cognitive, motivational, and emotional factors, for instance, as well as test the conditions under which hypnotic delusions—like clinical delusions—are maintained, acted upon or abandoned. With this work we hope to: (1) extend and apply the two-factor theory to hypnotic analogues of delusions, (2) provide the means to investigate false beliefs in the laboratory, and (3) generate new insights that can inform treatment of delusions.

In this paper we sketch the two-factor theory of delusions, explain what hypnosis is and how it works, describe previous research that has used hypnosis to model clinical phenomena, specify the parameters of our hypnotic delusion paradigm, discuss the implications and challenges posed by this research, and suggest future directions.

DELUSIONS AND THE TWO-FACTOR THEORY

Delusions are described as false beliefs based on incorrect inferences about reality, which are firmly sustained despite what almost everyone else believes and despite what constitutes incontrovertible and obvious proof to the contrary (Coltheart, 2007). They are common in dementia, schizophrenia, and after traumatic brain injury. Langdon and Coltheart proposed a two-factor theory of delusions (for more details see Coltheart, 2007; Langdon & Coltheart, 2000) where two independent factors, or breaks in information processing, combine to create delusions. Factor 1 explains why the false belief is generated in the first place. Factor 2 explains why the person fails to reject it as untrue. Each delusion is associated with (usually) a different Factor 1, explaining the specific content of the delusion. But Factor 2, impaired belief evaluation, is common across delusions. For instance, Breen, Caine, Coltheart, Hendy, and Roberts (2000) described patient FE who, in the early stages of dementia, suffered from mirrored-self misidentification delusion—he believed he saw a stranger in the mirror, not himself. FE's Factor 1 impairment was prosopagnosia; part of his brain was damaged so he had difficulty identifying familiar versus unfamiliar faces. Since people can have prosopagnosia without developing a delusion, a second factor must be involved. The proposed Factor 2 was impairment in FE's ability to evaluate beliefs.

In its original formulation, Langdon and Coltheart's theory focused on neuropsychological impairments (a two-*deficit* theory). More recently, Langdon, Coltheart, and colleagues have acknowledged that these breaks in information processing are often, but not necessarily, neuropsychological in origin. In other words, Factor 1 may involve a motivated or "functional" disruption in information processing (Coltheart, Langdon, & McKay, 2007; McKay, Langdon, & Coltheart, 2005, 2007). However, the Factor 2 impairment still requires specification. It may involve biased reasoning or attributions and/or disrupted reality monitoring (Coltheart, 2007; Johnson & Raye, 1998). It may be influenced by motivation (McKay & Kinsbourne, 2010 this issue), mood and/or situations that discourage critical evaluation (Coltheart, 2007; Fotopoulou, Conway, Griffiths, Birchall, & Tyrer, 2007; Young, 2000).

By developing hypnotic analogues of delusions, we aim to provide the means to efficiently and effectively conduct basic, theoretically driven work, which can then be applied to clinical cases. This is consistent with a cognitive neuropsychology approach in general. Before describing our methods for creating these hypnotic versions of clinical delusions, it is useful first to understand a little of the nature of hypnosis.

BACKGROUND TO HYPNOSIS

What is hypnosis?

Hypnosis has been defined as:

> a process in which one person, designated the hypnotist, offers suggestions to another person, designated the subject, for imaginative experiences entailing alterations in perception, memory and action. In the classic case, these experiences are associated with a degree of subjective conviction bordering on delusion and an experienced involuntariness bordering on compulsion. As such, the phenomena of hypnosis reflect alterations in consciousness that take place in the context of a social interaction. (Kihlstrom, 2008, p. 21)

This widely accepted definition captures two key elements of hypnosis: (1) *hypnosis-as-procedure*, what the hypnotist does, and (2) *hypnosis-as-product*, what the subject experiences.

The hypnotic procedure begins with an *introduction* where the hypnotist tells the subject that she will receive suggestions to experience herself and the world differently and that she should respond in whatever way feels comfortable. Next, the hypnotist administers an *induction*, which instructs the subject to close her eyes, to relax and to focus on the hypnotist's words. Exhortations within the induction to focus attention and to become absorbed in the (typically) monotonous communications of the hypnotist engender in the subject a "motivated cognitive commitment" to respond (Sheehan, 1991, p. 526). Following the induction, the hypnotist administers *suggestions* for alterations in perception, memory, action, thought, or emotion. The hypnotist administers, tests, and cancels each suggestion in turn. Following a series of such suggestions, the hypnotist administers a *deinduction*, which instructs the subject to terminate the experience of hypnosis.

These elements of introduction, induction, suggestions, and deinduction constitute hypnosis-as-procedure. But what makes hypnosis so interesting is the subject's reaction to them—hypnosis-as-product. In response to hypnotic suggestions, the subject may experience: (1) an altered sense of reality and/or volition associated with motor actions (e.g., she may be unable to bend her arm after a suggestion for it to feel stiff and rigid); (2) hallucinations (both positive and negative, including analgesia and perceptual distortion; e.g., she may feel no pain when exposed to a painful stimulus); (3) age regression and dreams (e.g., she may behave as if she were a small child); (4) amnesia and hypermnesia (e.g., she may have trouble remembering things that just occurred); and (5) posthypnotic suggestion (e.g., she may scratch her ear after hypnosis every time she hears a particular word).

Who does it work for and how does it work?

Responding to hypnotic suggestions feels very unusual. Hypnotised subjects experience hypnotic phenomena with "involuntariness bordering on compulsion" and "conviction bordering on delusion" (Kihlstrom, 2008, p. 21). However, it is not just that hypnotic responses happen easily or seem real. To a hypnotised person, they feel *surprisingly easy* and *surprisingly real* (see Barnier & Oakley, 2009).

It is worth noting that not everyone responds to hypnotic suggestions. Hypnotisability is normally distributed in the population (E. Hilgard, 1965). Approximately 10–15% of the population are very susceptible to hypnosis (called "high hypnotisable" or "highs"). Another 10–15% respond to few if any hypnotic suggestions (called "low hypnotisable" or "lows"). The remaining 70–80% experience some suggestions but not others (called "medium hypnotisable" or "mediums") (for more discussion of these issues, see Barnier & Oakley, 2009).

High hypnotisable people may enjoy daydreaming (J. Hilgard, 1965), may be creative and imaginative (Barber & Wilson, 1978), may be able to focus their attention very well (Crawford, 1994; Raz, Shapiro, Fan, & Posner, 2002), and may become easily absorbed in activities (Tellegen & Atkinson, 1974). Attitudes also play an important role in determining a person's hypnotisability. Although a positive attitude to hypnosis is a necessary condition for successful responding, it is not sufficient. Many low hypnotisable individuals have positive attitudes but cannot experience hypnosis. In contrast, a negative attitude generally guarantees poor or no hypnotic experiences (for more on individual differences in hypnotisability, see Barnier & McConkey, 2004; Barnier & Oakley, 2009). Despite these potential indicators of hypnotic ability, the only reliable way to measure hypnotisability is to administer a standardised test (for a summary of measures, see Barnier & McConkey, 2004).

We noted earlier that hypnotic responding feels surprisingly easy and surprisingly real. Hypnotised people typically describe their hypnotic experiences in ways that suggest that the normal processing or control of cognitive events and motor actions has been disrupted. One view of hypnosis says that this is merely an illusion; that hypnosis disrupts only the subject's introspective awareness of her internal states (e.g., following a suggestion for hypnotic analgesia she reports feeling no pain when exposed to a painful stimulus) with no effect on her actual internal states (e.g., her heart rate when exposed to the painful stimulus). Another view says that this is not an illusion; that hypnosis may disrupt the actual state of cognitive or physical systems. According to the first view, hypnotic responses are controlled in essentially normal, nonhypnotic ways but executive monitoring is disrupted. According to the second view, hypnotic responses reflect actual disruptions in the normal, nonhypnotic control of memory, perception and action systems (for detailed discussion, see Barnier & Oakley, 2009; Woody & Sadler, 2008). Both possibilities have value for using hypnosis to recreate and explore clinical conditions in the laboratory.

Hypnotic analogues of clinical conditions

Experimental hypnotic analogues aim to recreate the features of clinical conditions in the laboratory. Once this has been achieved, hypnosis researchers use these analogues in an attempt to model the processes that contribute to clinical disorders. Hypnosis has a long history of modelling a number of conditions including functional blindness, functional amnesia, conversion hysteria, and auditory hallucinations (Barnier, 2002; Bryant & McConkey, 1989a,b; Cox & Barnier, 2003; Haggard, Cartledge, Dafydd, & Oakley, 2004; Halligan, Athwal, Oakley, & Frackowiak, 2000; Szechtman, Woody, Bowers, & Nahmias, 1998; Zimbardo, Andersen, & Kabat, 1981; for a review, see Oakley & Halligan, 2009). Consider research on conversion disorder paralysis where a person experiences unexplained limb paralysis in the absence of any physical cause (that is, their nerves and muscles are intact). Marshall, Halligan, Fink, Wade, and Frackowiak (1997) used PET to examine brain activation in a woman with unexplained paralysis of her left leg. When the woman was asked to move her left leg, activation in her brain (in the premotor cortex and cerebellum) suggested she was genuinely attempting to move her leg. However, she lacked activation in brain areas responsible for motor action (primary sensorimotor areas) and displayed increased activation in two other brain areas (anterior cingulate cortex and right orbitofrontal cortex), suggesting an unconscious inhibition of intended leg movements (see also Oakley & Halligan, 2009).

These researchers then explored whether hypnotically suggested paralysis produced the same neural patterns as conversion disorder paralysis. They used PET to examine the brain of a high hypnotisable man who had received a hypnotic suggestion for left leg paralysis (Halligan et al., 2000). Following the suggestion, they asked the hypnotised man to try to move his left leg. Interestingly, his brain scans showed similar patterns of activation to the woman with conversion disorder paralysis, with a similar lack of activation in brain areas responsible for motor action. This suggests that the same brain mechanisms were involved in the clinical and hypnotic paralysis. More importantly, it suggests that hypnosis is a powerful technique for exploring and potentially treating conversion disorder symptoms (see Oakley & Halligan, 2009).

These studies using neuroimaging during hypnosis also challenge notions that hypnosis can be explained as mere faking or compliance. Indeed, researchers (Ward, Oakley, Frackowiak, & Halligan, 2003) have compared brain activations of high hypnotisable individuals during hypnotically suggested left leg paralysis and during attempts to fake left leg paralysis. Independent observers could not discern when participants were faking. However, there were clear differences in brain activation. Faked paralysis produced activation in areas not seen in hypnotically suggested paralysis.

These findings of genuine changes in brain activation during hypnotically suggested experiences reinforce the value of using hypnosis to model clinical conditions, especially conditions that have been traditionally difficult to study in the laboratory. This makes hypnosis particularly suited to the task of studying delusions, which are complex, multifaceted, and difficult to study in isolation. We now discuss early research that used hypnosis to study clinical delusions.

HYPNOSIS IN THE STUDY OF DELUSIONS

Hypnosis is particularly suitable for studying delusions because hypnosis and delusions share a number of features. Both are: (1) believed with absolute conviction, (2) resistant to rational counterargument, and (3) maintained regardless of overwhelming evidence to the contrary. These shared features are illustrated by a series of experiments by McConkey and colleagues who used hypnosis to create a sex-change delusion (Burn, Barnier, & McConkey, 2001; McConkey, Szeps, & Barnier, 2001; Noble & McConkey, 1995).

Based on work by Sutcliffe (1961), in their first study (Noble & McConkey, 1995), high and low hypnotisable participants received a hypnotic suggestion to become the opposite sex. Following this suggestion, high hypnotisable participants gave themselves a new name (consistent with being the opposite sex), described themselves as the opposite sex, and resisted challenges to the suggested delusion. In a second study, these researchers explored the impact of a hypnotic sex change delusion on information processing (Burn et al., 2001). Following a hypnotic suggestion to become the opposite sex, participants listened to a story about a male and female character. High hypnotisable participants later recalled more information from the story about the character consistent with their suggested sex, and this was not influenced by the character they identified with. In their third study, McConkey and colleagues investigated whether high hypnotisable participants could experience a sex-change delusion in their normal, waking state (McConkey et al., 2001). They gave high and low hypnotisable participants a hypnotic sex change suggestion, but half of these participants received the suggestion during hypnosis, and half received it whilst not hypnotised. Although McConkey et al. (2001) found that high hypnotisable participants could experience a suggested sex change in their waking state, the delusion was more compelling for high hypnotisable participants who received the suggestion during hypnosis. Together, these studies indicate that hypnosis is particularly effective at modelling the features of a sex-change delusion and that the hypnotic context plays an important role in facilitating these delusions.

In addition to modelling the features of clinical delusions, hypnosis may also be able to model some of the underlying processes. Recall that Langdon and Coltheart (2000) proposed a two-factor theory of delusions where Factor 1 is responsible for producing the delusional belief in the first place and Factor 2 explains why the belief isn't rejected as untrue. According to this theory, the cognitive disruptions involved in delusions are often neuropsychological in origin. However, there are other ways to disrupt normal information processing. One such way is with hypnosis (Kihlstrom & Hoyt, 1988). From the research described previously and the broader hypnosis literature, there is substantial evidence that hypnotic suggestions can create compelling, albeit temporary breaks in basic cognitive processes (e.g., perception, memory, action) of the kind argued to be involved in delusions (as Factor 1). There are numerous hypnotic phenomena with Factor 1-like features that can be used to create hypnotic versions of Factor 1. Table 1 presents a list of seven delusions.

In addition to modelling these Factor-1 impairments, it is also likely that hypnosis can model Factor 2, which is thought to involve a deficit or disruption to normal belief evaluation. The general view of hypnosis is that the hypnotic state reduces critical thinking and distorts reality monitoring akin to the proposed Factor 2. For instance, hypnotised people will focus on suggested experiences (e.g., when a male subject receives a hypnotic sex-change suggestion to become female) and can ignore contradictory information or challenges (e.g., what he really looks like when he views himself on a videomonitor; Noble & McConkey, 1995). Also, hypnotised people attribute as much reality to suggested events (e.g., that a ball they are holding is heating up) as they do to real events (e.g., when the ball has

TABLE 1
Monothematic delusions and relevant hypnotic phenomena

Delusion	*Hypnotic phenomena*
Capgras and Fregoli	Emotional numbing and familiarity
Cotard	Sex-change and identity delusions
Mirrored-self misidentification	Hypnotic mirrored-self misidentification
Reduplicative paramnesia	Trance logic and visual hallucination
Alien control	Anomalous control
Thought insertion	Posthypnotic suggestion

chemicals inside it that do heat up; McConkey, 2008). Thus, specific suggestions in hypnosis produce controllable disruptions and distortions to recreate the impact of Factor 1 and Factor 2 in delusions.

The hypnotic sex-change experiments described earlier, involved suggestions for a fully formed delusion. That is, they suggested the complete delusional experience (of being the opposite sex). In contrast, one study has used hypnosis to suggest Factor-1-like deficits. Zimbardo et al. (1981) explored the role of hypnotically induced deafness in paranoia. They gave two groups of high hypnotisable participants a suggestion for posthypnotic deafness. One group was aware of the source of this deafness (i.e., hypnotic suggestion) but the second group received an additional hypnotic instruction to forget the deafness suggestion (accompanying amnesia suggestion). After hypnosis, two confederates in the same room as participants engaged in a conversation with each other that could be misperceived as antagonistic. Both groups of participants reported a hearing deficit but those who received deafness-without-awareness (i.e., those who received the extra amnesia suggestion) became paranoid about the nature of the confederates' conversation and reported more irritation, agitation, hostility, and unfriendliness than participants who received deafness-with-awareness. In this study, the suggestion for deafness can be interpreted as a Factor 1 suggestion. When it was combined with amnesia for the source of the difficulty, it produced a delusion-like experience of paranoia. However, it is worth noting that Zimbardo and colleagues did not directly ask participants about their beliefs. Rather, they used participants' responses to questionnaire measures of paranoia as evidence of their beliefs.

OUR HYPNOTIC DELUSION PARADIGM

Our current work using hypnosis to model delusions was inspired by the previous research just described. Generally, to recreate delusions we begin by administering suggestions for a fully formed delusion. Once we have achieved this, and successfully recreated the features of clinical delusions, we explore underlying processes by administering suggestions for Factor 1 plus Factor 2 impairments. As noted earlier, Factor 1 explains the generation of the false belief or memory; it is responsible for the content of the delusion. Our experiments mimic this with a "Factor 1" hypnotic suggestion that recreates the different, specific break (in perception, action, emotion, agency, or memory) involved in different delusions. Factor 2 explains why the person fails to reject the false belief as untrue; it is responsible for impaired evaluation. Our experiments mimic this with a "Factor 2" hypnotic suggestion that recreates the specific break in evaluation. We based our Factor 2 suggestion on work by Turner (2006) who suggested that Factor 2 in delusions may involve a disruption to the normal process of checking beliefs for plausibility. Specifically, our hypnotic Factor 2 suggestion involves an instruction that any explanations that might account for the Factor-1 experience will seem plausible. To illustrate, Table 2 provides two examples of delusions. For each, we specify: (1) the Factor 1 impairment proposed in the literature, (2) the Factor 1 suggestion we use, and (3) the common Factor 2 suggestion we use. In our research we give participants either a fully formed delusion, only the Factor 1 suggestion (Factor 1 alone), or both the Factor 1 and Factor 2 suggestions (Factor 1 + Factor 2). Previous research indicates that a suggestion for a fully formed delusion generates experiences remarkably similar to clinical delusions. By comparing these three groups we test whether Factor 1 and Factor 2 suggestions—separately and combined—are more effective in generating hypnotic delusions (because they more closely model the proposed underlying mechanisms) than a suggestion for a fully formed delusion. We now describe our research in detail, including the types of suggestions we use, the impact of these suggestions, our challenge procedures, and work examining the impact of a delusion on autobiographical memory.

Types of suggestions

Our work has focused on developing hypnotic suggestions that recreate: (1) reverse intermetamorphosis—the belief that I am someone else, (2) mirrored-self misidentification—the belief that I see a stranger when I look in the mirror, (3) somatoparaphrenia—the belief that my arm belongs to someone else, and (4) alien control—the belief that my movements are caused by someone else. To create credible hypnotic delusions we began by developing fully formed suggestions that would make sense to a hypnotised person and would closely mimic the features of clinical delusions. For example, clinical delusions of misidentification involve a false belief about the identity of oneself or others. A subtype of this delusion is reverse intermetamorphosis which involves personal identity change. Clinical cases of reverse intermetamorphosis indicate that this identity change can occur across a variety of different identities. These individuals may adopt the identity of someone similar to themselves, someone dissimilar to themselves, someone familiar, or someone unfamiliar. Such delusions may encompass beliefs about real, existing individuals, as in the case of a woman known as RZ who believed that she was her father (Breen et al., 2000), or beliefs about nonexistent individuals, as in the case of a woman known as EN who believed that she had a nonexistent twin sister (Baddeley, Thornton, Chua, & McKenna, 1996).

TABLE 2
Hypnotic delusions and confabulations

	Proposed Factor 1	*Hypnotic Factor 1 suggestion*	*Hypnotic Factor 2 suggestion*	*Fully formed suggestion*
Delusions				
Mirrored-self misidentification	Prosopagnosia	Your face looks and feels unfamiliar	You'll have difficulty evaluating the reality of your experiences; any explanation will seem plausible	You see a stranger in the mirror
Somatoparaphrenia	Limb paralysis from brain lesion	Your left hand is paralysed		Your left hand does not belong to you
Confabulations				
Inefficient/disrupted retrieval	Amnesia for event and production of irrelevant memories	You won't remember this event but will fill in gaps in memory	You'll have difficulty evaluating the reality of your memories; any memory you retrieve will seem accurate	You'll remember irrelevant memories and believe them to be true
Temporal confusion	Amnesia for correct event sequence and temporally disorganised retrieval	You won't remember the order of events and will reorder them in any way		You'll remember this event out of order but believe it to be accurate

To map this range of delusional beliefs, we have written and tested a number of fully formed suggestions for reverse intermetamorphosis. These include suggestions for high hypnotisable participants to become real individuals, such as a friend or relative who is very similar, a friend or relative who is very dissimilar, a same-sex sibling who is presumably familiar, or a friend's sibling who is presumably less familiar. We have also administered suggestions for participants to have an extra (nonexistent) same-sex sibling. Although we thought it might be easier for people to experience a hypnotic delusion about someone real, similar, or familiar, we found that all of these suggestions were equally effective in producing a credible hypnotic delusion of reverse intermetamorphosis in high hypnotisable individuals (Cox, 2007; Cox & Barnier, 2009a, 2009b; Cox & Bryant, 2008).

In our work on hypnotic mirrored-self misidentification (Barnier et al., 2008; see also Bortolotti, Cox, & Barnier, 2009), we have administered fully formed suggestions to highs to either: (1) see a stranger in the mirror, (2) see the mirror as a window, or (3) see the mirror as a window with a view of a stranger on the other side. We used these suggestions to map the different pathways from neuropsychological impairment to clinical cases of mirrored-self misidentification. Langdon, McKay, and Coltheart (2008) have suggested that delusions may be seeded by various implausible thoughts so we used these three suggestions to explore the initial thoughts that might "seed" mirrored-self misidentification delusion. We found that whereas participants given the stranger in the mirror suggestion and the mirror as a window with a view of a stranger suggestion reported seeing a stranger in the mirror (and not themselves), participants given the mirror as a window suggestion simply reported that they saw themselves. In other words, the specifics of the suggestion influenced its success and the resulting pattern of delusional performance. This finding is similar to research on hypnotic sex-change delusions, where suggestions to become "more and more like the opposite sex" lead to a more compelling delusional experience than suggestions to become "less and less like your actual sex" (Noble & McConkey, 1995).

We have also developed a fully formed suggestion designed to recreate somatoparaphrenia (Rahmanovic, Barnier, & Cox, 2009). In this suggestion, we touched participants' nondominant arm, and suggested that the arm belonged to someone else. To avoid participants attributing their delusion experience to the hypnotic suggestion, we also gave them accompanying amnesia for the suggestion. This amnesia suggestion maps onto clinical cases where individuals frequently deny that there is anything wrong with their arm. However, this lack of awareness or insight does not necessarily occur in all delusions. Clinical patients may say that they know their beliefs seem implausible but they have them none the less. Following the somatoparaphrenia suggestion, we touched their arm again, and asked "can you tell me about this arm? Whose arm is this?" In response to this question, 54% of high hypnotisable participants either did not acknowledge ownership of their arm, denied ownership of their arm, or said their arm belonged to someone else.

We have compared this fully formed somatoparaphrenia suggestion with a Factor 1 plus Factor 2 suggestion. In somatoparaphrenia, Factor 1 is arm paralysis, so our hypnotic Factor 1 suggestion was for arm paralysis. Once again, we did not want participants to attribute their arm paralysis to the hypnotic suggestion, so we also gave them accompanying amnesia for the arm paralysis suggestion. Our hypnotic Factor 2 suggestion was: "You will not know why this arm feels paralysed and you will search for explanations to account for it. Any explanation you come up with will seem plausible." Our findings indicated that highs who received Factor 1 plus Factor 2 generated a variety of explanations for their Factor 1 impairment. For example, participants explained their arm paralysis by saying that their arm had been severed, that they had been in an accident, or that they had slept on their arm and made it feel numb. However, no highs who received the Factor 1 plus Factor 2 suggestion denied ownership of their arm or said that their arm belonged to someone else. One possible explanation for this is that our Factor 1 plus Factor 2 suggestion may not have completely captured all the aspects of somatoparaphrenia.

In our work on alien control, we have given participants a fully formed suggestion that someone else was causing the movements of their dominant hand and arm (Scott, Barnier, & Cox, 2009). Participants were informed that their hand and arm would move to respond to the hypnotist's instructions, but someone else would be causing these movements. Following this suggestion, we asked participants to pick up a pen and sign their name. During this task, high hypnotisable participants displayed behaviours consistent with the suggestion. For instance, they had difficulty moving and coordinating the movements of their dominant hand and arm. They also reported feeling a lack of control over their dominant hand and arm.

We have also tested a Factor 1 plus Factor 2 alien control suggestion. In alien control, Factor 1 is the inability to monitor the source of one's own actions so our hypnotic Factor 1 suggestion was for participants to feel as though they were not causing the movements of their dominant hand and arm. This Factor 1 suggestion was combined with a hypnotic Factor 2 suggestion which said: "You will not know why it feels as though you are not causing the movements of your hand and arm and you will search for explanations to account for it. Any explanation you come up with will seem plausible." However, similar to the Factor 1 plus Factor 2 somatoparaphrenia suggestion, this Factor 1 plus Factor 2 alien control suggestion was less successful than the fully formed suggestion at producing experiences of alien control.

In their hypnotic deafness study, Zimbardo et al. (1981) found that a hypnotic Factor 1 suggestion alone could produce delusion-like experiences. Based on this work, we were interested in whether a suggestion for Factor 1 alone would lead to a complete delusional experience. Further, in their hypnotic sex-change studies, McConkey et al. (2001) found that high hypnotisable individuals could experience a hypnotic sex change delusion outside of hypnosis. However, highs who received the suggestion in hypnosis experienced a more compelling delusion. Therefore, we investigated the impact of a suggestion for Factor 1 alone, with and without hypnosis. Here, we were particularly interested in whether the hypnotic state, which is known to disrupt belief evaluation, might play the role of Factor 2.

We applied this design to mirrored-self misidentification delusion (Connors, Cox, & Barnier, 2008). High hypnotisable participants received either a Factor 1 alone suggestion or a Factor 1 plus Factor 2 suggestion. Half of the participants received the suggestion during hypnosis (hypnosis condition), and the other half received the suggestion while awake (waking condition). The Factor 1 alone suggestion informed participants that when they opened their eyes and looked into the mirror they would not be able to recognise the person they saw. This was based on Coltheart and colleagues' suggestion that Factor 1 in mirrored-self misidentification may involve a deficit in face processing (Breen et al., 2000; Coltheart, 2007). The Factor 1 plus Factor 2 suggestion involved the same Factor 1 suggestion plus a Factor 2 suggestion that any explanations they came up with to account for their inability to recognise the person in the mirror would seem plausible. Figure 1 illustrates the percentage of participants who passed the suggestion (i.e., reported seeing a stranger in the mirror). Focusing first on the hypnosis condition, 73% of participants who received the Factor 1 alone suggestion and 58% of participants who received the Factor 1 plus Factor 2 suggestion reported seeing a stranger in the mirror. This suggests that a separate Factor 2

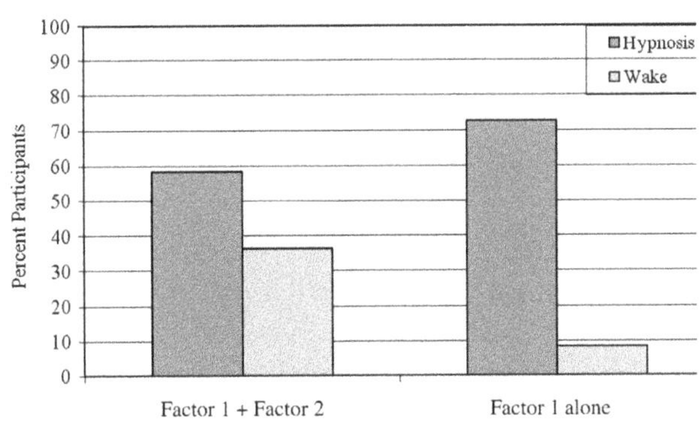

Figure 1. Percentage of highs in hypnosis and waking conditions who passed delusion according to suggestion.

suggestion did not appear to be necessary for creating hypnotic mirrored-self misidentification. In contrast, in the waking condition, only 8% of participants who received the Factor 1 alone suggestion and 36% of participants who received the Factor 1 plus Factor 2 suggestion reported seeing a stranger in the mirror. These results suggest that hypnosis may produce a disruption in belief evaluation akin to the proposed Factor 2. Also, the hypnotic context appears to play an important role in creating delusional experiences.

Impact of suggestions

We have used a variety of measures to index the impact of our hypnotic delusion suggestions. We begin by testing whether participants pass the suggestion (i.e., whether they display evidence of experiencing the suggestion). For example, to test the impact of a suggestion for somatoparaphrenia, we placed a tray of objects next to participants and asked them to pick up each object. Factor 1 in somatoparaphrenia involves arm paralysis so we placed the tray next to the arm targeted by the suggestion and we noted which arm they used to pick up each object. If participants did not use the arm targeted by the suggestion they passed this particular test. As expected, highs displayed difficulty moving this limb and reached across their body to pick up the objects with their other hand. One of the objects on the tray was a bottle which we asked participants to open. Interestingly, many highs managed to open the bottle using just one hand!

To index the impact of a hypnotic suggestion for mirrored-self misidentification, we asked highs to open their eyes, look in a mirror and describe what they could see. In this initial test of the suggestion we were interested in whether participants could recognise themselves in the mirror. If participants did not recognise themselves they passed the suggestion. We found that the majority of highs passed the suggestion and described seeing a stranger in the mirror. The following excerpt illustrates one participant's compelling experience (from Barnier et al., 2008, pp. 417–418):

Hypnotist: Tell me, what do you see?
Participant: *(Participant looks in the mirror and then looks behind him).* Who's that?
Hypnotist: Tell me about what you see.
Participant: Another person.
Hypnotist: Tell me about the person.
Participant: They're wearing a purple shirt, they've got a big nose, got a mole on their neck.
Hypnotist: Is the person you see a male or a female?
Participant: Male *(Participant looks behind him).*

Hypnotist: Tell me more about what they look like.
Participant: They've got short, curly hair, brown eyes, brown hair.
Hypnotist: Have you ever seen this person before?
Participant: No *(Participant looks behind him)*.
Hypnotist: Does this person remind you of anyone?
Participant: I think I've seen him before at school.
Hypnotist: Tell me about that ... where you might have seen him.
Participant: I think he was in the year below me ... yeah I knew there was something.
Hypnotist: What do you think his name is?
Participant: Anthony *(not the participant's name)*.
Hypnotist: In what ways does this person look like you?
Participant: Same coloured hair. I've got hazel eyes.
Hypnotist: And what colour eyes does he have?
Participant: Brown.
Hypnotist: In what ways does the person you can see look different to you?
Participant: Different coloured eyes. I think my nose is smaller ... got bigger lips.
Hypnotist: He has or you have?
Participant: I have ... and I've got more freckles.
Hypnotist: What is he doing at the moment?
Participant: Looking into the mirror. I don't know where he is though *(participant looks behind him and around the room)*.
Hypnotist: Is he doing anything in particular or saying anything in particular?
Participant: Just looking at me. He's saying something but I can't understand.
Hypnotist: Why can't you understand?
Participant: Because I can't lip read.
Hypnotist: Can you hear him?
Participant: No.
Hypnotist: How come?
Participant: Because I can only see him.

This illustrates the compelling reality of the hypnotic delusion as well as highs' ability to maintain the delusion in response to detailed questioning, long after the initial test of the suggestion.

In addition to indexing whether participants pass these suggestions, we have developed a range of other measures to assess the impact of our hypnotic delusions on participants' beliefs and experiences. For example, following a suggestion for reverse intermetamorphosis, which involves a change in self, we measured the impact of the suggestion on identity. We asked participants to say their name, describe themselves, and to list some personal likes and dislikes for their (deluded) identity. We also administered two different self-concept tasks before and during the suggested delusion. The first task was a modified version of Higgins' (1987) self-discrepancy task. In this task, participants provided five words to describe their actual self and five words to describe their ideal self. The second task was an "I am" task (Kuhn &

McPartland, 1954; Rathbone, Moulin, & Conway, 2008). In this task, participants completed five sentences, each beginning with the words "I am". Participants completed these tasks at the beginning of the session and then again following the delusion suggestion when they were experiencing themselves as a different identity. We were interested in the extent to which highs' and lows' self-concept might change following the delusion suggestion so we calculated the number of different self-descriptions provided (i.e., different words and different sentence completions) after the delusion suggestion, compared to before the suggestion. We found that across six experiments, 90% of highs provided a new name and described themselves differently during the suggested delusion. Highs also generated approximately 4.90 personal likes and dislikes for their deluded identity, whereas lows generated 3.09 personal likes and dislikes. Additionally, highs completed the self-concept tasks with approximately 4.39 different self-descriptions, whereas lows completed the self-concept tasks with only 2.57 different self-descriptions (Cox, 2007; Cox & Barnier 2009a, 2009b). Using multiple tasks in this way gives us a more complete understanding of any temporary changes in self following a suggestion for reverse intermetamorphosis.

We have also developed a test to index the impact of a hypnotic alien control delusion suggestion on self-monitoring (Scott et al., 2009). A number of authors have proposed that individuals with alien control delusions have a deficit in self monitoring (Frith & Done, 1989; Stirling, Hellewell, & Ndlovu, 2001; Stirling, Hellewell, & Quraishi, 1998). For example, Stirling et al. (1998) asked schizophrenic and control participants to complete a self-monitoring task where they made three different types of drawings on a computer graphics tablet: (1) eight abstract drawings with their eyes closed, (2) eight drawings of shapes (e.g., triangles, squares) with their eyes closed, and (3) eight drawings of shapes with their eyes open. According to Stirling et al., abstract drawings with eyes closed are the most demanding on self-monitoring and drawings of shapes with eyes open are the least demanding on self-monitoring. After completing each drawing, participants were presented with four images. These included their original drawing and the same drawing rotated 90°, 180°, and 270°. Their task was to select the one they originally drew. Stirling et al. found that schizophrenic patients with alien control symptoms were poorer at recognising their own drawings than controls and their performance worsened as demands on self-monitoring increased.

In our hypnotic analogue, following a suggestion for alien control of the dominant hand and arm, we first asked participants to pick up a pen and sign their name. We then asked them how it felt to sign their name. Many high hypnotisable participants commented that their arm movements felt outside of their control and a number of participants also expressed the belief that an external agent was responsible for their arm movements. Next, we administered Stirling et al.'s (1998) self-monitoring task. Our results indicated that high hypnotisable participants had more difficulty than low hypnotisable participants at recognising their self-drawn images when they were asked to draw abstract pictures with their eyes closed (the task that was most demanding on self-monitoring). This is consistent with Stirling et al.'s findings and suggests that the hypnotic alien control suggestion lead to an impairment in self-monitoring among high hypnotisable individuals.

Challenge procedures

To examine whether hypnotic delusions are maintained with the conviction displayed by clinically deluded individuals, we have developed challenge procedures inspired by previous research and clinical techniques. We have modified these challenges and tailored them to our hypnotic analogues.

In the hypnotic sex-change research described earlier, McConkey and colleagues introduced two useful challenge procedures: a contradiction and a confrontation. In the contradiction, they asked participants what they would say if a doctor (a hypothetical authority figure) came in and said they were not their suggested sex. In the contradiction, they asked participants to open their eyes, look at themselves on a monitor, and describe what they were experiencing as they did so. McConkey and colleagues found that highs maintained their deluded identity in the face of these challenges. In response to the contradiction they defended their delusional belief, by saying for instance, that the doctor was a "quack". In response to the confrontation, they defended their delusional belief by saying they could see someone else on the monitor (Noble & McConkey, 1995).

We adapted these challenge procedures in our work on reverse intermetamorphosis. In a contradiction, we asked participants what they would say if their mother came into the room and said they were not their suggested identity. In a confrontation, we asked participants to open their eyes, look at themselves on a monitor, and describe what they were experiencing as they did so. Across three experiments, approximately 81% of our highs maintained their suggested identity in the face of these challenges (Cox, 2007; Cox & Barnier 2009a, 2009b; Cox & Bryant, 2008). In response to the contradiction, they made comments such as "mum's gone crazy ... she's lost the plot." In response to the confrontation, they made comments such as "it was very blurry at first. Then my eyes focused and I thought that's my brother on the TV." Notably, in one experiment involving real, high hypnotisable participants (hereafter referred to as "reals") and simulating, low hypnotisable participants (hereafter referred to as "simulators") tested with Orne's (1959, 1962) real-simulating paradigm, we found that more than twice as many reals than simulators maintained their identity following the confrontation (Cox, 2007; for similar findings, see Noble & McConkey, 1995). This indicates that the delusional experiences of real, high hypnotisable individuals cannot be explained solely in terms of the demand characteristics of the hypnotic setting; that is, participants are not simply faking in order to please the hypnotist. Rather, their responses are a genuine reaction to the delusion suggestion.

We have recently examined the impact of similar challenge procedures on a hypnotic suggestion for somatoparaphrenia (Rahmanovic et al., 2009). In a contradiction we asked participants what they would say if a doctor walked into the room, examined their arm, and said that it belonged to the participant. In response, a number of highs claimed that the doctor was mistaken. In a confrontation, we asked participants to look at themselves in a mirror, focus on their arms, wiggle their fingers, and describe what they could see and how they felt. Some high hypnotisable participants claimed that their arm looked different and that they found it difficult to wiggle their fingers. We also developed a video challenge where we showed participants a video of a person with somatoparaphrenia. After watching the video we asked participants to describe their reactions to the person. Rather than saying that the person in the video was mistaken, some of our highs said that the video reinforced their deluded beliefs and helped them make sense of their experience.

In our hypnotic analogues of mirrored-self misidentification, we have used a graded series of first person, second person and third person challenges designed to map the challenges used by clinical neuropsychologists with delusional clients. Our first person challenges include questions about appearance such as "how is it possible that you and the person you see in the mirror look so similar?" Second person challenges involve the experimenter appearing in the mirror beside participants and asking "who else do you see in the mirror", and "if there are two people in the room and two people in the mirror, who must the people in the mirror be?" Third person challenges involve behavioural tasks such as asking participants to touch their nose while looking in the mirror and asking "what did the person in the mirror do?, "why did they do that?, and "how do you explain that the person you can see always does exactly what you do?" The following excerpt illustrates one participant's response to this particular challenge:

Hypnotist: I'd like you to touch your nose with your finger.
Participant: He's copying me *(participant laughs)*.
Hypnotist: What did he do?
Participant: He touched his nose *(participant laughs and looks behind him)*.
Hypnotist: What do you think he did that?
Participant: Maybe he's trying to make me seem like I'm crazy or something.

In response to this nose-touching challenge, 94% of high hypnotisable participants maintained their delusion. The most effective challenge involved the hypnotist appearing in the mirror alongside participants. This challenge breached the delusion for approximately 33% of highs (Connors et al., 2008). One reason why this challenge may be so effective is because it diverts participants' attention away from the mirror and asks them to calculate the number of people in the room. Subsequently, they seem to infer that the two people in the mirror must be the same as the two people in the room. However, we found that some highs will maintain their suggested mirror delusion across an entire series of graded challenges. Just like clinical patients, highs can provide a myriad of explanations when confronted with evidence that contradicts their delusional beliefs.

Overall, these challenge procedures indicate that hypnotic delusions are credible, realistic, and held with strong conviction. Highs do not ignore information that contradicts their suggested experiences. Rather, when confronted with challenging information, they appear to interpret it in a way that is consistent with their delusion by generating explanations that support their delusion (see also Burn et al., 2001).

Autobiographical memory during hypnotic delusions

In addition to establishing a hypnotic paradigm that closely maps the features of clinical delusions we have also been interested in the impact of reverse intermetamorphosis on autobiographical memory. Empirical work on autobiographical remembering during delusions has been both limited and mixed (see Baddeley et al., 1996, Corcoran & Frith, 2003, and Kaney, Bowen-Jones, & Bentall, 1999, for mixed findings on memory specificity among deluded individuals). However, clinical cases suggest that autobiographical memories are often distorted during delusions (Baddeley et al., 1996; Breen et al., 2000). Deluded individuals appear to recall memories that "serve" their delusional beliefs. For example, Breen et al. (2000) described the case of a woman known as RZ who suffered from reverse intermetamorphosis and believed she was her father. When RZ's delusion was challenged, she continued to maintain that she was a man and recalled a memory about having an operation to make her look like a woman. She said "I have a man's voice and I've got a man's legs so I can't be female, because Dr R gave me injections in the arm to grow breasts and they castrated me about, in the hospital … I just remember going with Wayne and whoever is out on the farm, Doug, I remember going with him to C_____ and having an operation and I woke up … and I said 'oh yes, it's been done.' Those were my first words when I woke up" (p. 96). This memory served RZ's delusional belief because it explained why she had man's voice and a woman's body.

To investigate how a hypnotic suggestion for reverse intermetamorphosis influences autobiographical remembering, we asked participants to elicit memories during a suggested delusion. We used participants' responses to an "I am" task to cue specific memories (Kuhn & McPartland, 1954; Rathbone et al., 2008). For example, if participants said "I am confident" we asked them to describe a specific event from their (deluded identity's) past that illustrated this. Across four experiments we found that highs were more likely to generate specific memories than lows: 86% of highs' memories were specific, whereas only 43% of lows' memories were specific (where specific memories were unique events with an identifiable beginning and end as defined by Conway & Pleydell-Pearce, 2000). Also, when challenged, highs provided more justification for having personally experienced their memories than lows. Notably, highs rarely fabricated memories but 30% of lows' memories were fabrications. Highs preferred to recall memories of previously experienced events, but reinterpreted these in light of their delusion and viewed them from the perspective of their deluded identity (Cox, 2007; Cox & Barnier, 2009a).

Together, these findings suggest that during a hypnotic delusion for reverse intermetamorphosis memories consistent with the suggested identity are facilitated. In our work, highs selectively recalled, reinterpreted and built upon memories that supported their deluded identity rather than completely fabricating new events. This is similar to many clinically deluded patients such as RZ (Breen et al., 2000) who appear to remember events that serve their delusions. RZ had been hospitalised on a number of previous occasions and also suffered from hirsutism (excessive hair growth), which was so severe that she needed to shave her face. It is possible that she conflated, reinterpreted, and built upon these experiences, resulting in a "memory" of a sex-change operation. Such memories may provide deluded individuals with evidence for their delusional beliefs. This type of selective and reconstructive remembering may reinforce a delusion and thereby contribute towards its maintenance. Conway and Tacchi (1996) have made a similar argument in their discussion of autobiographical confabulations. They suggest that such confabulations may be reconstructions of existing autobiographical memories rather than entirely new memories. They argue that these reconstructions may help individuals maintain a positive sense of self. The degree to which clinically deluded patients and hypnotic subjects reinterpret and build upon existing memories versus fabricate entirely new memories is an area for future research. However, it is typically difficult to judge the accuracy of autobiographical memories unless they are bizarre or contradicted by other individuals who were present at the time.

INTERPRETATIONS, IMPLICATIONS, CHALLENGES, AND FUTURE DIRECTIONS

Our programme of research indicates that a hypnotic suggestion can produce credible, compelling delusions with features similar to their clinical counterparts (Bortolotti et al., 2009). Hypnotic delusions are most effective for high hypnotisable individuals who receive a formal hypnotic induction (the suggestion can be experienced by highs who receive imagination instructions, but their experience is less compelling; Cox & Barnier, 2009a). Importantly, response to the hypnotic delusion cannot be explained simply in terms of the demands of the experimental procedure because we have consistently found differences in the reactions of real, hypnotised participants and simulating participants (e.g., in response to challenges and in autobiographical memories elicited during the delusion; Burn et al., 2001; Cox, 2007; Noble & McConkey, 1995). In striving to recreate clinical delusions, we have found three striking similarities between clinical cases and our hypnotic analogues. These include: (1) the phenomenological features of clinical and hypnotic delusions, (2) the resistance to challenge displayed by hypnotic and clinically deluded individuals, and (3) the features of autobiographical memory during hypnotic and clinical delusions.

First, in terms of phenomenological features, all our fully formed hypnotic delusion suggestions and our hypnotic Factor 1 alone suggestion for mirrored-self misidentification have successfully recreated features displayed by clinically deluded patients. For example, in reverse intermetamorphosis, clinical patients may believe themselves to be a variety of different identities. Likewise, our hypnotic paradigm was effective across a range of identities—real and nonexistent, similar and dissimilar, familiar and unfamiliar (Cox, 2007; Cox & Bryant, 2008). Also, in mirrored-self misidentification, both clinically and hypnotically deluded individuals make attempts to converse with the person in the mirror and may express frustration at not being able to converse normally with the person (Breen et al., 2000). In our hypnotic analogue, one participant said, "he's saying something but I can't understand". When asked why he couldn't understand he said, "because I can't lip read" (Barnier et al., 2008). Notably, our hypnotised individuals, like their clinical counterparts, often expressed discomfort at seeing a stranger in the mirror. They made comments such as: "I felt kind of weird seeing someone just stare at me that close", and "I didn't trust the other person". This suspicion is reminiscent of clinical patients who may cover all the mirrors in their house because they dislike the idea of a stranger peering out at them (Breen et al., 2000).

Second, in terms of resistance to challenge, both clinical and hypnotic delusions are maintained with conviction even in the face of rational counterarguments or evidence to the contrary. During our challenge procedures for reverse intermetamorphosis, somatoparaphrenia, and mirrored-self misidentification (e.g., contradiction, confrontation, graded challenges), the majority of highs maintained their deluded beliefs. For example, in hypnotic reverse intermetamorphosis subjects claimed that they could see someone else when asked to look at themselves on a monitor. And, in the hypnotic mirrored-self misidentification delusion, subjects claimed that their family would have no trouble distinguishing them from the stranger in the mirror and said that the stranger was copying their actions (e.g., touching their nose). Thus, just like clinical patients, our hypnotically deluded individuals had no difficulty generating reasons to explain and justify their (temporary) deluded beliefs.

Third, in terms of autobiographical memory, in both clinical and hypnotic delusions that influence identity (e.g., reverse intermetamorphosis), individuals recall autobiographical memories that serve their delusion. Like clinically deluded individuals, hypnotic subjects recall these autobiographical events from the perspective of their deluded identity. For example, the patient RZ who believed she was her father, adopted her father's perspective when recalling a memory that involved both her father and herself, making comments such as "I kicked RZ out of the house when she was living there." This change in perspective during a delusion (whether clinical or hypnotic) may help to reinforce the conviction that memories are of self-experienced events, which in turn may help to render these delusions resistant to challenge.

It is worth noting here that across all our studies, the comments and reactions of our hypnotically deluded participants were essentially spontaneous. The delusion suggestions to become another person or to see a stranger in the mirror, for instance, provided very little information about how to react and what such an experience might be like. Our participants were first- and second-year undergraduate students and it is unlikely that they would have knowledge about the delusions that we were attempting to recreate. It is therefore quite remarkable that their reactions so closely mimicked those of clinically deluded individuals. It indicates that a hypnotic suggestion, when coupled with less stringent criteria for evaluating beliefs (produced by the hypnotic state), is sufficient to create a complex and compelling delusional experience. Whereas our hypnotic delusions are able to model many features of clinical delusions, there are important differences between clinical and hypnotic delusions, which we must acknowledge and address in future research.

First, there are differences in the longevity of clinical and hypnotic delusions. Typically, hypnotic effects are confined to the hypnotic setting. In contrast, clinical delusions persist over time, and often in the face of much stronger challenges (e.g., persistent challenges from family and friends).

However, some hypnotic effects can continue outside of the hypnotic context. For instance, Barnier and McConkey (1998) gave participants a posthypnotic suggestion that they would feel compelled to mail a postcard every single day to the experimenter and indeed, some high hypnotisable individuals mailed postcards everyday for up to 16 weeks! It remains to be tested whether hypnotically suggested beliefs, especially delusions, can be maintained outside the hypnotic context and over long periods of time.

Second, the intensity and behavioural consequences of clinical and hypnotic delusions are markedly different (Kopelman, 2007). For instance, in mirrored-self misidentification, the belief that one's reflection is that of a stranger might be so overwhelming that the person avoids looking in the mirror and covers up all the mirrors in the house (as in the case of TH; Breen et al., 2000). In Capgras delusion, the belief that someone emotionally close, such as a family member, has been replaced by an impostor, is occasionally accompanied by acts of violence (Bourget & Whitehurst, 2004; for discussion of the classic case of a son who decapitated his father in the belief that the father was a robot, see Stone & Young, 1997). However, the range of behavioural responses to the Capgras delusion is variable (for discussion, see Davies et al., 2002). Although we think it unlikely that hypnotic suggestions would ever engender beliefs that lead to such extreme or criminal behaviour, there is strong evidence from clinical applications of hypnosis that hypnotic suggestions can lead to significant and long lasting cognitive and behavioural changes, at least until they are cancelled and perhaps even after cancellation (Nash & Barnier, 2008).

Third, clinical and hypnotic delusions may differ in their aetiology. A number of clinical delusions are thought to arise when a neuropsychological impairment (e.g., brain injury) produces perceptual and/or affective deficits, combined with faulty belief evaluation processes (Langdon & Coltheart, 2000). In contrast, hypnotic delusions arise due to a combination of cognitive (e.g., dissociative) and social/motivational processes. Notably, however, Langdon, Coltheart, and colleagues have acknowledged that some clinical delusions may involve a motivated or functional disruption in information processing (McKay et al., 2005), rather than a neuropsychological impairment (e.g., persecutory delusions). Hypnosis may be best suited to modelling these sorts of delusions. This is supported by research we described earlier on hypnotic analogues of conversion disorder paralysis. Halligan, Oakley, and colleagues reported that the patterns of brain activation in a clinical case of conversion disorder paralysis were remarkably similar to the patterns in a hypnotic analogue. They argued that these clinical and hypnotic versions shared the same neural underpinnings (Halligan et al., 2000; see also Barnier & Oakley, 2009; Oakley, 2006). In a similar way, hypnotic analogues may be able to model both the features and underlying neural processes involved in certain types of delusions.

Fourth, clinical and hypnotic delusions differ in the extent to which individuals may be aware of the source of their difficulties. After giving participants a hypnotic Factor 1 suggestion for somatoparaphrenia, we administered accompanying amnesia for this Factor 1 suggestion. We administer this amnesia suggestion to model neuropsychological cases where clinical patients may have a Factor 1 deficit that they are unaware of. For instance, a clinical patient with mirrored-self misidentification may have lost the ability to recognise faces (Factor 1) and will also be unaware of this Factor 1 deficit. Our hypnotic amnesia suggestion creates a similar lack of awareness in hypnotically deluded subjects for the content of their hypnotic experience. However, we acknowledge that during hypnotic delusions, individuals are potentially aware of the source of their deficits. This is because the hypnotic amnesia is reversible, they may have implicit awareness of the hypnotic suggestion (Schacter, 1987), and they are likely to be motivated to experience the suggested effects (Sheehan, 1991).

Extending our hypnotic analogues to confabulation

We can extend this instrumental use of hypnosis to explore whether hypnosis can model other pathological conditions (see Oakley & Halligan, 2009). One condition we are currently focusing on is clinical confabulation. Just like delusional patients, confabulators may believe and remember extraordinary, clearly false things. Confabulating patients might mistakenly remember, for instance, that "I had a huge argument with my [long dead] father yesterday" (Downes & Mayes, 1994) or "I met my friend's mother; she had the head of a bee" (Turner & Coltheart, 2010 this issue). Although both delusions and confabulations involve distortions of reality, they are generally considered distinct pathologies, demanding different explanations and treatments (Kopelman, Guinan, & Lewis, 1995). But Langdon, Coltheart, and colleagues recently proposed that confabulations can be understood by extending their influential two-factor theory of delusions (Metcalf et al., 2007). By their view, we don't need to distinguish between the two pathologies. We just need to answer the same two questions: (1) What generates the false proposition (belief or memory) in the first place? (2) Once generated, why isn't it rejected as untrue? This positioning of the two-factor theory as a common explanatory framework has generated much interest and controversy, and needs to be tested. To do this, we can use hypnosis to create temporary versions of confabulations.

Confabulations involve the "production of fabricated, distorted, or misinterpreted memories about one's self or the world without the conscious intention to deceive" (Fotopoulou et al., 2007, p. 6). Like delusions, they are common in dementia, schizophrenia, and after traumatic brain injury. The richness and specificity of these false memories is illustrated by a male patient, who started to confabulate after brain surgery. In the following excerpt from Fotopoulou et al. (2007), he describes seeing an ophthalmologist.

Patient:	I used to come and he used to try my eyes and say "that eye, the lens is not working properly". He used to take the lens off, polish it, or replace it.
Examiner:	The lens in your spectacles?
Patient:	No, my eyes.

There is no single theory of confabulations but they may involve: (1) inefficient/disrupted memory retrieval leading to the inability to adequately specify a sought after memory (Moscovitch & Melo, 1997), (2) temporal confusion, where fragments of different memories are inappropriately conjoined, or where previous memories are reexperienced as current (Dalla Barba, Cappelletti, Signorini, & Denes, 1997), and/or (3) poor reality monitoring, where elements of imagination and memory are inappropriately combined and never experienced events are misattributed as real (Johnson, Hashtroudi, & Lindsay, 1993). Some argue that motivation combines with these processes to influence the content of confabulations (Fotopoulou et al., 2007). Laying aside these explanations, there is a strong view that delusions and confabulations are distinct pathologies (Kopelman et al., 1995). Delusions are supposed to be fixed, held with conviction, resistant to counterargument, and acted on, whereas confabulations are supposed to be fleeting, quickly abandoned, and generally not acted on. But recent clinical reports highlight overlap and confusion. For instance, whereas a delusional patient's conviction in their false belief may wax and wane, a confabulator may report the same false memory day after day (Turner & Coltheart, 2010 this issue; see also Coltheart, 2007). And some people show both delusion and confabulation according to established criteria, which makes diagnosis extremely challenging. In light of these overlaps, Langdon, Coltheart, and colleagues proposed that confabulations may be understood by extending the two-factor theory (Metcalf et al., 2007). By their view, both delusions and confabulations involve a distinct Factor 1, a broken process that generates the false belief or memory, and a common Factor 2, a broken process that impairs evaluation.

We have identified three pathways—potential Factor 1s—to confabulation. With hypnosis we can recreate these Factor 1 impairments and the common Factor 2 impairment. As in our delusion paradigm, we can compare fully formed confabulation suggestions, Factor 1 plus Factor 2 suggestions, and Factor 1 alone, inside and outside hypnosis. Confabulators are also typically amnesic to varying extents, suggesting that amnesia may be a necessary component of clinical confabulation. Using hypnosis, we can recreate the three versions of confabulation described previously (see Table 2 for examples): (1) To recreate the inability to adequately specify a sought-after memory, we can suggest complete or partial amnesia for a life period or event, combined with a suggestion to fill in any gaps in memory (while we note that the inability to specify a sought-after memory occurs as a consequence of a retrieval disruption, our current suggestion is an attempt to convert this hypothesised retrieval disruption into a hypnotic suggestion); (2) to recreate temporal confusion we can suggest confusion for the sequence of events or suggest the inappropriate conjunction of two events; and (3) to recreate the inappropriate combination of imagination and memories due to poor reality monitoring, we can suggest imagination inflation for never experienced events. Additionally, as a control condition, we can examine the impact of amnesia alone as Factor 1 and combine this with a Factor 2 suggestion for difficulty evaluating the reality and accuracy of memories.

In our current work, we are giving participants a hypnotic suggestion to either: (1) forget everything that has happened to them since they started university, (2) forget everything that has happened to them since they started university plus a suggestion to fill in gaps in their memory, or (3) forget the correct order of events that have happened since they started university. We are indexing response to the suggestions by asking highs to complete a modified confabulation battery (Dalla Barba et al., 1997) consisting of personal semantic information (e.g., name, age), episodic memories, and impossible questions (where the answer should be "I don't know"). After hypnosis, highs indicate whether they confabulated and rate the qualities (e.g., vividness, emotionality) and source their memories.

CONCLUSION

Research indicates that hypnosis is a powerful technique to investigate (as well as treat) complex clinical phenomena. Our instrumental use of hypnosis allows us to explore aspects of delusions that have been either neglected in research or difficult to study in the laboratory. Our hypnotic techniques offer a new way to explore the separate and combined effects of Factor 1 and Factor 2 in delusions. They also offer a novel technique for examining Langdon and Coltheart's (2000) two-factor theory of delusions and its controversial extension to confabulation. By developing hypnotic versions of delusions and confabulations, this research can improve our understanding of these conditions and provide an important link between the clinic and the laboratory. In this way, our research adds to a long tradition in the field of hypnosis, and will have both theoretical and practical benefits for the fields of delusion and confabulation.

REFERENCES

Baddeley, A. D., Thornton, A., Chua, S. E., & McKenna, P. (1996). Schizophrenic delusions and the construction of autobiographical memory. In D. C. Rubin (Ed.), *Remembering our past: Studies in autobiographical memory* (pp. 384–428). Cambridge, UK: Cambridge University Press.

Barber, T. X., & Wilson, S. C. (1978). The Barber Suggestibility Scale and the Creative Imagination Scale: Experimental and clinical applications. *American Journal of Clinical Hypnosis, 21*, 84–108.

Barnier, A. J. (2002). Posthypnotic amnesia for autobiographical episodes: A laboratory model of functional amnesia? *Psychological Science, 13*, 232–237.

Barnier, A. J., Cox, R. E., O'Connor, A., Coltheart, M., Langdon, R., Breen, N., & Turner, M. (2008). Developing hypnotic analogues of clinical delusions: Mirrored-self misidentification. *Cognitive Neuropsychiatry, 13*, 406–430.

Barnier, A. J., & McConkey, K. M. (1998). Posthypnotic responding: Knowing when to stop helps to keep it going. *International Journal of Clinical and Experimental Hypnosis, 46*, 204–219.

Barnier, A. J., & McConkey, K. M. (2004). Defining and identifying the highly hypnotisable person. In M. Heap, R. J. Brown, & D. A. Oakley (Eds.), *The highly hypnotizable person: Theoretical, experimental and clinical issues* (pp. 30–61). Hove, UK: Brunner-Routledge.

Barnier, A. J., & Oakley, D. A. (2009). Hypnosis and suggestion. In W. P. Banks (Ed.), *Encyclopaedia of consciousness* (pp. 351–368). Oxford, UK: Elsevier.

Bortolotti, L., Cox, R. E., & Barnier, A. J. (2009). Can we create delusions in the laboratory? *Manuscript submitted for publication.*

Bourget, D., & Whitehurst, L. (2004). Capgras syndrome: A review of the neurophysiological correlates and presenting clinical features in cases involving physical violence. *Canadian Journal of Psychiatry, 49*, 719–725.

Breen, N., Caine, D., Coltheart, M., Hendy, J., & Roberts, C. (2000). Towards an understanding of delusions of misidentification: Four case studies. *Mind and Language, 15*(1), 74–110.

Bryant, R. A., & McConkey, K. M. (1989a). Hypnotic blindness: A behavioural and experiential analysis. *Journal of Abnormal Psychology, 98*, 71–77.

Bryant, R. A., & McConkey, K. M. (1989b). Hypnotic blindness, awareness, and attribution. *Journal of Abnormal Psychology, 98*, 443–447.

Burn, C., Barnier, A. J., & McConkey, K. M. (2001). Information processing during hypnotically suggested sex change. *International Journal of Clinical and Experimental Hypnosis, 49*, 231–242.

Coltheart, M. (2007). The 33rd Bartlett Lecture: Cognitive neuropsychiatry and delusional belief. *Quarterly Journal of Experimental Psychology, 60*, 1041–1062.

Coltheart, M., Langdon, R., & McKay, R. (2007). Schizophrenia and monothematic delusions. *Schizophrenia Bulletin, 33*, 642–647.

Connors, M., Cox, R. E., & Barnier A. J. (2008, October). *A stranger in the looking glass: Challenging hypnotic delusions of mirrored-self misidentification.* Paper presented at the annual conference of the Society for Clinical and Experimental Hypnosis, King of Prussia, PA, USA.

Conway, M. A., & Pleydell-Pearce, C. W. (2000). The construction of autobiographical memories in the self-memory system. *Psychological Review, 107*, 261–288.

Conway, M. A., & Tacchi, P. C. (1996). Motivated confabulation. *Neurocase, 2*, 325–339.

Corcoran, R., & Frith, C. D. (2003). Autobiographical memory and theory of mind: Evidence of a relationship in schizophrenia. *Psychological Medicine, 33*, 897–905.

Cox, R. E. (2007). Autobiographical memory during hypnotic identity delusions. Unpublished doctoral dissertation, University of New South Wales, Australia.

Cox, R. E., & Barnier, A. J. (2003). Posthypnotic amnesia for a first romantic relationship: Forgetting the entire relationship versus forgetting selected events. *Memory, 11*, 307–318.

Cox, R. E., & Barnier, A. J. (2009a). Hypnotic illusions and clinical delusions: A hypnotic paradigm for investigating delusions of misidentification. *International Journal of Clinical and Experimental Hypnosis, 57*, 1–32.

Cox, R. E., & Barnier, A. J. (2009b). Selective information processing in hypnotic identity delusion: The impact of time of encoding and retrieval. *Contemporary Hypnosis, 26*, 65–79.

Cox, R. E., & Bryant, R. A. (2008). Advances in hypnosis research: Methods, designs, and contributions of intrinsic and instrumental hypnosis. In M. R. Nash & A. J. Barnier (Eds.), *The Oxford handbook of hypnosis: Theory, research and practice* (pp. 311–336). Oxford, UK: Oxford University Press.

Crawford, H. J. (1994). Brain dynamics and hypnosis: Attentional and disattentional processes. *International Journal of Clinical and Experimental Hypnosis, 42*, 204–232.

Dalla Barba, G., Cappelletti, J. Y., Signorini, M., & Denes, G. (1997). Confabulation: Remembering "another" past, planning "another" future. *Neurocase, 3*, 425–436.

Davies, M., Coltheart, M., Langdon, R., & Breen, N. (2002). Monothematic delusions: Towards a two-factor account. *Philosophy, Psychiatry, and Psychology, 8*, 133–158.

Downes, J. J., & Mayes, A. R. (1994). How bad memories can sometimes lead to fantastic beliefs and strange visions. In R. Campbell & M. A. Conway (Eds.), *Broken memories: Case studies in the neuropsychology of memory* (pp. 115–123). Oxford, UK: Blackwell.

Fotopoulou, A., Conway, M. A., Griffiths, P., Birchall, D., & Tyrer, S. (2007). Self-enhancing confabulation: Revisiting the motivational hypothesis. *Neurocase, 13*, 6–15.

Frith, C. D., & Done, D. J. (1989). Experiences of alien control in schizophrenia reflect a disorder in the central monitoring of action. *Psychological Medicine, 19*, 359–363.

Haggard, P., Cartledge, P., Dafydd, M., & Oakley, D. A. (2004). Anomalous control: When "free will" is not conscious. *Consciousness and Cognition, 13*, 646–654.

Halligan, P. W., Athwal, B. S., Oakley, D. A., & Frackowiak, R. S. J. (2000). Imaging hypnotic paralysis: Implications for conversion hysteria. *The Lancet, 355*, 986–987.

Higgins, E. T. (1987). Self-discrepancy: A theory relating self and affect. *Psychological Review, 94*, 319–340.

Hilgard, E. R. (1965). *Hypnotic susceptibility*. New York: Harcourt, Brace & World.

Hilgard, J. R. (1965). Personality and hypnotisability: Inferences from case studies. In E. R. Hilgard (Ed.), *Hypnotic susceptibility* (pp. 343–374). New York: Harcourt, Brace & World.

Johnson, M. K., Hashtroudi, S., & Lindsay, D. S. (1993). Source monitoring. *Psychological Bulletin, 114*, 3–28.

Johnson, M. K., & Raye, C. L. (1998). False memories and confabulation. *Trends in Cognitive Sciences, 2*, 137–145.

Kaney, S., Bowen-Jones, K., & Bentall, R. P. (1999). Persecutory delusions and autobiographical memory. *British Journal of Clinical Psychology, 38*, 97–102.

Kihlstrom, J. F. (2008). The domain of hypnosis, revisited. In M. R. Nash & A. J. Barnier (Eds.), *The Oxford handbook of hypnosis: Theory, research and practice* (pp. 21–52). Oxford, UK: Oxford University Press.

Kihlstrom, J. F., & Hoyt, I. P. (1988). Hypnosis and the psychology of delusions. In T. F. Oltmanns & B. A. Maher (Eds.), *Delusional beliefs* (pp. 66–109). Oxford, UK: Wiley.

Kopelman, M. (2007, July). *Varieties of confabulation and delusion*. Invited talk presented at the Delusions and Confabulations workshop, Macquarie Centre for Cognitive Science, Sydney, Australia.

Kopelman, M. D., Guinan, E. M., & Lewis, P. D. R. (1995). Delusional memory, confabulation and frontal lobe dysfunction. In R. Campbell & M. A. Conway (Eds.), *Broken memories: Case studies in memory impairment* (pp. 137–153). Oxford, UK: Blackwell.

Kuhn, M. H., & McPartland, T. S. (1954). An empirical investigation of self attitudes. *American Sociological Review, 19*, 68–76.

Langdon, R., & Coltheart, M. (2000). The cognitive neuropsychology of delusions. *Mind and Language, 15*, 184–218.

Langdon, R., McKay, R., & Coltheart, M. (2008). The cognitive neuropsychological understanding of persecutory delusions. In D. Freeman, R. Bentall, & P. Garety (Eds.), *Persecutory delusions: Assessment, theory and treatment* (pp. 221–236). Oxford, UK: Oxford University Press.

Marshall, J. C., Halligan, P. W., Fink, G. R., Wade, D. T., & Frackowiak, R. S. J. (1997). The functional anatomy of a hysterical paralysis. *Cognition, 64*, B1–B8.

McConkey, K. M. (2008). Generations and landscape of hypnosis: Questions we've asked, questions we should ask. In M. R. Nash & A. J. Barnier (Eds.), *The Oxford handbook of hypnosis: Theory, research and practice* (pp. 53–77). Oxford, UK: Oxford University Press.

McConkey, K. M., Szeps, A., & Barnier, A. J. (2001). Indexing the experience of sex change in hypnosis and imagination. *International Journal of Clinical and Experimental Hypnosis, 49*, 123–138.

McKay, R., & Kinsbourne, M. (2010). Motivational factors and false claims. *Cognitive Neuropsychiatry, 15*(1/2/3), 288–318.

McKay, R., Langdon, R., & Coltheart, M. (2005). Sleights of mind: Delusions, defences, and self-deception. *Cognitive Neuropsychiatry, 10*, 305–326.

McKay, R., Langdon, R., & Coltheart, M. (2007). The defensive function of persecutory delusions: An investigation using the implicit association test. *Cognitive Neuropsychiatry, 12*, 1–24.

Metcalf, K., Coltheart, M., & Langdon, R. (2007). Models of confabulation: A critical review and a new framework. *Cognitive Neuropsychology, 24*, 23–47.

Moscovitch, M., & Melo, B. (1997). Strategic retrieval and the frontal lobes: Evidence from confabulation and amnesia. *Neuropsychologia, 35*, 1017–1034.

Nash, M. R., & Barnier, A. J. (2008). *The Oxford handbook of hypnosis: Theory, research and practice.* Oxford, UK: Oxford University Press.

Noble, J., & McConkey, K. M. (1995). Hypnotic sex change: Creating and challenging a delusion in the laboratory. *Journal of Abnormal Psychology, 104*, 69–74.

Oakley, D. A. (2006). Hypnosis as a tool in research: Experimental psychopathology. *Contemporary Hypnosis, 23*, 3–14.

Oakley, D. A., & Halligan, P. W. (2009). Hypnotic suggestion and cognitive neuroscience. *Trends in Cognitive Sciences, 13*, 264–270.

Orne, M. T. (1959). The nature of hypnosis: Artifact and essence. *Journal of Abnormal and Social Psychology, 58*, 277–279.

Orne, M. T. (1962). On the social psychology of the psychological experiment: With particular reference to demand characteristics and their implications. *The American Psychologist, 17*(11), 776–783.

Rahmanovic, A., Barnier, A. J., & Cox, R. E. (2009). An hypnotic analogue of the somatoparaphrenia delusion: Recreating the delusion, testing the proposed factors, and challenging experiences. *Manuscript in preparation.*

Rathbone, C. J., Moulin, C. J. A., & Conway, M. A. (2008). Self-centred memories: The reminiscence bump and the self. *Memory and Cognition, 36,* 1403–1414.

Raz, A., Shapiro, T., Fan, J., & Posner, M. I. (2002). Hypnotic suggestion and the modulation of Stroop interference. *Archives of General Psychiatry, 59*, 1155–1161.

Schacter, D. L. (1987). Implicit memory: History and current status. *Journal of Experimental Psychology: Learning, Memory, and Cognition, 13*(3), 501–518.

Scott, A., Barnier, A. J., & Cox, R. E. (2009). Creating an hypnotic analogue of a delusion of alien control. *Manuscript in preparation.*

Sheehan, P. W. (1991). Hypnosis, context, and commitment. In S. J. Lynn & J. W. Rhue (Eds.), *Theories of hypnosis: Current models and perspectives* (pp. 520–541). New York: Guilford Press.

Stirling, J. D., Hellewell, J. S. E., & Ndlovu, D. (2001). Self-monitoring dysfunction and the positive symptoms of schizophrenia. *Psychopathology, 34*, 198–202.

Stirling, J. D., Hellewell, J. S. E., & Quraishi, N. (1998). Self-monitoring and schizophrenic symptoms of alien control. *Psychological Medicine, 28*, 675–683.

Stone, T., & Young, A. (1997). Delusions and brain injury: The philosophy and psychology of belief. *Mind and Language, 12*, 327–364.

Sutcliffe, J. P. (1961). "Credulous" and "skeptical" views of hypnotic phenomena: Experiments on esthesia, hallucination, and delusion. *Journal of Abnormal and Social Psychology, 62*, 189–200.

Szechtman, H., Woody, E., Bowers, K., & Nahmias, C. (1998). Where the imaginal appears real: A positron emission tomography study of auditory hallucinations. *Proceedings of the National Academy of Sciences, 95*, 1956–1960.

Tellegen, A., & Atkinson, G. (1974). Openness to absorbing and self-altering experiences ("absorption"), a trait related to hypnotic susceptibility. *Journal of Abnormal Psychology, 83*, 268–277.

Turner, M. (2006, July). *Confabulations, delusion, and déjà vu*. Paper presented at the fourth international conference on Memory, Sydney, Australia.

Turner, M., & Coltheart, M. (2010). Confabulation and delusion: A common monitoring framework? *Cognitive Neuropsychiatry, 15*(1/2/3), 346–376.

Ward, N. S., Oakley, D. A., Frackowiak, R. S. J., & Halligan, P. W. (2003). Differential brain activations during intentionally simulated and subjectively experienced paralysis. *Cognitive Neuropsychiatry, 8*, 295–312.

Woody, E. Z., & Sadler, P. (2008). Dissociation theories of hypnosis. In M. R. Nash & A. J. Barnier (Eds.), *The Oxford handbook of hypnosis: Theory, research and practice* (pp. 189–221). Oxford, UK: Oxford University Press.

Young, A. W. (2000). Wondrous strange: The neuropsychology of abnormal beliefs. *Mind and Language, 15*, 47–73.

Zimbardo, P. G., Andersen, S. M., & Kabat, L. G. (1981). Induced hearing deficit generates experimental paranoia. *Science, 212*, 1529–1531.

COGNITIVE NEUROPSYCHIATRY
2010, 15 (1/2/3), 233–260

The misidentification syndromes as mindreading disorders

William Hirstein
Elmhurst College, Elmhurst, IL, USA

The patient with Capgras' syndrome claims that people very familiar to him have been replaced by impostors. I argue that this disorder is due to the destruction of a representation that the patient has of the mind of the familiar person. This creates the appearance of a familiar body and face, but without the familiar personality, beliefs, and thoughts. The posterior site of damage in Capgras' is often reported to be the temporoparietal junction, an area that has a role in the mindreading system, a connected system of cortical areas that allow us to attribute mental states to others. Just as the Capgras' patient claims that that man is not his father, the patient with asomatognosia claims that his arm is not really his. A similar account applies here, in that a nearby brain area, the supramarginal gyrus, is damaged. This area works in concert with the temporoparietal junction and other areas to produce a large representation of a mind inside a body situated in an environment. Damage to the mind-representing part of this system (coupled with damage to executive processes in the prefrontal lobes) causes Capgras' syndrome, whereas damage to the body-representing part of this system (also coupled with executive damage) causes asomatognosia.

Keywords: Capgras' syndrome; Misidentification; Asomatognosia; Theory of mind; Mindreading; Executive processes.

INTRODUCTION

Capgras' syndrome is a misidentification disorder in which people deny the identities of people close to them, claiming that they have been replaced by impostors. Patients with *anosognosia* deny having a disability that they obviously have, and may even deny that an injured arm or leg is their own, a condition called *asomatognosia* (or sometimes *somatoparaphrenia*). These are the two oddest members of the family of confabulation syndromes, and the most difficult to assimilate to what is known about the others. A comprehensive theory of confabulation that encompasses these syndromes as well as the others could shed light on some extremely puzzling responses

Correspondence should be addressed to William Hirstein, Cognitive Science Laboratory, Elmhurst College, Elmhurst, IL 60126-3296, USA. E-mail: williamh@elmhurst.edu

 DOI: 10.1080/13546800903414891

to brain injury. Neurologist Todd Feinberg (2001) has proposed a hypothesis designed to encompass both the misidentification syndromes and asomatognosia, according to which they are disorders of the patient's sense of personal relatedness to other people and to his own body. In the subsequent sections, I will offer an alternative to Feinberg's view that brings these two syndromes under the tent of a two-factor hypothesis of confabulation (Hirstein, 2005). I will start by briefly describing the hypothesis, and conjoining it with a definition of the term "confabulation". Aside from showing that these two syndromes fit the suggested definition of "confabulation", and its accompanying two-factor hypothesis, my point in this paper is that we can understand why people have these strange beliefs if we understand the nature of the representation systems that, when damaged, produce them.

TWO-FACTOR HYPOTHESES OF CONFABULATION AND DELUSION

In 1787, speaking of confabulatory patients with Korsakoff's amnesia, John Coakley Lettsom (1789) said, "They talk freely in the intervals of mitigation, but of things that do not exist; they describe the presence of their friends, as if they saw realities, and reason tolerably clearly upon false premises." One year later, speaking of Cotard's syndrome patients (see later), Charles Bonnet said, "They usually draw apparently logical conclusions unfortunately on a completely unsubstantiated premise" (cited in Förstl & Beats, 1992). Both quotations imply a distinction between the "premises" of the reasoning process and that process itself. Perception and the memory store supply the premises for cognition, which then operates on them to produce effective actions. Indeed, one might argue that folk psychology itself, our everyday way of describing our minds, contains this distinction, since it applies separate concepts to perception and memory on the one hand (*see, hear, feel, recall*) and cognition on the other (*think, decide, plan*). Maher (1988) has a modern version of the accounts of Bonnet and Lettsom, arguing that certain delusions are false beliefs produced by a normal response to strange experiences. There is a powerful objection to this approach, however: Why doesn't the person simply use his ability to reason to reject the strange experience? We all experience strange thoughts on occasion, the feeling that someone is watching us; the odd notion that we had a causal influence on something where no reasonable physical explanation is available (e.g., I flip a light switch and a car horn honks outside); the idea that others can read our thoughts. But we are able to reject these, and not let them establish themselves as beliefs because we have the cognitive processes required to assess their plausibility. So it seems that in order for such thoughts to become beliefs, there needs to be a second problem at the cognitive level. A two-factor hypothesis of delusions finds its first full explicit form in 2000 (Langdon & Coltheart), followed a year later by a more general version of the hypothesis (Davies, Coltheart, Langdon, & Breen, 2001). More recently, Coltheart (2007) describes in greater detail the nature of the executive problems leading to the failure to reject anomalous beliefs. Those authors were focusing on delusions, but confabulation and delusion are closely related, at least in some syndromes, including Capgras' and asomatognosia. Confabulation and delusion cannot be entirely equated, since a confabulation is a claim made by person, whereas a delusion is a mental state, typically thought of as a belief. However, a confabulation can be made on the basis of a delusion, and this seems to be what happens in the case of Capgras' syndrome. The patient has the delusion that his father, for example, is an impostor, then produces a confabulation when he explicitly makes that claim. Metcalf, Langdon, and Coltheart (2007) broached the idea that a single, common monitoring framework fails at the second phase in both confabulation and delusion. Turner and Coltheart (2010 this issue) provide convincing evidence for this hypothesis.

Contemporary writers attempting to construct a definition of "confabulation" have despaired of the fact that some of the classical syndromes involve memory disorders (Korsakoff's, and a similar syndrome: aneurysm of the anterior communicating artery), whereas others involve problems of perception (anosognosia, split-brain syndrome, the misidentification disorders). Since memory and perception are both knowledge domains, however, perhaps a broader sense of "confabulation" applies to knowledge itself, or more specifically, to the making of knowledge claims. According to this approach, to confabulate is to confidently make an ill-grounded (and hence probably false) claim that one should know, but does not know, is ill-grounded (Hirstein, 2005). So envisaged, the confabulation syndromes do form a natural category, which can be further specified. Confabulations are the result of two different phases of error. The first occurs in one of the brain's epistemic systems, either mnemonic or perceptual. This produces an ill-grounded memory or perception. These malfunctioning perceptual or mnemonic processes tend to be located in the back half of the brain's cortex, in the temporal or parietal lobes. Second, even with plenty of time to assess the situation and with urging from doctors, therapists, and relatives, the patient fails to realise that his claim is flawed, due to a malfunction of higher level brain processes known collectively as executive processes, located in the prefrontal lobes. Nonconfabulating brains sometimes create flawed perceptions or memories, but we are able to correct them, using these executive processes. If I ask you whether you have ever seen the Eiffel Tower, for instance, your brain is happy to provide an image of the Tower, even if you've never been near it. But you are able to reject this as a real memory because you catch the mistake at the second phase before claiming that you have seen the Tower. Thus, the typical aetiology of confabulation involves damage in the posterior of the brain to some perceptual or mnemonic process, causing the first error stage, coupled with damage to some prefrontal process, causing the second error stage. The two events of damage need not occur at the same time; there are numerous cases in the literature in which patients with an existing site of brain damage began confabulating after damage to a second site.

If we understand confabulation as an epistemic problem then, the confabulation syndromes can be categorised as disorders of the brain's knowledge domains:

1. Knowledge of the body and its surroundings: anosognosia.
2. Knowledge of recent events involving oneself, i.e., autobiographical memories: Korsakoff's syndrome, anterior communicating artery syndrome.
3. Knowledge of other people: the misidentification syndromes.
4. Knowledge of our minds: split-brain syndrome.
5. Knowledge derived from visual perception: Anton's syndrome (denial of blindness).

Stated in terms of individually testable criteria, the recommended definition of "confabulation" is: S confabulates (that *p*) if and only if (Hirstein, 2005):

1. S claims that *p*.
2. S believes that *p*.
3. S thought that *p* is ill-grounded.
4. S does not know that her thought is ill-grounded.
5. S should know that her thought is ill-grounded.
6. S is confident that *p*.

The concept of *claiming* (rather than, for instance, *saying* or *asserting*) is broad enough to cover a wide variety of responses, including nonverbal responses such as drawing or pointing. The second criterion captures the sincerity of confabulators: They are not lying, and if explicitly asked, "Do you believe that *p*?" they will answer affirmatively. The third criterion refers to the problem that caused the flawed response to be generated in the first place (the first factor): Processes within the relevant knowledge domain were not acting optimally. The fourth criterion refers to a cognitive failure at a second phase (the second factor), the failure to check and reject the flawed response. The fifth criterion captures a normative element in our concept of confabulation: If the confabulator's brain were functioning properly, she would know that the claim is ill-grounded, and not make it. The claims made are about things any normal person would easily get right. This criterion also prevents the definition from applying too broadly. We do not consider theologians to be confabulating, for instance, even though their claims sometimes seem to be made on the basis of little evidence, because we do not expect people to know the answers to their questions. We do, however, expect people to know whether they can see, or move their arms, and we expect them to be able to recognise people they know. The sixth and last criterion refers to another important characteristic of confabulators routinely observed in the clinic: the serene certainty they have in their claims, even in the face of obvious disbelief by their listeners (see Langdon & Bayne, 2010 this issue, who discuss a similar quality of subjective certainty in patients with delusions). Research from multiple groups indicates that there may be an additional component at work in at least some cases of confabulation: The confabulator has a motive to believe that *p* (Feinberg, 2009; Fotopoulou, 2009, 2010 this issue; McKay & Kinsbourne, 2010 this issue).

This epistemic approach eliminates a problem endemic to the falsity criterion in the original; narrower definition of "confabulation", according to which confabulations are false memory reports (Berlyne, 1972). If a patient answers correctly, but out of luck, we still consider her to be confabulating. The problem is not the falsity of the patients' claims but rather their ill-groundedness and unreliability, at least in the affected domain. In shorter form then, in this epistemic view, to confabulate is to confidently make an ill-grounded claim that one should know, but does not know, is ill-grounded.

Capgras' syndrome

Neurological patients with Capgras' syndrome claim that people close to them, typically spouses, parents, or children, have been replaced by similar-looking impostors. When asked how they can tell that the person is an impostor, Capgras' patients will often confabulate. One patient claimed that she could tell her husband had been replaced because the new person tied his shoelaces differently; another patient said that the impostor of her son "had different-colored eyes, was not as big and brawny, and that her real son would not kiss her" (Frazer & Roberts, 1994, p. 557). A blind Capgras' patient said that the impostor's hand felt softer than his mother's (Rojo, Caballero, Iruela, & Baca, 1991). The patient's attitude towards the "impostor" can vary. The majority of Capgras' patients are suspicious of the "impostor" at the very least. Many are paranoid about the "impostor", and attribute intent to harm to him, but there are also cases where the patient's attitude is positive. Capgras' syndrome patients will sometimes even misidentify themselves as seen in photos, or even in a mirror (Hirstein

& Ramachandran, 1997; Silva & Leong, 1994, review 30 cases of Capgras' for oneself). Capgras' syndrome fits the pattern of damage seen in the memory syndromes: damage to some knowledge system, in this case a perceptual one, paired with frontal damage (Signer, 1994).

Asomatognosia

"Anosognosia" means lack of knowledge, or unawareness, of illness. First described in detail by Babinski in 1914, this unawareness can accompany certain types of paralysis caused by damage to the right inferior parietal cortex, and seems to play a role in causing an intriguing response known as *denial* in some patients. When asked about their disabilities, they will calmly and firmly deny that they are paralysed or weakened. The typical denial patient, interviewed as he rests in bed after a stroke that has paralysed his left arm, will claim that both arms are fine. When asked to touch the doctor's nose with his left arm the patient will move his torso slightly, then stop. When asked whether they touched the doctor's nose, some patients will say that they did; others will admit that they didn't but confabulate a reason why, such as that they are tired, don't feel like following commands right now, always had a weak left arm, and so on. Some of these patients will further deny that their brain injury has hampered or limited them in any way.

Although there is evidence that some anosognosic patients have some types of somatosensation, typically important higher level somatosensory areas are damaged. These posterior areas of damage, especially in the inferior parietal cortex, create the first malfunction needed for confabulation, but until recently no clear pattern of frontal damage had emerged in the study of anosognosia. In 2005, however, Berti et al. showed that patients who denied paralysis differed from those with paralysis but no denial in that the denial patients had additional damage in the frontal portions of a large brain network involved in the planning of motor actions. These frontal areas are directly connected to the damaged inferior parietal areas. Apparently, the frontal areas are capable of monitoring representations of intended actions generated by posterior areas in the same network. As Berti and her colleagues say, "monitoring systems may be implemented within the same cortical network that is responsible for the primary function that has to be monitored" (p. 488). Davies, Davies, and Coltheart (2005) contains a sustained defence of a two-factor hypothesis applied to all types of anosognosia.

Asomatognosia is regarded as a subtype of anosognosia. Patients with this syndrome will deny ownership of their own limbs. The patient will typically confabulate that the limb belongs to the doctor, or sometimes to a spouse or relative. They may claim that the arm "belongs to a fellow patient previously transported by ambulance, or that it had been forgotten in bed by a previous patient" (Bisiach & Geminiani, 1991). Patients tend not to elaborate these claims into more coherent stories, about how exactly a limb came to be left in bed, for instance, and they may stop responding and turn away if pressed further. The arm involved is almost always the left arm, and asomatognosia also occurs at a high frequency among patients whose right hemisphere is temporarily anaesthetised. Feinberg and his colleagues tested 12 patients with right hemisphere stroke damage for asomatognosia, by holding up the patient's left hand so that it was visible to him and asking, "What is this?" (Feinberg, Haber, & Leeds, 1990). The most common misidentification was calling the limb "your [the doctor's] hand", or "your arm". One patient referred to her limb as "a breast" and a "deodorant". One patient called it "my mother-in-law's" hand (Feinberg et al., 1990). Another patient called his arm a piece of "dead wood" (Weinstein, 1991); yet another called his "a piece of dead meat" (Critchley, 1974). "The idea that the arm is 'dead' in some sense, literally or figuratively, is common in anosognosia" according to Feinberg (2006, p. 75). Some patients claim that their flesh is rotting away (Fine, 2006). As Feinberg notes, asomatognosia may be regarded as a species of misidentification, in that the patients fail to acknowledge the true identity of their own arms.

Theories of the crucial neural locus for asomatognosia have focused on the inferior parietal lobes, particularly on the right side. The inferior parietal lobes are constituted by two gyri, the supramarginal gyrus (Brodmann's Area 40) and the angular gyrus (Brodmann's Area 39). Nielsen was the first to argue, in 1938, that the crucial site of damage leading to asomatognosia is the right supramarginal gyrus or its connections to subcortical areas. The study mentioned earlier by Feinberg et al. (1990) involving 12 asomatognosic patients supported this localisation.

THREE HYPOTHESES

In the cases of both Capgras' syndrome and asomatognosia, something very close and very familiar, a loved one or a body part, is claimed to be distant and unfamiliar. Jacques Vié (1930) was the first to explicitly mention this similarity (Feinberg & Roane, 1997). In this section, I will examine three candidate explanations for the misidentification syndromes and asomatognosia. According to what is known as the affective responsiveness hypothesis of Capgras' syndrome, the patient fails to experience the normal affective reaction to the sight of a familiar person, and this causes him to form the belief that the person is an impostor. This hypothesis seems to originate with Capgras' and Reboul-Lachaux's seminal article, in which they write, "the delusion of doubles is not ... really a sensory delusion, but rather the conclusion of an emotional judgment" (1923/1994). Many subsequent writers have argued that in Capgras' syndrome there is a disconnection between the representation of a face and what Ellis and Young refer to as "the evocation of affective memories" (1990, p. 243) (see also Bauer, 1986; Hirstein & Ramachandran, 1997; Staton, Brumback, & Wilson, 1982). The patients recognise a face, but do not feel the expected emotions, and confabulate to explain this: "When patients find themselves in such a conflict (that is, receiving some information which indicates the face in front of them belongs to X, but not receiving confirmation of this), they may adopt some sort of rationalisation strategy in which the individual before them is deemed to be an impostor, a dummy, a robot, or whatever extant technology may suggest" (Ellis & Young, 1990, p. 244).

What is the link, however, between the absence of an emotion and the creation of the impostor story? Why doesn't the patient merely say that people seem strange or unfamiliar to him? Stone and Young (1997, p. 344) add another ingredient, the patient's prior personality, suggesting that once the patient loses the normal affective reaction to faces and, "because of a co-existing suspicious mood, or maybe a premorbid disposition, the person arrives at the idea that the source of these strange experiences must lie in a change in the external world, and the possibility of some kind of a trick, perhaps involving a substitution presents itself". But why would so many different patients with different personalities, and different premorbid dispositions arrive at the same highly unlikely story about the same trick? It is also hard to see how the affective responsiveness hypothesis could be applied to asomatognosia (something its authors have not attempted). When applied to asomatognosia, the affective responsiveness hypothesis would generate the claim that we normally experience an affective reaction at the sight of our own arms, then confabulate that the arm is not our own in order to explain the absence of this reaction, which seems implausible.

The second hypothesis is the *personal relatedness* hypothesis of Feinberg. The Capgras' patient has lost his sense of personal relatedness to his father, while the asomatognosic has lost his sense of personal relatedness to his arm. "Asomatognosia can be understood as a Capgras syndrome for the arm in which the personal relationship with the body part is lost" (Feinberg, DeLuca, Giacino, Roane, & Solms, 2005, p. 103). Feinberg points out an intriguing asymmetry between Capgras' and asomatognosia on one hand, and another misidentification syndrome, Frégoli's syndrome. A patient with this syndrome will claim that a familiar person is capable of manifesting different physical appearances, so that the patients might complain that a certain person is following them or spying on them while taking on the outward appearance of different people. Feinberg observes that both Capgras' patients and asomatognosic patients claim that something or someone personally related to them is unfamiliar and distant, while the patient with Frégoli's syndrome sees unfamiliar people as familiar, or more broadly, falsely sees people as being personally related to him. Feinberg argues that the distinction between seeing something as personally related and seeing something as distant and foreign allows us to form a taxonomy of the misidentification disorders and other syndromes. As he puts it, "the essential dichotomization of these various disorders is on the basis of an alteration in personal relatedness or significance" (Feinberg & Roane, 1997, p. 80). Syndromes such as Capgras' and asomatognosia that involve a decreased sense of relatedness in the patient "should be thought of as a disavowal, estrangement, or alienation from persons, objects, or experiences". Syndromes such as Frégoli's are on the "the opposite side of the spectrum" and "are manifestations of an over-relatedness with persons, objects, or experiences" (Feinberg & Roane, 1997, p. 80).

Feinberg acknowledges, though, that not all patients can be described as claiming solely under- or over-relatedness to people and things. Some of them do both at the same time, with the same person. "Many of the important misidentifications seen in neurological patients actually represent a *co-occurrence* of both Capgras and Fregoli types of misidentifications" (1997). Many confabulations by asomatognosics, for example, do not involve the patient claiming that the arm or person is completely unrelated to him. One patient of Feinberg's said that her hands were not hers but her husband's, saying that, "He left them ... just like he left his clothes" (2006, p. 74). She believes that her hands are not her own, but nevertheless sees them as having a closeness to her. Because of this third, mixed type, Feinberg and his colleagues phrase their hypothesis in its final form thus: Syndromes such as Capgras', Frégoli's, and asomatognosia "represent either an increase, a decrease, or simultaneous increase and decrease in the patient's personal relatedness to objects, persons, places, or events in the patient's environment" (Feinberg & Roane 1997, p. 80).

Personal relatedness might be too broad of a concept, however. A very high percentage of the representations in our brains are of things personally related to us, for obvious reasons. The entirety of episodic-autobiographical memory, for instance, contains representations of events personally related to us. There are many different ways in which we represent things, properties, and facts that are important to us. In addition to episodic memory, we use somatotopic maps to represent several different properties of our bodies, and our semantic memories contain a self-concept that knits together all sorts of biographical information about us, and is immediately connected to our concepts of people and things of significance to us. Feinberg also seems to overlook an important distinction between representing something as literally me or a part of me, e.g., my arm, and representing something as very closely related to me, e.g., a spouse. The presence of "mixed" patients, who show both an increase and a decrease in their senses of personal relatedness for an object or person, is also troubling, since it indicates that the patients do not line up neatly on a single personal relatedness continuum. One way to respond to these criticisms would be to further specify the types of personal relatedness involved.

The following hypothesis offers a more specific explanation of Capgras' syndrome, Frégoli's syndrome, asomatognosia, and other disorders of person and limb recognition that fits the basic two-factor approach. It provides an alternative account for why these syndromes exhibit the interesting variations in personal relatedness that Feinberg and his colleagues observed. Our brains represent people both allocentrically and egocentrically. Allocentric representations of people are viewpoint-independent representations of their external bodily features. Our representations of peoples' faces are a paradigmatic example of allocentric representations. One sign that they are viewpoint - independent is that we can recognise people from many different angles. Egocentric representations, in contrast, encode the positions of things and spaces relative to a central "ego". Our representations of the spaces we inhabit are usually egocentric; they represent the distance of objects from us, the trajectories of objects with regard to our location, the possible effects on us of nearby objects, and so on. Egocentric representations contain an intrinsic point of view, whereas allocentric representations are viewpoint independent. Egocentric representations give the ego a privileged place in the representations system, whereas a person's allocentric system can represent him as one person among many. Among the faces we are able to visually recognise is our own, usually seen in a mirror, but the same allocentric visual recognition processes are used whether we are looking at ourselves or at our friends.

When I represent you from my perspective, I am representing you allocentrically. When I represent you from your perspective, by using my brain's natural mindreading or simulation functions, I am typically representing you egocentrically. One type of egocentric representation of an agent is a (spatial) analogue representation from the unique point of view of that agent, from inside that agent's head, of processes and events within that agent's body, including that person's thoughts. We represent people egocentrically by simulating their current experiences from their points of view, I suggest. The brain achieves this with an egocentric representation system that functions to represent a mind situated in a body, which is in turn situated in an environment, according to the representational hypothesis. This egocentric representation system is responsible for part of our normal sense that we are embodied minds, moving about an environment. This system does not always represent us, however. It has two modes of functioning that we might call *self-mode* and *other-mode*. In self-mode, this system represents my mind, situated in my body, situated in my environment. When this system functions in other-mode it represents other people as minds situated in bodies situated in environments. In either mode, the system is egocentric; but different individuals can occupy the ego position of the system. In self-mode, I am the ego at the centre of this system; in other-mode, the egocentric system represents or simulates the egocentric system of a person of interest.

The allocentric system represents people from the outside, including detailed facial representations, as well as representations of entire bodies, or characteristic modes of dress or movement. The skin seems to mark the boundary of what the allocentric system represents, whereas the mental component of the egocentric system represents events occurring inside the skin, as experienced from the point of view of that body's owner. These egocentric representations involve somatosensory representations, but also involve our awareness of our conscious perceptions, thoughts and emotions. Allocentric representations are primarily visual, but also involve auditory representations, as well as representations generated by other sense modalities.

REPRESENTATIONS OF MINDS

We read several different features of minds using several different brain processes, one of which, I suggest, is the egocentric mindreading system described here. The problem of the misidentification patients on this hypothesis is due to a failure of their brains to activate the correct egocentric representation of the person they are looking at. Once we get to know a person well, we develop an individualised egocentric representation of her mind. I will argue later that we also possess generic egocentric representations that can be applied to people we do not yet know well. These generic representations show themselves in our psychologies as character stereotypes, the loud obnoxious person, the shy, quiet person, and many more. We employ our own egocentric representation system in other-mode, or as a simulation, to understand the actions of other people. This is a variety of simulation theory (Goldman, 2006) in which an egocentric representation system is employed as an analogue model of that same system in another person. The misidentification syndromes can be understood as caused by damage to the mind-representing part of this large egocentric representation system. According to this hypothesis, both Capgras' and Frégoli's syndromes are mindreading disorders (Hirstein, 2005), due to failures of one of our mindreading systems, a set of brain processes we use to understand and predict the behaviour of others. Capgras' syndrome occurs when egocentric representations of a particular person are damaged or inaccessible and are replaced by other, incorrect representations. One piece of data that is at least consistent with the claim that malfunction exists in a system that is involved in representing both ourselves and others is the cooccurrence in patients of both self-misidentifications and misidentifications of others (see, e.g., Hirstein & Ramachandran, 1997; several of the 30 patients with Capgras' for self reviewed by Silva & Leong, 1994, also had Capgras' syndrome directed at others).

The representational hypothesis takes what the patients say seriously, unlike the other approaches which dismiss it as a convenient creation. These hypotheses do not account for why so many patients tell the same story. There is nothing specific about an absence of affective arousal, or of a sense of personal relatedness, that would lead someone to posit an impostor. But the experience of an unfamiliar mind situated within a familiar body, with a familiar face, is exactly what would lead to assertions about impostors. According to Feinberg's hypothesis, the Capgras' patient experiences a lack of a sense of personal relatedness, and this causes him to claim that the person he sees is an impostor. But the patient does not merely see someone familiar as unfamiliar, he perceives that person as having a different identity. The patient does not merely treat the "impostors" as less related than they were before; he treats them as different people. This is because he sees them as no longer having the same mind, the same motives, moods, and emotions. For example, paranoid Capgras' patients attribute evil intentions to the impostors.

To claim that someone is not in fact your father, but rather some stranger pretending to be your father, is to make a claim about the identity of that person, and also to disavow the personal relatedness of that person. Logically, the identity of someone is independent of that person's degree of personal relatedness to us, but in practicality, when the identity of loved ones is at stake, alterations in perceived identity will also involve alterations in perceived personal relatedness. Conversely, alterations in the patient's sense of personal relatedness need not also involve alternations in perceived identity. One might experience a loss in the sense of personal relatedness to a person, yet not doubt the identity of that person, even if that person is one's father, so that the person might say, "Dad seems strangely unfamiliar to me." Thus, an alteration in one's sense of personal relatedness alone is not sufficient to produce a misidentification patient. Similar logic applies to the affective responsiveness hypothesis. Failing to register a certain affective response at the sight of a person would not in itself lead one to doubt the identity of that person. One might rather think something like, "I don't love my mother as much as I used to." If I believe that the person in front of me is an impostor, however, strongly resembling my mother but with a different mind and identity, this would certainly lead me to have different affective responses. Thus, the representational hypothesis is logically prior to the other two, with greater explanatory power.

The personal relatedness factor one sees in the misidentification syndromes may be due to the way that the egocentric system is not merely egocentric, and typically used to represent ourselves, but used also to represent people, objects, and events of personal significance. Rather than explaining the patient's beliefs by way of a malfunction in her person-representation systems, Feinberg attributes them partly to affective/motivational factors. The tendency of patients to cling to the delusional belief, according to Feinberg, "suggests that there is an impediment or resistance to the truth" (Feinberg et al., 2005; see also Feinberg, 2009). Feinberg posits various motivational factors as a way to explain this tenacity, but another explanation for the patients' insistence on their beliefs is that they are experiencing a distinct perception of an unfamiliar person (see also Langdon & Bayne, 2010 this issue). This perception is coming from a normally trustworthy source, and the patients lack the ability to critically assess its groundedness. The idea that affective or motivational factors are doing the work also does not square with the frequently reported blandness of the patients. They are not shocked that a foreign arm is attached to their shoulder, or that impostors keep visiting them in the hospital.

In order to produce an accurate simulation of another person, we need an extensive and detailed representation. We need to build a complete scale model of an aeroplane in order to test it in a wind tunnel, for example, because of the holistic way in which changes in one property of the aeroplane affect others. If we change the airflow over one part of the plane, we have then changed the airflow over the parts of the plane behind this part. Similarly, we need a full model of a minded, embodied person in an environment in order to perform effective simulations of people in alternative situations. The way we know what to expect from a person is to create a simulation of him or her. This simulation should include the person's emotions. Knowing someone means knowing what makes her happy and what makes her angry, as well as how she behaves when she's angry or happy. Some types of simulations of minds can be thought of as functions from perceptions to actions. Two different people will respond differently to the same perceptions. One person may do what another person merely considers then inhibits, in the same situation. There are also cases where a perception causes a certain emotion that in turn causes an action. In order to represent these personalities, these functions, we would also need to simulate these emotions. We are not normally aware of our mind-representations as representations because we simply see ourselves as perceiving people with emotions and personalities and characters. We do not realise that we are not directly perceiving their emotions, intentions, or motives; we are reproducing them within ourselves, usually spontaneously.

One objection here is that the Capgras' patients tend to mention external features, not mental features, when asked how they can tell that the person in question is an impostor. I suggested earlier that Capgras' patients' claims about how they detect the imposter by slight differences in appearance might be a kind of confabulation. Breen, Caine, Coltheart, Hendy, and Roberts (2000) offer a quotation from author Clifford Beers, in which he describes his experiences after his recovery from the Capgras delusion. When relatives came to see him, he said, "I was able to detect some slight difference in look or gesture or intonation of voice, and this was enough to confirm my belief that they were impersonators" (Beers, 1953, pp. 62–63). Beers thought he detected slight differences, as many patients do, but notice that during the delusional phase, he regarded these as *confirmatory* of a preexisting belief that the person he was looking at was a different person, some stranger who was "impersonating" his relative. One good example of this is the blind patient with Capgras' who said that the impostor's hand felt softer than his mother's (Rojo et al., 1991). It seems improbable that he determined that she was an impostor by feeling her hand. Rather, he believed she was an impostor prior to touching her hand, most likely when hearing her voice.

EXECUTIVE PROCESSES

According to the two-factor hypothesis of confabulation, once a person or limb is misidentified (Factor 1), the brains of the patients fail to employ executive processes to correct the error (Factor 2). What exactly are executive processes, though? Cognition requires both representations and processes for manipulating those representations—these latter are executive processes. Executive processes perform many different operations on representations. One clear illustration of executive processes at work managing representations occurs when we recall some past event from our lives. Your memory itself is just a huge collection of representations; executive processes must control the search and reconstruction processes that take place when we remember. Executive processes also control mental activity by allowing us to shift our focus from perception to memory or back, or to rearrange items held in working memory (e.g., in the digit span task, where a sequence of numbers is read out loud to the subject, who must then report the sequence in reverse order).

A great deal of what we normally call thinking, deciding, planning, and remembering is accomplished primarily by the brain's executive processes. One introspectively accessible measure of the amount of executive activity is our sense of mental effort. Increased mental effort correlates with increased usage of oxygen by executive areas, which is detectable by brain imaging. In such studies, tasks are devised that require the intervention of executive functions; brain activity is then monitored as the subject attempts the task. Most executive processes reside in the prefrontal lobes, including the dorsolateral frontal lobes on the side of the brain, the ventrolateral frontal lobes below them, the medial prefrontal lobes, on the inner surfaces of the two hemispheres, and the orbitofrontal lobes located on the brain's undersurface just above the eye sockets (Moscovitch & Winocur, 2002). One area that is frequently active during effortful processing is the anterior cingulate, in the medial prefrontal cortex. The anterior cingulate is thought to play a role in resolving conflicts between routine actions that are not relevant to the present task, and novel actions that are relevant. It also activates strongly when the subject detects an error in his response (Carter, Botvinick, & Cohen, 1999).

The executive processes can participate in the act of recognition itself, and they normally have the power to overrule our initial perceptual identifications. We all experience strange misperceptions at times, but we are able to correct them using executive processes. I believe I see my friend in a hotel lobby in Nairobi, but then I realise how improbable that is—this friend never travels, has no interest in Africa, etc.—so I tell myself that it is just someone who resembles my friend. The decision must be made at the executive level as to whether the presence in consciousness of a given representation truly means that the represented object is there. For example, the existence of phantom limbs involves an active egocentric representation of the missing limb, but at the executive level that activity is not taken as a veridical representation, mainly because the allocentric system strongly confirms the absence of the limb. Conversely, severing of the nerve to an arm can produce the impression that the arm is not there, due to the removal of somatosensation, which is part of the egocentric system. But executive processes are able to let the continued correctness of the external, allocentric representations of the arm overrule this impression: The arm is still there, merely numb, the patient concludes. The executive systems thus have the ability to let either the allocentric system or the egocentric system win out over the other, in the event of discord between them. When we first become aware of a person's presence, two different streams of processing, one egocentric and one allocentric, commence their work. In neurological patients, failure of either the allocentric stream or the egocentric stream, coupled with the relevant executive failure, should produce a confabulation if the patient is asked the right question.

PROSOPAGNOSIA, COTARD'S SYNDROME, AND FRÉGOLI'S SYNDROME

One way to test and further elucidate the representational hypothesis and its larger two-factor approach is to apply it to other syndromes in which recognition of persons fail. Neurological patients with *prosopagnosia* can no longer visually recognise the people they know, and their faces do not look familiar to the patient, but the patients continue to attribute the same personalities and other mental traits to them once they recognise them, typically by the sounds of their voices. Prosopagnosics can sometimes recognise people using specific visual cues, such as a person's distinctive nose or ears, or even the type of glasses or tie someone typically wears. For the prosopagnosic, the familiar face is not present, but the person is; once the patient hears his mother speak, he recognises her, and will treat her as his mother. For the Capgras' patient, the familiar face is present, but the person is not. The Capgras' patient's allocentric system is intact, but his normal egocentric representation of that person is damaged or inaccessible. The Capgras' patient's relevant executive processes are malfunctioning, and this prevents him from realising how implausible the impostor claim is and rejecting it. The typical prosopagnosic does not have executive damage, but according to the hypothesis described here, a prosopagnosic with executive damage should confabulate when asked to identify people. The two patients of Rapcsak, Polster, Comer, and Rubens (1994) seem to fit this profile. They were both unable to recognise familiar faces, and when asked to identify faces in photographs, they employed the style typically seen in prosopagnosics of attempting to identify faces by focusing on distinctive features. The use of this strategy, together with executive failure, caused the patients to confabulate that unfamiliar people were familiar, because the unfamiliar person shared some facial feature with the familiar person. One of the patients pointed to a fellow patient on the ward, for instance, and exclaimed, "There's my father! I'd recognise that hooked nose anywhere!" The authors seem to favour a two-factor approach, noting that, "the frontal lobes are also likely to be responsible for detecting and resolving potential ambiguities arising in connection with the operations of perceptual recognition systems" (Rapscak et al., 1994, p. 577). They further observe that, "the dysfunction of the decision making process in our patients was evidenced by the fact that they rarely if ever attempted to verify the correctness of their initial impressions regarding a person's identity. Instead, they seemed to accept the output generated by the impaired face recognition system unconditionally." We might call this syndrome *dysexecutive prosopagnosia*. It causes misidentifications based on superficial similarities of facial features that patients lack the executive processes to correct.

The patient with Cotard's syndrome says that he is dead, hollow, or empty. These patients perceive their own body and face well enough, but see no mind at home there, rather like a dense neurological version of depersonalisation. Cotard's original patient said that she had "no brain, nerves, chest, or entrails, and was just skin and bone" (Berrios & Luque, 1995). One Cotard's patient described "feeling nothing inside" (Wright, Young, & Hellawell, 1993); another patient "felt that her brain was dead"

(Young, Leafhead, & Szulecka, 1994). Although strictly speaking, Cotard's syndrome is not a misidentification syndrome, since the person is correctly identified but thought to be dead, an explanation of it can be derived from the account given here. According to the representational hypothesis, Cotard's syndrome is caused by complete destruction of the mind-representing part of the egocentric representation system. Patients with Cotard's and Capgras' for themselves recognise themselves externally, but attribute either no mind at all to themselves, and hence speak of themselves as "dead" or "robots" (Cotard's), or they perceive themselves to have strange, unknown minds (Capgras'). Some Capgras' patients see an unfamiliar mind behind the face in photos of themselves or even in their own mirror images, and hence may speak of the persons seen in photos or mirrors as impostors. The Frégoli's syndrome patient sees a certain significant person as somehow inhabiting several different bodies. According to the representational hypothesis, what happens in Frégoli's syndrome is that the patient's egocentric representation of a familiar person is paired with allocentric representations of unfamiliar faces and bodies. This produces in the patient the impression of a single familiar person disguising herself as a succession of strangers.

The crucial posterior damage site for misidentification syndromes (in addition to prefrontal damage causing executive failures) may be a cortical area just inferior to the supramarginal gyrus, the temporoparietal junction (TPJ). Two Cotard's patients studied by Young and his colleagues (Young et al. 1994; Young, Robertson, Hellawell, de Pauw, & Pentland, 1992) had temporoparietal contusions along with bilateral frontal damage. The Capgras' patient of Staton et al. (1982, p. 26) showed "a discrete area of moderate atrophy deep in the [right] posterior-superior temporal lobe at the temporo-parietal junction". Similarly, a Capgras' patient seen by Johnson and Raye (1998) had a right temporoparietal hematoma. A Frégoli's patient described by Feinberg, Eaton, Roane, and Giacino (1999) also had damage at the temporoparietal junction. The temporoparietal junction has been found to be active during several "theory of mind" tasks, in which subjects attempt to understand the actions and motives of others. In a typical task, the brain of a subject is scanned as she observes people performing certain actions, or displaying certain emotions. The right TPJ's activity level was observed to be high when "participants read stories that describe a character's beliefs but low during stories containing other socially relevant information" (Young & Saxe, 2009). It is also relevant that the right TPJ activates more strongly when the target person has beliefs that are known by the subject to be false (Young & Saxe, 2009). Saxe (2006, p. 235) describes the TPJ as an "area for representing mental states" that responds selectively to "the attribution of mental states" (Saxe & Wexler, 2005, p. 1391) and plays a role in developing an "integrated impression" of people (Saxe & Wexler, 2005, p. 1396).

There are two gaps in the representational hypothesis which still need filling, however. First, the findings of Saxe and others concern real-time attributions of mental states to strangers, whereas at least some of the misidentification syndromes involve people very well known to the patient. A second gap is that the mindreading system findings concern real-time, single events of mental state attribution, whereas I am postulating that these events are accumulated in a type of memory into a mental representation of someone's mind. A first step in meeting this objection is to point out that there is evidence of a TPJ link to the autobiographical memory system; Maguire (2001) and Fink et al. (1996) found TPJ activity during a task in which subjects recalled emotional autobiographical events. There is still a gap here, though, in that autobiographical memory is about me, whereas I am postulating that there is a related type of memory centred on significant other people; i.e., that the ego in the egocentric position of the autobiographical memory system is not always that of the owner of that system.

Recall that the egocentric representation represents not merely a mind, but a mind housed in a body, which is itself situated in an environment. We use this system to understand the intentional actions of people in environments. Saxe notes that the TPJ is also "selectively recruited for determining how the spatial relations between two objects would appear from a character's point of view versus the subject's own position" (2006, p. 236). The role in computing perspective differences and the role in computing mental states may actually involve different but adjacent portions of the TPJ. Aichhorn, Perner, Kronbichler, Staffen, and Ladurner (2006) recommend that the TPJ be divided into two areas, arguing that its dorsal portion is "responsible for representing perspective differences and making behavioural predictions", whereas its ventral part—along with the medial prefrontal cortex—is responsible for "predicting behavioural consequences" of another person's mental states. The egocentric system may well have other modes, including what we might call an alternative self-mode, which we use to imagine ourselves in possible scenarios. Blanke and his colleagues found that one can produce a vivid out-of-body experience involving what they refer to as an "abnormal egocentric visuospatial perspective" (Blanke et al., 2005) by electrically stimulating the temporoparietal junction (Blanke & Arzy, 2005), something that again is consistent with its use to represent not only our own location in space, but also locations that we are not currently in. Notice that even though these out-of-body experiences are vivid and realistic, the person does not actually believe that he is, e.g., flying around the room. According to the two-factor approach, this is because her executive processes are intact and are able to overrule the experience. This predicts, however, that it these experiments were tried on someone with the right executive processes damaged, she would actually take the experience to be veridical. Recent research on what is called the brain's default network supports the idea that a single large system functions to represent both ourselves when navigating through space or imagining ourselves in other possible situations, as well as functioning to achieve mindreading tasks when our attention is directed at others, and to achieve autobiographical memory (Buckner & Carroll, 2007). This would also make sense of the finding by Mitchell (2008) that the right TPJ is active both when we are attributing beliefs to others and when we are reorienting our attention to a different location in space: Normally the TPJ represents our space, but sometimes it represents the simulated space of a person of interest.

EPISODIC MEMORIES OF OTHERS

A person's episodic memories are memories of that person from her point of view. The representations that are stored in episodic memory are egocentric because they represent events as we experienced them; hence they are also called autobiographical memories. Autobiographical episodic memories combine several different subrepresentations including representations of our bodies moving through different spaces and environments and representations of the people and objects we have significant interactions with. We carefully represent each aspect of a particularly significant interaction, exactly what was said, and in which tone of voice. In addition to representations of emotions, episodic memories may also contain representations of other conscious states, such as our thoughts, motives, and intentions at the time of the event. Hence, a full autobiographical memory representation is of a person with a conscious mind, moving through space, interacting with people and objects.

The episodic memory system is also able to aggregate its information into our existing concepts of important people and things. Once this information enters the system of concepts it becomes part of the semantic memory system also, and is then accessible to the process of thinking. Thus, the episodic memory system can feed the semantic memory system. For instance, if I travel to Paris, the episodic memories I amass as I see important sites in the city also add information to my semantic representation of Paris, the Eiffel Tower, the Arc de Triomphe, etc. All of this information tends to be either semantic/conceptual or allocentric in form, but I suggest that the egocentric realm has its own ability to aggregate its representations into a full-blown simulation of persons' minds. As I accumulate information about someone over the course of many interactions with her, I also accumulate information about her thoughts, moods, and emotions, using the egocentric representations system in other-mode. We might call such accumulated memories, "biographical memories". They contain information that is extremely valuable to us, so I suspect that we do not discard it, but rather carefully organise and maintain it, in the form of accumulations of simulated mental states that are representations of the minds of the significant people in our lives. If this is right, our full representation of a significant person contains an allocentric component with representations of how he looks and sounds, and an egocentric representation of his mind, body, and environments from his viewpoint. Our awareness of the minds of others when the egocentric system is operating in other-mode seems to be nonexplicit and faint in our minds. Perhaps this is a reason why distinguishing whether an emotion or a simulation of a mind is missing (as may happen in Capgras' syndrome) is difficult for the patients. One hypothesis for why the activity level of the egocentric system needs to be low when it is operating in other-mode is that vivid conscious representation leads to actual external actions, not merely to represented actions, in much the same way that the dreaming mind malfunctions during REM sleep disorder, when perceptions that are merely dreamed cause real actions. Simulations cannot fully and explicitly employ this representation system without danger of causing real actions, with potentially disastrous consequences.

If correct, this view implies that we possess representations of specific individual minds, but surely we also have some ability to understand the minds of strangers. There is also evidence that we possess a set of generic mind representations that we can employ with people who we don't know well enough yet to have created a mind representation of. It seems obvious that we create generic representations of significant *things*. All of my episodic memories of visits to grocery stores, for instance, organise themselves into generic memories of certain grocery store types, which I access when I decide where to go to purchase certain foods, or where to look once I'm in a grocery store. I employ different accumulations of autobiographical memories if I am in a huge chain store, a country grocery, or the corner convenience mart. If the Capgras' patient has lost his representation of his father's individual mind, but uses a generic representation when he now looks at him, this is precisely what would produce the impression of an impostor—his father's body and face, but alloyed with the mind of some other, unfamiliar person. On this hypothesis, then, when both individual and generic egocentric representations are unusable, Cotard's syndrome results. The patient can only represent himself externally, using the allocentric system, and this causes him to see himself as empty and without a mind. This can also explain why some patients, such as that of Wright et al. (1993), alternate between Cotard's and Capgras' syndromes: The patient's egocentric representations are inaccessible, while his generic egocentric representations are intermittently on- and offline, perhaps due to irregular blood flow, or to remapping of the damaged neural networks. When they are functioning, the patient has Capgras' syndrome, when they are not functioning, he has Cotard's syndrome.

One objection to this account is that it locates the problem in the misidentification syndromes at too high a level. Misidentification is much closer to being a lower level perceptual problem than a higher level problem representing the mind of the target person, according to this objection. Think of what it would be like, however, if you became convinced that someone you knew well had been replaced by an impostor. As you see her coming towards you, you recognise the familiar face, and conclude that it is your friend. But when she becomes closer and begins to speak to you, something seems wrong. As you continue to interact with her, it seems to you that she doesn't have the same beliefs, thoughts, moods, and preferences of the person you originally knew. You start to get the impression that this is actually someone else. If you were a normal person, with intact executive processes, you would not allow yourself to form this conclusion, however. You would be much more likely to conclude that your friend has undergone some sort of change in personality, or even to attribute the problem to yourself, concluding perhaps that you hadn't really known her as well as you thought you did. If this account is true to the phenomenology of Capgras' syndrome, the problem is not immediately perceptual. It is also important not to tie Capgras' too closely to visual perception at least, since as noted earlier it has been observed in blind people (Dalgalarrondo, Fujisawa, & Banzato, 2002; Hermanowicz, 2002; Rojo et al., 1991).

ASOMATOGNOSIA AND PHANTOM LIMBS

If Capgras' syndrome is in one sense the opposite of Frégoli's syndrome, then what is the opposite of asomatognosia? The vast majority of people who undergo amputation of a limb have a clear sensation that the limb is still there—a phantom limb. Their experience of the limb seems to be the same as before. They experience it as being in a certain position, as being hot or cold, as being in pain, as being paralysed, and sometimes even as moving in response to their intentions, for instance reaching out to shake hands with someone (Ramachandran & Hirstein, 1998). The asomatognosic's arm is there, but it seems to him that it is not; the phantom limb patient's arm is not there, but it seems to him that it is. The arms of phantom limb patients feel the same from the inside, as it were, but obviously do not look the same on the outside. Asomatognosia is just the opposite: The patient's limb looks the same externally but lacks certain internal sensations. There is a great difference in conviction, of course; the asomatognosic is certain that the arm is not his arm, whereas the phantom limb patient is able to overrule the vivid impression of the arm's presence and acknowledge that his limb is gone.

If the two-factor hypothesis of confabulation is correct, however, the difference between the two is that the asomatognosic has damaged prefrontal processes—processes that should prevent his odd impression from establishing itself as a belief, and this explains the difference in conviction. Those cases of asomatognosia in which the patient claims that his arm is dead may be the bodily analogue of Cotard's syndrome in the case of mindreading. In both cases, a complete destruction of the relevant portions of the egocentric representation system causes the patient to feel that his arm, or he himself, is empty or dead. There is an asymmetry here, however: With Capgras' or Cotard's syndrome, the representation of the entire mind is compromised, whereas in asomatognosia, a representation of only a portion of the body is compromised. This may be due to a difference in the sort of representations the brain employs. Body representations occur in the form of somatotopic maps, spread out over cortical areas, so that damage might affect just a portion of the map. Perhaps mind representations are in some more holistic form, so that damage to a portion of them affects the entire representation.

What would a phantom limb patient *with* compromised executive processes say about his limb? There is an analogy here with dysexecutive prosopagnosia in the realm of limbs. Amputee patients with phantom limbs have not normally also sustained brain damage, but if a person lost a limb *and* damaged the relevant frontal processes, would he actually deny that his limb was gone? The Capgras' patient DS described in Hirstein and Ramachandran (1997) was just such a person. His right arm needed to be amputated, just below the elbow, after a car accident in which he also sustained serious brain damage. At several points in our interactions with him, he denied that his arm was gone.

MISIDENTIFICATION AND THE THIRD VISUAL STREAM

In spite of not being able to consciously recognise familiar people, prosopagnosics will register a larger average skin-conductance response (SCR) to familiar faces than to unfamiliar faces. Bauer (1984) and Ellis and Young (1990) suggested that Capgras' syndrome is the mirror-image of prosopagnosia, and hypothesised that Capgras' patients would lack the normal SCR to familiar faces, and this was later verified in several patients (Ellis, Young, Quayle, & de Pauw, 1997; Hirstein & Ramachandran, 1997). Prosopagnosics typically show damage to the fusiform gyrus, on the undersurface of the temporal lobes, so it was generally thought that damage to this more ventral route destroys the ability to recognise familiar faces, while some other processing stream was intact, and still able to produce an SCR to the seen faces. It is not clear where the other processing stream is, however. Bauer initially suggested that the SCR route was in the dorsal cortex, but this seemed implausible given that this cortex specialises not in face recognition, but in representing the body, and in coordinating the computations needed for spatial navigation, reaching for objects, and such tasks.

In 2003, Rizzolatti and Mattelli proposed that the traditional division of visual streams leaving the occipital lobe into a ventral and a dorsal one (Ungerleider & Mishkin, 1982) is inadequate, and that the dorsal stream of visual processing should be divided into two separate streams which they call the dorsodorsal stream, and the ventrodorsal stream. The dorsodorsal stream has all of the characteristics traditionally attributed to the dorsal stream: It terminates in the superior parietal lobe and functions to provide the information required to execute actions involving, e.g., reaching for nearby objects. The idea of a ventrodorsal stream is a new concept, though, and that stream has been found to have some interesting characteristics. Area PF in the rhesus monkey, which corresponds to the supramarginal gyrus in humans, is the primary recipient area of visual input for this stream. Area PF is now known to contain mirror neurons, neurons that respond when the subject executes a particular, e.g., arm action, or when the subject sees another person execute that same action (Rizzolatti & Craighero, 2004). In my earlier terminology, PF is able to operate in both self-mode and other-mode. This raises the intriguing possibility that the recipient areas of the ventrodorsal stream are the ones damaged in Capgras' patients, as well as other misidentification patients.

The mindreading system and the mirror neuron system are different systems, however, and several writers have pointed out that they are disjoint (Decety & Lamm, 2006; Jackson & Decety, 2004; Saxe, 2005). The mindreading system is currently thought to consist of the left and right TPJ, an area of dorsomedial prefrontal cortex, an area of the superior temporal sulcus (STS), and a portion of the posterior cingulate gyrus (Saxe, 2005). The mirror neuron system consists of three cortical areas, one that corresponds to PF, a portion of the superior temporal sulcus, and a frontal component, located in the ventral portion of Brodmann's Area 6 (Rizzolatti & Craighero, 2004). The STS does not contain mirror neurons, but does respond to biological motion, i.e., movements by living organisms, including human eye movements (Hoffman & Haxby, 2000; Puce & Perrett, 2003). Perhaps the superior temporal sulcus links the mindreading and mirror systems. One would expect to find such a link, on the hypothesis that we use the mirror neuron system to understand what action a person is performing, leading naturally to the use of the mindreading system to understand the beliefs, motives, and intentions behind the action.

CONCLUSION

The brain's right hemisphere appears to contain areas, such as the supramarginal gyrus and the temporoparietal junction just below it, that serve the dual function of representing ourselves on certain occasions, and other people on other occasions. I suggest that areas such as the supramarginal gyrus and the TPJ, working in concert with interconnected areas in the temporal and prefrontal lobes, are responsible for the sense of oneself as an embodied being with a mind situated in an environment. Out-of-body experiences, for instance, contain representations of what one's phenomenology, one's mental life, would be like, as well the changes in one's body and its environment. When we understand the intentional actions of others, these areas serve as an egocentric representation of them.

The debates here raise deeper issues about how we represent things and people, independently of the properties that they have only contingently. Descartes (1632/1967) famously noted that a ball of wax can change every one of its properties, its shape, colour, texture, smell, and hardness, when brought near a flame and melted, and yet we still represent it as the same thing. Philosophers in the middle ages spoke of things as containing a sort of core essence that they called a "haecceity", that maintains their identities despite changes in their properties. Perhaps haecceities or something like them exist not in things themselves (indeed, where would they be, and what sort of material existence could they have?) but rather in our brains. Perhaps the central "ego" in the egocentric system functions as a sort of haecceity, in that it is tied to the identity of a specific person (which may vary over time), no matter what the other parts of the egocentric system represent, while itself having no representational content.

The account here, if correct, brings the misidentification syndromes and asomatognosia into line with the rest of the confabulation syndromes by showing how they also fall under a two-factor hypothesis. Confabulation is caused by two events: (1) Damage to some perceptual or mnemonic process in the posterior of the brain, typically the cortex; and (2) damage to some prefrontal executive process that monitors and can correct the output of that perceptual or mnemonic process. In the case of asomatognosia, the posterior lesion tends to occur in the inferior parietal lobe, often in the supramarginal gyrus. The lesion that causes misidentifications of people seems to be just below that one, in the temporoparietal junction. We build large, detailed representations of the minds of those close to us, according to this hypothesis. We create these representations so automatically, and they operate so subtly, that when they are damaged we have trouble understanding what has happened. Capgras' patients perceive a familiar face and body, but inhabited by an unfamiliar mind. With no executive processes to resolve the contradiction, the odd impression forms into a delusional belief which, when expressed, becomes a confabulation about an impostor.

REFERENCES

Aichhorn, M., Perner, J., Kronbichler, M., Staffen, W., & Ladurner, G. (2006). Do visual perspective tasks need theory of mind? *Neuroimage, 30*, 1059–1068.

Babinski, J. (1914). *Contribution a l'etude des troubles mentaux dans l'hemiplegie organique cerebrale (anosognosie). Revue Neurologique (Paris), 27*, 845–848.

Bauer, R. M. (1984). Autonomic recognition of names and faces in prosopagnosia: A neuropsychological application of the Guilty Knowledge Test. *Neuropsychologia, 22*, 457–469.

Bauer, R. M. (1986). The cognitive psychophysiology of prosopagnosia. In H. Ellis, M. A. Jeeves, F. Newcombe, & A. Young (Eds.), *Aspects of face processing.* (pp. 235–267) Dordrecht, The Netherlands: Nijhoff.

Beers, C. W. (1953). *A mind that found itself: An autobiography* (7th ed.). New York: Doubleday.

Berlyne, N. (1972). Confabulation. *British Journal of Psychiatry, 120*, 31–39.

Berrios, G. E., & Luque, R. (1995). Cotard's syndrome: Analysis of 100 cases. *Acta Psychiatrica Scandia, 91*, 185–188.

Berti, A., Bottini, G., Gandola, M., Pia, L., Smania, N., Stracciari, A., et al. (2005). Shared cortical anatomy for motor awareness and motor control. *Science, 309*, 488–491.

Bisiach, E., & Geminiani, G. (1991). Anosognosia related to hemiplegia and hemianopia. In G. P. Prigatano & D. L. Schacter (Eds.), *Awareness of deficit after brain injury: Clinical and theoretical issues.* (pp. 17–39) Oxford, UK: Oxford University Press.

Blanke, O., & Arzy, S. (2005). The out-of-body experience: Disturbed self-processing at the temporo-parietal junction. *Neuroscientist, 11*, 16–24.

Blanke, O., Mohr, C., Michel, C. M., Pascual-Leone, A., Brugger, P., Seeck, M., et al. (2005). Linking out-of-body experience and self processing to mental own-body imagery at the temporoparietal junction. *Journal of Neuroscience, 25*, 550–557.

Breen, N., Caine, D., Coltheart, M., Hendy, J., & Roberts, C. (2000). Towards an understanding of delusions of misidentification: Four case studies. In M. Coltheart & M. Davies (Eds.), *Pathologies of belief.* (pp. 75–110) Oxford, UK: Blackwell.

Buckner, R. L., & Carroll, D. C. (2007). Self-projection and the brain. *Trends in Cognitive Sciences, 11*(2), 49–57.

Capgras, J., & Reboul-Lachaux, J. (1923). L'illusion des "sosies" dans un délire systématisé chronique. *Bulletin de la Société Clinique de Médecine Mentale, 11*, 6–16. Reprinted in H. D. Ellis, J. Whitley, & J. P. Luauté (Eds.). (1994). Delusional misidentifications: The three original papers on the Capgras, Fregoli and intermetamorphosis delusions. *History of Psychiatry, 5*, 117–146.

Carter, C. S., Botvinick, M. M., & Cohen, J. D. (1999). The contribution of the anterior cingulate cortex to executive processes in cognition. *Reviews in the Neurosciences, 10*, 49–57.

Coltheart, M. (2007). The 33rd Bartlett lecture: Cognitive neuropsychiatry and delusional belief. *Quarterly Journal of Experimental Psychology, 60*, 1041–1062.

Critchley, M. (1974). Misoplegia or hatred of hemiplegia, *Mt. Sinai Journal of Medicine, 41*, 82–87.

Dalgalarrondo, P., Fujisawa, G., & Banzato, C. E. M. (2002). Capgras syndrome and blindness: Against the prosopagnosia hypothesis. *Canadian Journal of Psychiatry, 47*(4), 387–388.

Davies, M., Coltheart, M., Langdon, R., & Breen, N. (2001). Monothematic delusions: Toward a two-factor account. *Philosophy, Psychiatry, and Psychology, 8*(2–3), 133–158.

Davies, M., Davies, A. A., & Coltheart, M. (2005). Anosognosia and the two-factor theory of delusions. *Mind and Language, 20*(2), 209–236.

Decety, J., & Lamm, C. (2006). Human empathy through the lens of social neuroscience. *Scientific World Journal, 6*, 1146–1163.

Descartes, R. (1967). *Meditations on first philosophy.* Trans. E. Haldane & D. Ross. Cambridge, UK: Cambridge University Press. (Original work published 1632)

Ellis, H. D., & Young, A. W. (1990). Accounting for delusional misidentifications. *British Journal of Psychiatry, 157*, 239–248.

Ellis, H. D., Young, A. W., Quayle, A. H., & de Pauw, K. W. (1997). Reduced autonomic responses to face in Capgras delusion. *Proceedings of the Royal Society of London, Series B, 264*, 1085–1092.

Feinberg, T. E. (2001). *Altered egos: How the brain creates the self.* Oxford, UK: Oxford University Press.

Feinberg, T. E. (2006). Our brains, our selves. *Daedelus*, Fall, 72–80.

Feinberg, T. E. (2009). Confabulation and ego functions: The ego dysequilibrium theory. In W. Hirstein (Ed.), *Confabulation: Views from neuroscience, psychiatry, psychology, and philosophy* (pp. 91–108). Oxford, UK: Oxford University Press.

Feinberg, T. E., DeLuca, J., Giacino, J. T., Roane, D. M., & Solms, M. (2005). Right hemisphere pathology and the self: Delusional misidentification and reduplication. In T. E. Feinberg & J. P. Keenan (Eds.), *The lost self: Pathologies of brain and identity.* Oxford, UK: Oxford University Press.

Feinberg, T. E., Eaton, L. A., Roane, D. M., & Giacino, J. T. (1999). Multiple Fregoli delusions after brain injury. *Cortex, 35*, 373–387.

Feinberg, T. E., Haber, L. D., & Leeds, N. E. (1990). Verbal asomatognosia. *Neurology, 40*, 1391–1394.

Feinberg, T. E., & Roane, D. M. (1997). Anosognosia, completion and confabulation: The neutral-personal dichotomy. *Neurocase, 3*, 73–85.

Fine, C. (2006). *A mind of its own: How your brain distorts and deceives.* New York: W. W. Norton.

Fink, G. R., Markowitsch, H. J., Reinkemeier, M., Bruckbauer, T., Kessler, J., & Heiss, W. D. (1996). Cerebral representation of one's own past: Neural networks involved in autobiographical memory. *Journal of Neuroscience, 16*, 4275–4282.

Förstl, H., & Beats, B. (1992). Charles Bonnet's description of Cotard's delusion and reduplicative paramnesia in an elderly patient. *British Journal of Psychiatry, 160*, 416–418. (Original work published 1788)

Fotopoulou, A. (2009). Disentangling the motivational hypotheses in confabulation. In W. Hirstein (Ed.), *Confabulation: Views from neuroscience, psychiatry, psychology, and philosophy* (pp. 263–290). Oxford, UK: Oxford University Press.

Fotopoulou, A. (2010). The affective neuropsychology of confabulation and delusion. *Cognitive Neuropsychiatry, 15*(1/2/3), 38–63.

Frazer, S. J., & Roberts, J. M. (1994). Three cases of Capgras' syndrome. *British Journal of Psychiatry, 164*, 557–559.

Goldman, A. (2006). *Simulating minds: The philosophy, psychology, and neuroscience of mind-reading*. Oxford, UK: Oxford University Press.

Hermanowicz, N. (2002). A blind man with Parkinson's disease, visual hallucinations, and Capgras syndrome. *Journal of Neuropsychiatry and Clinical Neuroscience, 14*(4), 462–463.

Hirstein, W. (2005). *Brain fiction: Self-deception and the riddle of confabulation*. Cambridge, MA: MIT Press.

Hirstein, W., & Ramachandran, V. S. (1997). Capgras syndrome: A novel probe for understanding the neural representation of the identity and familiarity of persons. *Proceedings of the Royal Society of London, Series B, 264*, 437–444.

Hoffman, E. A., & Haxby, J. V. (2000). Distinct representations of eye gaze and identity in the distributed human neural system for face perception. *Nature Neuroscience, 3*, 80–84.

Jackson, P. L., & Decety, J. (2004). Motor cognition: A new paradigm to study self-other interactions. *Current Opinion in Neurobiology, 14*, 259–263.

Johnson, M. K., & Raye, C. L. (1998). False memories and confabulation. *Trends in Cognitive Sciences, 2*, 137–145.

Langdon, R., & Bayne, T. (2010). Delusion and confabulation: Mistakes of perceiving, remembering and believing. *Cognitive Neuropsychiatry, 15*(1/2/3), 319–345.

Langdon, R., & Coltheart, M. (2000). The cognitive neuropsychology of delusions. *Mind and Language, 15*, 184–218.

Lettsom, J. C. (1789). *History of some of the effects of hard drinking*. London: Henry Fry.

Maguire, E. A. (2001). Neuroimaging studies of autobiographical memory. In A. Baddeley, J. Aggleton, & M. A. Conway (Eds.), *Episodic memory: New directions in research* (pp. 165–180). Oxford, UK: Oxford University Press.

Maher, B. A. (1988). Anomalous experience and delusional thinking: The logic of explanations. In T. F. Oltmanns & B. A. Maher (Eds.), *Delusional beliefs* (pp. 15–33). Chichester, UK: Wiley.

McKay, R., & Kinsbourne, M. (2010). Confabulation, delusion, and anosognosia: Motivational factors and false claims. *Cognitive Neuropsychiatry, 15*(1/2/3), 288–318.

Metcalf, K., Langdon, R., & Coltheart, M. (2007). Models of confabulation: A critical review and a new framework. *Cognitive Neuropsychology, 24*(1), 23–47.

Mitchell, J. P. (2008). Activity in the right temporo-parietal junction is not selective for theory-of-mind. *Cerebral Cortex, 18*, 262–271.

Moscovitch, M., & Winocur, G. (2002). The frontal cortex and working with memory. In D. T. Stuss & R. T. Knight (Eds.), *Principles of frontal lobe functions* (pp. 188–209). Oxford, UK: Oxford University Press.

Nielsen, J. M. (1938). Gerstmann syndrome; finger agnosia, agraphia, confusion of right and left, acalculia; comparison of this syndrome with disturbances of body scheme resulting from lesions of right side of brain. *Archives of Neurological Psychiatry, 39*, 536–560.

Puce, A., & Perrett, D. (2003). Electrophysiology and brain imaging of biological motion. *Philosophical Transactions of the Royal Society of London, Series B: Biological Sciences, 358*, 435–445.

Ramachandran, V. S., & Hirstein, W. (1998). The perception of phantom limbs: The D. O. Hebb lecture. *Brain, 121*, 1603–1630.

Rapcsak, S. E., Polster, M. R., Comer, J. F., & Rubens, A. B. (1994). False recognition and misidentification of faces following right hemisphere damage. *Cortex, 30*, 565–583.

Rizzolatti, G., & Craighero, L. (2004). The mirror neuron system. *Annual Reviews of Neuroscience, 27*, 169–192.

Rizzolatti, G., & Mattelli, M. (2003). Two different streams form the dorsal visual system: Anatomy and function. *Experimental Brain Research, 153*, 146–157.

Rojo, V. I., Caballero, L., Iruela, L. M., & Baca, E. (1991). Capgras' syndrome in a blind patient. *American Journal of Psychiatry, 148*(9), 1271–1272.

Saxe, R. (2005). Against simulation: The argument from error. *Trends in Cognitive Sciences, 9*, 174–179.

Saxe, R. (2006). Uniquely human social cognition. *Current Opinion in Neurobiology, 16*, 235–239.

Saxe, R., & Wexler, A. (2005). Making sense of another mind: The role of the right temporo-parietal junction. *Neuropsychologia, 43*, 1391–1399.

Signer, S. F. (1994). Localization and lateralization in the delusion of substitution. *Psychopathology, 27*, 168–176.

Silva, J. A., & Leong, G. B. (1994). Delusions of psychological change of the self. *Psychopathology, 27*, 285–290.

Staton, R. D., Brumback, R. A., & Wilson, H. (1982). Reduplicative paramnesia: A disconnection syndrome of memory. *Cortex, 18*, 23–36.

Stone, T., & Young, A. W. (1997). Delusions and brain injury: The philosophy and psychology of belief. *Mind and Language, 12*, 327–364.

Turner, M., & Coltheart, M. (2010). Confabulation and delusion: A common monitoring framework. *Cognitive Neuropsychiatry, 15*(1/2/3), 346–376.

Ungerleider, L. G., & Mishkin, M. (1982). Two visual streams. In D. J. Ingle, M. A. Goodale, & R. J. W. Mansfield (Eds.), *Analysis of visual behavior* (pp. 549–586). Cambridge, MA: MIT Press.

Vié, J. (1930). Un trouble de l'identification des personnes: l'illusion des sosies. *Annals of Medical Psychology, 88*, 214–237.

Weinstein, E. A. (1991). Anosognosia and denial of illness. In G. P. Prigatano & D. L. Schacter (Eds.), *Awareness of deficit after brain injury: Clinical and theoretical issues* (pp. 240–257). Oxford, UK: Oxford University Press.

Wright, S., Young, A. W., & Hellawell, D. J. (1993). Sequential Cotard and Capgras delusions. *British Journal of Clinical Psychology, 32*, 345–349.

Young, A. W., Leafhead, K. M., & Szulecka, T. K. (1994). Capgras and Cotard delusions. *Psychopathology, 27*, 226–231.

Young, A. W., Robertson, L. H., Hellawell, D. J., de Pauw, K. W., & Pentland, B. (1992). Cotard delusion after brain injury. *Psychological Medicine, 22*, 799–804.

Young, L., & Saxe, R. (2009). An fMRI investigation of spontaneous mental state inference for moral judgment. *Journal of Cognitive Neuroscience, 21*(7), 1396–1405.

COGNITIVE NEUROPSYCHIATRY
2010, 15 (1/2/3), 261–287

Abductive inference and delusional belief

Max Coltheart[1], Peter Menzies[2], and John Sutton[1,2]
[1]*Macquarie Centre for Cognitive Science,* [2]*Department of Philosophy, Macquarie University, Sydney, Australia*

Delusional beliefs have sometimes been considered as rational inferences from abnormal experiences. We explore this idea in more detail, making the following points. First, the abnormalities of cognition that initially prompt the entertaining of a delusional belief are not always conscious and since we prefer to restrict the term "experience" to consciousness we refer to "abnormal data" rather than "abnormal experience". Second, we argue that in relation to many delusions (we consider seven) one can clearly identify what the abnormal cognitive data are which prompted the delusion and what the neuropsychological impairment is which is responsible for the occurrence of these data; but one can equally clearly point to cases where this impairment is present but delusion is not. So the impairment is not sufficient for delusion to occur: a second cognitive impairment, one that affects the ability to evaluate beliefs, must also be present. Third (and this is the main thrust of our paper), we consider in detail what the nature of the inference is that leads from the abnormal data to the belief. This is not deductive inference and it is not inference by enumerative induction; it is abductive inference. We offer a Bayesian account of abductive inference and apply it to the explanation of delusional belief.

Keywords: Delusion; Abductive inference; Cognitive neuropsychiatry; Bayesian inference; Experience.

INTRODUCTION

William James—that uncannily prescient forefather of cognitive science—had this to say about delusional beliefs: "The delusions of the insane are apt to affect certain typical forms, very difficult to explain. But in many cases they are certainly theories which the patients invent to account for their bodily sensations" (1890/1950, chap. XIX). We think this is correct. So did one of the most influential recent thinkers about delusions, Brendan Maher: "A delusion

Correspondence should be addressed to Max Coltheart, Macquarie Centre for Cognitive Science, Macquarie University, Sydney NSW 2019, Australia. E-mail: max@maccs.mq.edu.au

We thank Ryan McKay and an anonymous reviewer for very helpful critiques of earlier drafts of this paper, and Robyn Langdon for her editorial work.

 DOI: 10.1080/13546800903439120

is a hypothesis designed to explain unusual perceptual phenomena" (1974, p. 103).

Our paper is about how deluded people go about generating the "theories" (James) or "hypotheses" (Maher) by which they can explain the unusual "bodily sensations" (James) or "perceptual phenomena" (Maher) with which they are confronted.

James was also correct in his view that delusions come in certain typical forms, and these forms have begun to be well-characterised since the birth, a century after the publication of his *Principles* (1890/1950), of the discipline of cognitive neuropsychiatry. The forms of delusion include the Cotard delusion (the belief that you are dead), the Frégoli delusion (the belief that you are constantly being followed around by people you know, whom you can't recognise because they are in disguise), somatoparaphrenia (the belief that some part of your body—your arm, for example—belongs to someone else rather than you), mirrored self-misidentification (the belief that the person you see when you look in the mirror is not you, but some stranger who happens to look like you), and others. What we have to say in this paper about how patients generate hypotheses that give rise to delusional beliefs is intended to apply to all of these forms of delusion. But we will mainly expound these ideas in relation to just one form of delusion, the one that has been most extensively studied.

THE CAPGRAS DELUSION

This is the belief that someone who is emotionally close to you—often a spouse, for example, let's say your wife—has been replaced by someone else, someone whom you consider a stranger even while acknowledging that this person does look very like your wife.

What could possibly suggest to someone the idea that the woman he is looking at (who is in fact his wife) is not his wife but some complete stranger? We believe the answer to this question is: a neuropsychological impairment that has disconnected the face recognition system (itself intact) from the autonomic nervous system (itself intact).

The evidence for this view is now very strong. In healthy control subjects, and in nondelusional psychiatric subjects, familiar faces evoke much larger responses of the autonomic nervous system, indexed by the skin conductance response (SCR) evoked by the presentation of a face, than do unfamiliar faces. But four different studies of Capgras patients (Brighetti, Bonifacci, Borlimi, & Ottaviani, 2007; Ellis, Lewis, Moselhy, & Young, 2000; Ellis, Young, Quayle, & de Pauw, 1997; Hirstein & Ramachandran, 1997) have shown that this differential autonomic responsivity to familiar faces compared to unknown faces is absent in people with Capgras delusion. In Capgras sufferers, the autonomic responses to faces are small, and are no greater for familiar than for unfamiliar faces. Hence, for the Capgras patient the autonomic response to his wife's face is just as it would be if the face he is looking at *were* the face of a stranger; and the patient does indeed say—and, we believe, *believe*—that this is the face of a stranger.

Imagine that you suffered a sudden stroke whose only effect on your brain was to disconnect your face recognition system (itself intact) from your autonomic nervous system (itself intact). Consider what will happen the next time you encounter your wife, in some context where you are expecting to see her (in the kitchen of your house, for example) and see her face. When you do encounter her, you will expect the usual consequence—a response by your autonomic nervous system. But this does not happen. Why not?—and see her face. How are you to explain this violation of expectation?

James, and Maher, would say that the task confronting the deluded person here is to formulate a hypothesis, which, if true, would account for the failure of an autonomic response to occur. Maher was very explicit concerning how this happens. His view was that the types of inferences from observations to the explanations of those observations that are performed by the deluded patient in the genesis of the delusion are no different from the types of inferences routinely made by the folk, and indeed those made by the scientist ("the explanations [i.e., the delusions] of the patient are derived by cognitive activity that is essentially indistinguishable from that employed by non-patients, by scientists, and by people generally"; 1974, p. 103).

Proponents of the view that delusions arise via a normal inferential process applied to abnormal data, a view originating with James and Maher and currently being developed further (see, e.g., Coltheart, 2007; Coltheart, Langdon, & McKay, 2007; Langdon & Coltheart, 2000) have not considered what particular form of inference is involved; but it is clear that what's involved is not deductive or (enumerative) inductive inference—it is a third type of inference, one known as *abductive* inference. So this view of delusional belief might benefit from a consideration of the philosophical conception of abductive inference. The main aim of our paper is to offer such a consideration. Before pursuing that theme, however, we need to elaborate upon what might be meant by the term "abnormal data" used at the beginning of this paragraph, and the corresponding terms used by James ("bodily sensations") and Maher ("unusual perceptual phenomena"). What's particularly important here is the use of the word "experience" in this context.

DELUSIONS AND EXPERIENCES

The James-Maher idea about delusional belief is often expressed by proposing that delusions arise via the application of normal reasoning processes to abnormal experiences. Maher himself often expressed matters in this way, e.g., "these experiences demand explanation which the patient develops through the same cognitive mechanisms that are found in the normal and scientific theory-building" (1974, p. 111).

The problem we see here is that it is common to treat experiences as by definition conscious, so that nothing of which a person is not conscious can be called an "experience", and the term "conscious experience" is a tautology. If that is how the term "experience" is being used when one proposes that delusions are rational responses to abnormal experiences, then that theory of delusion is false for many kinds of delusions—the Capgras delusion, for example. The reason is that people are not conscious of the activities of their autonomic nervous systems, and so a man would not be conscious of a failure of his autonomic nervous system to respond when he encountered his wife. Hence, what happens here is not an abnormal experience, because it is not an experience. It is an abnormality; and the application of processes of abductive inference so as to generate a hypothesis to explain this abnormality is, we consider, the source of the delusion; but we don't want to say that it is an abnormality of experience, because if we do then either (a) we must allow that experiences can be unconscious (which we don't want to do) or else (b) we must conclude that the James-Maher explanation of delusional belief fails to account for the Capgras delusion and kindred delusions (which we also don't want to do).

Of course, there is no doubt that people with Capgras delusion *do* have abnormal (conscious) experiences: Having a stranger living in your house without any explanation is an abnormal experience. So is having some stranger pretending to be your wife. But these experiences are not the cause of the delusion; they are *consequences* of the delusion.

Hence, we want to take the view that the abnormality in Capgras delusion, which prompts the exercise of abductive inference in an effort to generate a hypothesis to explain this abnormality, is not an abnormality of which the patient is *aware*. Nor is the patient aware of the application of abductive inference that occurs here. In the sudden-stroke example we gave earlier, we argue that the first delusion-relevant event of which the patient is aware is the belief "That isn't my wife". Everything that preceded the occurrence of that belief and was responsible for the belief having come about—the stroke, the neuropsychological disconnection, the absence of an autonomic response when the wife is next seen, the invocation of a process of abductive inference to yield some hypothesis to explain this, and the successful generation of such a hypothesis—all of these processes are unconscious. What's conscious is only the *outcome* that this chain of processes generated: the conscious belief "This person isn't my wife."

We consider that this kind of analysis holds true for many forms of delusion, not just for Capgras delusion. That is, in many forms of delusion, something abnormal occurs of which a person is not conscious, unconscious processes of abductive inference are invoked to seek a hypothesis which, if true, would explain that abnormality, and a hypothesis is found which is judged satisfactory by these unconscious inferential processes. After all of that unconscious processing has been completed, the hypothesis is accepted as a (delusional) belief, and enters consciousness.

Consider, for example, the Frégoli delusion—the belief that people whom you know are constantly following you around, and that the reason you don't recognise which of your acquaintances are doing this is that they wear disguises. One speculative explanation of the Frégoli delusion (Ramachandran & Blakeslee, 1998) is that it is due to neuropsychological damage that has caused abnormal hyperresponsivity of the face recognition system. That would cause the faces of unfamiliar people to activate representations of known faces in the face recognition system, and hence to generate the degree of autonomic response normally occurring only when a familiar face has been seen. This in turn generates the hypothesis that strangers you encounter in the street are often people with whom you are familiar, in disguise. All of this cognitive processing would be unconscious; the hypothesis thus formed unconsciously would subsequently arise in consciousness as a (delusional) belief.

Suppose you suffered a form of brain damage that impaired the autonomic nervous system itself. Now you would not respond autonomically to any form of stimulation. What hypothesis might abductive inference yield that would be explanatorily adequate here? The hypothesis "I am dead" is one such (because dead people are autonomically unresponsive). The delusional belief "I am dead" is known as Cotard delusion.

These specific ideas about the genesis of delusional beliefs are consistent with the general theory of unconscious processing developed in considerable detail by Mandler (1975). For example, "The analysis of situations and appraisal of the environment ... goes on mainly at the unconscious level" (p. 241); "There are many systems that cannot be brought into consciousness, and probably most systems that analyse the environment in the first place have that characteristic. In most cases, only the products of cognitive and mental activities are available to consciousness" (p. 245); "unconscious processes ... include those that are not available to conscious experience [such as] affective appraisals" (p. 230).

We do not mean to suggest that in *every* type of delusion the abnormality whose detection triggers processes of abductive inference is always an abnormality of which the deluded person is unconscious. Delusions of reference and delusions of persecution may be examples of forms of delusion in which the initial abnormality, which triggers an abductive-inference process, is a conscious experience. Maher (1974, p. 110) gives some persuasive examples of delusions of reference which, from the patients' own accounts, seem to have been triggered by abnormal perceptual experiences such as a recurrent crackling sound in the wall, or the light coming through a window seeming to be abnormally bright. Our point is that we wish to make it clear that, when we are discussing the role of abductive inference in the genesis of delusional belief, we will be allowing that the entire chain of processes, from the initial abnormality up to the identification via abductive inference of a hypothesis to explain why that abnormality has occurred, may all be unconscious. That is the reason why we will not be using the term "abnormal experience" to refer to the initial event that triggers the chain of processes that culminates in the formation of a delusional belief. Instead, we will use the neutral term "abnormal data".

ABNORMAL DATA WITHOUT DELUSIONAL BELIEF

It seems difficult to deny that the failure of autonomic response to familiar faces that occurs in Capgras delusion plays a causal role in the genesis of the delusion. Surely it can't be the case that it is just an accident that Capgras patients exhibit this failure? We assume it is not, and so we take the view that this failure is necessary for the Capgras delusion to occur. But is it *sufficient* to cause the delusion? The answer seems to be "No". Patients with damage to ventromedial regions of the frontal lobe also fail to show greater autonomic responsivity to familiar than to unfamiliar faces (Tranel, Damasio, & Damasio, 1995); but these patients still correctly identify spouses and other family members (D. Tranel, personal communication, 6 May 2008)—they are not delusional. Why not?

This conundrum is not confined to Capgras delusion; it arises in connection with a number of other delusions. Just as is the case with Capgras delusion, in other forms of delusion one can identify (or in some cases hypothesise) forms of abnormal data to which the patient is being exposed and which by their very nature would seem highly likely to be causally responsible for the content of the delusional belief. But for all of these other delusions, patients exist in whom the relevant form of abnormal data is present and yet there is no delusional belief, implying that even if the occurrence of the abnormal data is necessary for the delusion to arise, it is not sufficient.

Table 1 lists examples. The third column lists the forms of delusional belief being considered here. The first column lists the neuropsychological impairment documented as being present when the delusion is present (except for Frégoli and Cotard delusions, where the impairment has been presented as hypothesised by Ramachandran & Blakeslee, 1998; no empirical studies of autonomic responsivity in these two delusions have been reported). The second column describes the form of abnormal data that would be present as a consequence of the neuropsychological impairment.

TABLE 1
Neuropsychological impairments with and without delusion

Neuropsychological impairment	*Abnormal data generated by neuropsychological impairment*	*Hypothesis abductively inferred to explain the abnormal data*	*Cases where the neuropsychological impairment is present but there is no delusion*
Disconnection of face recognition system from autonomic system	Highly familiar faces (e.g. wife's face) no longer produce autonomic response	"That's not my wife; it is some stranger who looks like her" (Capgras delusion)	(Tranel, Damasio, & Damasio, 1995)
Autonomic system over-responsive to faces	Even the faces of strangers produce autonomic responses	"People I know are following me around; I don't recognize them; they are in disguise" (Fregoli delusion)	Patient experiences faces of strangers as highly familiar (Vuilleumier, Mohr, Valenza, Wetzel, & Landis, 2003)
Autonomic system under-responsive to all stimuli	No emotional response to one's environment	"I am dead" (Cotard delusion)	Pure autonomic failure: patient is not autonomically responsive to any stimuli (Heims, Critchley, Dolan, Mathias, & Cipolotti, 2004; Magnifico, Misra, Murray, & Mathias, 1998)
Mirror agnosia (loss of knowledge about how mirrors work)	Mirrors are treated as windows	"This person can't be me (because I am looking at him through a window, so he is in a different part of space than I)" (Mirrored-self misidentification)	Other cases of mirror agnosia (Binkofski, Buccino, Dohle, Seitz, & Freund, 1999)

Table 1 (*Continued*)

Neuropsychological impairment	*Abnormal data generated by neuropsychological impairment*	*Hypothesis abductively inferred to explain the abnormal data*	*Cases where the neuropsychological impairment is present but there is no delusion*
Impaired face processing	When the patient looks into a mirror, the mental representation constructed of the face that is seen there does not match the representation of the patient's face that is stored in long-term memory,	"The person I am looking at in the mirror isn't me" (Mirrored-self misidentification)	Many cases of prosopagnosia
Failure of computation of sensory feedback from movement	Voluntary movements no longer are sensed as voluntary	"Other people can cause my arm to move" (Delusion of alien control)	Haptic deafferentation: patient gets no sensory feedback from any actions performed (Fourneret, Paillard, Lamarre, Cole, & Jeannerod, 2002)
Damage to motor area of brain controlling arm	Left arm is paralysed; patient can't move it.	"This arm [the patient's left arm] isn't mine; it is [some specified other person]'s" (Somatoparaphrenia)	Many cases of left-sided paralysis

We wish to make two points about the contents of this table. The first point is that for all seven delusions the relationship between the specific form of the neuropsychologically generated abnormal data (Column 2) and the specific content of the delusional belief (Column 3) is such as to make highly plausible the view that the nature of the abnormal data is causally responsible for the content of the belief. So our claim is that each delusion results from applying a process of abductive inference to the abnormal data in an effort to explain why these data are occurring.

The second point is that for all seven delusions the neuropsychological impairment (Column 1) that we consider causally implicated in the delusion can nevertheless also be present in people who are not delusional (Column 4).

Thus, we have two things to explain. The first is the nature of the inferential processes which, when applied to the task of explaining the abnormal data, yield the delusional belief. The second is why it is the case that there are patients in whom the same forms of abnormal data are present but who are nevertheless not delusional.

So we turn first to a consideration of the abductive inference process itself, and exactly what role it might play in the generation of delusional beliefs.

ABDUCTIVE INFERENCE

Abductive inference, or inference to the best explanation, is the kind of inference that is used in selecting a hypothesis from a range of hypotheses on the basis of observations. Its governing idea is that explanatory considerations are a guide to inference: People infer from observations to the available hypothesis that best explains those observations. Many inferences in science and in everyday life are naturally characterised in this way. For example, when Newton inferred the truth of his theory of mechanics, he did so on the basis of the fact that it provided the best explanation of a vast range of terrestrial and celestial phenomena. When Sherlock Holmes inferred that it was Moriarty who committed the crime, he did so because this hypothesis best explained the fingerprints, the bloodstains, and other forensic evidence. Notwithstanding Holmes' claims to the contrary, this was not a matter of deduction. The evidence did not logically imply that Moriarty was the culprit, since it remained a logical possibility, formally consistent with the evidence, that someone else committed the crime. Nor was this a matter of enumerative induction that involves reasoning from observed instances of some phenomenon ("These observed swans are white") to the next instance of the phenomenon ("The next swan will be white"), or a generalisation about the phenomenon ("All swans are white"). Holmes did not infer Moriarty's guilt by inferring from Moriarty's commission of many crimes in the past to the conclusion that he has committed this crime, for this may have been the first crime that Moriarty ever committed. In any case, the evidence took the form of observations that were specific to this particular crime. Indeed, what is typical of abductive inference, unlike enumerative inductive inference, is that the conclusion introduces new concepts that are not present in the reports of the observational evidence. For example, Holmes arrived at a conclusion ("Moriarty is the culprit") that employed concepts not present on the reports of the observational data ("The murderer left fingerprints on the knife; and has a bloodstained shirt.")

As just remarked, explanation plays a key role in abductive inference. There are two standard accounts of abductive inference in the literature, drawing on different understandings of explanation. (In the philosophy of science literature, these accounts are sometimes called accounts of hypothesis or theory confirmation since they are accounts of when a hypothesis is confirmed or disconfirmed by observational evidence.) One account is the logical empiricist account and the other is the Bayesian account. Although differing in the way they understand explanation, the accounts can be understood as normative accounts of how subjects *should* reason and as descriptive accounts of how subjects *actually* reason.

We shall sketch both these accounts before turning to consider how deluded subjects might be seen as employing abductive inference to form their delusional beliefs.

The logical empiricist account of abductive inference turns on its distinctive understanding of explanation as logical implication. On this account, a hypothesis or theory H explains some observation O just in case H logically implies O. (This is consistent with the earlier remark that abductive inference is not a matter of deduction, for there we were saying that the inference of H from O is not a matter of deductively inferring H from O.) The logical empiricists concentrated on abductive inference or theory confirmation within an account of scientific theories that construed them as formal axiomatic structures. They maintained that while the scientific theories actually used by scientists might not have a formal axiomatic structure, all proper scientific theories could be reconstructed in terms of a characteristic set of axioms and rules of inference. So, within this account, a theory explains some observed phenomenon when a sentence describing the phenomenon can be deduced from the axioms of the regimented theory. For example, Newton's classical mechanics explains the orbit of a planet around the sun by virtue of the fact that the laws of the theory (in conjunction with sentences describing the initial conditions of masses and distances) logically imply a sentence describing the orbit of the planet around the sun. The first part of abductive inference or theory confirmation on the logical empiricist model consists in checking to see whether sentences describing observed phenomena can be deduced from the theory. However, this is not the whole story; there may be several hypotheses or theories that logically imply the same set of observation sentences. So the second part of abductive inference or theory confirmation consists in comparing the competing theories that explain some observational phenomena to see which of these theories provides the best explanation of the phenomena. Unfortunately, there was not a lot of consensus among the logical empiricists about which explanatory virtues make a theory the best explanation of some phenomena. It was said, for example, that of two rival hypotheses one is a better explanation than the other if it is simpler, or less ad hoc, or more coherent with a wider body of theory. It turned out to be surprisingly difficult to explicate these crucial explanatory virtues without introducing some subjective elements into theory choice.

This account of abductive inference or theory confirmation makes sense in the context of scientific theories that have a highly articulated formal structure enabling hypotheses to logically imply observational sentences. However, the theories or hypotheses that we are interested in do not have this kind of structure; and indeed they are not the kind of theories or hypotheses that logically imply observation sentences. For example, we want to be able to say that the hypothesis that Moriarty committed the crime explains the observed evidence to do with fingerprints, blood stains, etc., even though this hypothesis does not, strictly speaking, logically imply the evidence. Similarly, we want to be able to say that a deluded subject's hypothesis that his wife has been replaced by a stranger explains certain observations even though it does not, strictly speaking, logically entail the observations.

The second model of abductive inference we wish to discuss, the Bayesian model, is better suited to explaining this form of inference in the context of theories or hypotheses with little or no formal structure. For this reason we shall focus on this model in the rest of our discussion. The crucial mark of the model is that it marries a natural probabilistic account of explanation to the standard Bayesian model of rational belief systems. Let us start with the probabilistic account of explanation. As remarked earlier, we need to be able to say that hypotheses can explain observational data even when these hypotheses do not logically imply these data. It is possible to capture this idea of explanation if we allow that explanation is not an-all-or-nothing matter and that it can come in degrees. Let us say that the hypothesis H explains observations O to the degree x just in case the probability of O given H is x, i.e., $P(O|H)$ is x. The limiting case is one where H logically implies O, in which case $P(O|H)$ is 1. This definition links degree of explanation to the value of a conditional probability function. It follows from the definition that one hypothesis H_1 explains observations O better than another hypothesis H_2 just in case $P(O|H_1) > P(O|H_2)$. For example, the hypothesis that Moriarty committed the murder explains the observed phenomena better than an alternative hypothesis just in case the observed phenomena are more probable under the first hypothesis than under the second. Similarly, the deluded subject's hypothesis that his wife has been replaced by a stranger is a better explanation of the observed phenomena than an alternative hypothesis just in case these observed phenomena are more probable under the stranger hypothesis than under the alternative hypothesis.

The probabilistic definition of explanation has the virtue of providing a quantitative measure of a hypothesis' explanatory power (*vis-à-vis* some observations). It also has the virtue of being combinable with the standard Bayesian account of belief systems. The Bayesian account is supposed to be a model of the way a subject organises her belief system and the way she revises her belief system in the light of observational data. There are two basic representational assumptions made in the account. First, a subject's belief system is represented by the degrees of belief she has in certain propositions; and these degrees of belief can be represented as subjective probabilities that satisfy the axioms of the probability calculus. Second, a subject's degrees of belief or subjective probabilities change over time by the process of conditionalisation. Let us represent a subject's degrees of belief at an initial starting point in terms of the probability function P. The Bayesian model represents how this subject's belief system, as represented by her subjective probabilities, change after she has accepted a new observation O into her belief system. Let us suppose that her new degrees of belief continue to satisfy the axioms of the probability calculus; and let us symbolise them in terms of the *new* probability function P_n. Then the Bayesian thesis that belief change occurs by conditionalisation states that for any hypothesis H:

$$P_n(H) = P(H|O)$$

In other words, the value assigned by the new probability function P_n to any hypothesis H after the observational data O have been accepted is the same as the value assigned by the initial probability function P conditional on O.

The latter probability function can be expanded by Bayes' theorem into the following

$$P(H|O) = P(H).\ P(O|H)/P(O)$$

This equation tell us that a rational subject's conditional probability $P(H|O)$ (the *posterior probability* of H conditional on the observational data O) is a function of P(H) (the *prior probability* of H), the probability $P(O|H)$ (the *likelihood* of O given H), and P(O) (the initial probability of the evidence O).

The previous Bayesian formula breaks down the calculation of the conditional probability $P(H|O)$ into several steps. One step is the calculation of the likelihood function $P(O|H)$. According to the definition of explanation we have proposed, the value of this function should be given by how well the hypothesis H explains the observational data O. If it explains them well, then the likelihood function will be high; and if it doesn't explain them well, the likelihood function will be low. But the likelihood function does not by itself determine the posterior probability P(H|O). It may be that the likelihood function P(O|H) is high, but because the prior probability of H, P(H), is low, the posterior probability is also relatively low. David Hume's remarks about miracles illustrate this point. The hypothesis that a miracle has occurred (H) may explain, in the sense of being a good fit with, the fact that a witness has reported seeing the miracle (O). Indeed the likelihood function P(O|H) may be very high. But this does not mean that a person should give a high probability to the hypothesis that the miracle has occurred on the basis of the report of the witness. For the prior probability of the hypothesis that the miracle has occurred, P(H), is very low indeed: If a miracle is defined as a violation of a law of nature, then a person should assign the hypothesis that a law has been violated a very low prior probability. Given this low prior probability, the posterior probability will be low too even though the likelihood function has a high value. In Hume's view, a person should give minimal credence to the hypothesis that a miracle has occurred on the basis of a witness report. The Bayesian formula for calculating posterior probabilities vindicates Hume's plausible view.

In this exposition we have made no mention of the probability of the evidence O. In many Bayesian models of hypothesis confirmation, this probability does not play a central role. It is a commonplace of such accounts that hypothesis confirmation is almost always comparative in character: We are seldom interested in the question whether one hypothesis is confirmed by observational data in absolute terms, and almost always interested in the question which of two or more available hypotheses the observational data best confirm or support. When comparing the posterior probability of the hypothesis H with that of another hypothesis H′, Bayes' theorem implies the following equality holds

$$\frac{P(H|0)}{P(H'|0)} = \frac{P(H).\ P(O|H)}{P(H').\ P(O|H')}$$

In words, this says that the ratio of the posterior probabilities of H and H′ is a function of the ratios of the prior probabilities of these hypotheses and ratios of the likelihoods of the observational data given these two hypotheses. In this equation the probability of the observational data, P(O), has disappeared because it is cancelled out in the multiplication processes.

We have now assembled all the pieces needed to give the Bayesian account of abductive inference. As we noted at the outset, an account of abductive inference must supply an answer to the question: When is it reasonable to infer a hypothesis H on the basis of observational data O? Or perhaps the question may be more naturally expressed in comparative form: When is it reasonable to prefer one hypothesis H over another hypothesis H′ on the basis of the observational data O? The Bayesian model answers this question by saying that it is rational to prefer the hypothesis H to hypothesis H′ on the basis of the observed data O just when the conditional probability P(H|O) is higher than the conditional probability P(H′|O). When this condition holds, the model states that H is *better supported or confirmed* by these data than H′. An abductive inference to the hypothesis H from O is justified or reasonable, then, just when H is better supported by O than any other available hypothesis H′.

In this Bayesian account of abductive inference, we can see the two-step procedure evident in the logical empiricist account. The first step consists in the assessment of how well one or more hypotheses explain the observational data. In the logical empiricist account, this is decided by whether each hypothesis logically implies the observational data, whereas in the Bayesian account this is determined by a comparison of the likelihood functions associated with each hypothesis. The second step of the assessment procedure consists in comparing rival hypotheses on the basis of their general plausibility. In the logical empiricist account, the second step is effected by comparing rival hypotheses in terms of their simplicity, their level of "adhocness", and their coherence with background assumptions. In the Bayesian account, this assessment is made by comparing the prior probabilities of the rival hypotheses, where these probabilities express a measure of the general plausibility of the hypotheses based on their simplicity and overall coherence with background assumptions. The second step in each account seems to involve an irremediable element of subjectivity: There does not seem to be any objective measure of the general plausibility of a hypothesis in either account. The virtue of the Bayesian theory is that it gives us a quantitative measure of each element in the assessment procedure and a way of combining them (via Bayes' theorem) to yield an overall measure of the extent to which it is reasonable or justified to accept a hypothesis on the basis of certain observations.

It is worthwhile noting two important restrictions in scope of the Bayesian account of abductive inference. One restriction is that the account says nothing about where hypotheses come from. In the account, the provenance of hypotheses is not a matter for rational assessment. The account simply tells us when it is rational to accept a hypothesis on the basis of evidence, however the hypothesis is generated. The other restriction is that the Bayesian account says nothing systematic about the nature of observations, or the conditions of their rational acceptance into belief systems. The account is silent about questions such as what counts as an observation and to what extent observations are theory laden and so on. The account characterises observations as the starting points for the process of abductive reasoning: Observations are whatever propositions are taken for granted and treated as givens in the process of testing the explanatory adequacy of hypotheses and theories. However, the Bayesian account does presuppose it is rational for subjects in suitable circumstances to trust their senses and the testimony of others and to incorporate such observational data into their belief systems. If this was not rational, the Bayesian account of abductive reasoning could never explain belief change or revision: The procedure would simply describe the hypothetical process by which hypotheses would be confirmed if certain observations were made without ever implying that subjects actually revised their hypotheses on the basis of what they observed. Clearly, it is normal and usually rational to accept the deliverances of one's senses and the testimony of others; and the Bayesian account presupposes that this is rational even though it does not provide a systematic account of the specific circumstances in which it is rational. This second point will prove to be significant in our discussion of when the reasoning of Capgras subjects lapses into irrationality.

We must now apply the account of abductive inference we have sketched to our problems about delusional belief systems. But first we offer a more general observation about the very possibility of explaining delusions in this way, prompted by the pessimism of one philosopher of cognitive science about the idea of such explanations. In *The Mind Doesn't Work That Way*, Jerry Fodor argues that "by all the signs, the cognitive mind is up to its ghostly ears in abduction" (2000, p. 78). Fodor identifies holistic abductive reasoning as the characteristic form of belief fixation in human cognition. Computational processes in an autonomous and encapsulated peripheral module access only the information in that module's proprietary database. Such computational processes may in a sense be abductive in nature, but the fact that they draw only on local information makes them tractable to model. In contrast, our "central systems" typically employ a quite different kind of abductive reasoning: "global" or "context-sensitive" thinking, in which potentially any other background beliefs we hold may influence the current reasoning process. Even though such reasoning is, as we have suggested, fallible and defeasible, we rely entirely on it: As Paul Thagard puts it (2007, p. 226), "despite its inherent riskiness, abductive inference is an essential part of human mental life".

Fodor is pessimistic about the scope of cognitive science precisely because of the centrality of this global kind of abductive reasoning. For, he argues, "we do not know how abduction works. So we do not know how the cognitive mind works; all we know anything much about is modules" (2000, p. 78). The problem, in his view, is that the global, holistic forms of abductive reasoning that central systems typically employ seem to involve a paradox. When Sherlock Holmes inferred that the criminal is Moriarty, he drew on a scattered array of background assumptions about fingerprints, blood stains, human motivation, and so on, as well as his recent observational data: His effective use of this entire system of background beliefs was what gave his abductive reasoning its reliability. But Holmes didn't laboriously search through every single item in memory: To be effective, his abductive inference required the use of only a small subset of his beliefs. The paradox of this global form of abduction, then, is that on the one hand, in principle "the whole background of epistemic commitments [should] be somehow brought to bear in planning and belief fixation", while on the other hand it is only feasible in real time to access only the relevant information (Fodor, 2000, p. 37). Yet somehow, as if by magic, we ordinary reasoners, like Sherlock Holmes, successfully manage this selective access, judging relevance well enough to get by, most of the time. This is one version of the frame problem for artificial intelligence (Copeland, 1993, pp. 91–117; Fodor, 2000, pp. 37–38; Pylyshyn, 1987): Our models and theories offer no good formalism for specifying or delimiting in advance just how many and which other items of background knowledge should be included as relevant for any episode of reasoning. Fodor argues, in particular, that the computational theory of mind can't capture the way that we draw on the right beliefs for the current context (2000, pp. 23–53): Until someone has a good idea about how to model abductive inferences "which are sensitive to global properties of belief systems", we should hold off on studying the "more interesting and less peripheral parts of the mind" (pp. 98–99; cf. Fodor, 1975, pp. 197–205, on the limits of computational psychology).

But perhaps the prospects for computational accounts of global forms of abduction are not as gloomy as Fodor suggests. Some researchers seek to integrate computational and cognitive neuroscientific accounts of the mechanisms of inference (see Thagard, 2007, for a review; also Thagard & Shelley, 1997); and although they are not our topic here, there are also promising attempts to formalise models of inference in Bayesian networks and machine learning (Pearl, 1988). But more to the point in the current context is a direct response to Fodor. If we are right that the Bayesian model of abductive inference can help us both explain and evaluate the rationality of typical inferences made by delusional subjects, then the possibility of scientific study of central systems will be vindicated, and hence Fodor's "First Law of the Nonexistence of Cognitive Science" (Fodor, 1983) will be refuted.

In delusional subjects, we have argued, the balance between the whole background belief system and the particular evidence base is not successfully achieved. Capgras patients, for example, exhibit nonstandard reasoning in the sense that they do not efficiently use the right subset of background beliefs, or check their hypothesis effectively against other information available to them. As a result, their abductive reasoning isn't reliable. An account, within our Bayesian framework, of the peculiarities of their reasoning would go some way towards countering Fodor's pessimistic assessment. We now attempt to offer such an account.

THE APPLICATION TO DELUSIONAL BELIEF

We are now in a position to explain how the account of abductive inference we have sketched vindicates Maher's basic contention that delusional beliefs arise via rational inferential responses to highly unusual data. We shall evaluate the rationality of typical inferences made by delusional subjects within the Bayesian model of abductive inference.

Let us consider the situation of a person with Capgras delusion who is confronted with some highly unusual data: in seeing the person who claims to be his wife, the heightened activity in his autonomic nervous system that occurred on previous encounters with his wife now does not occur. Let O be the proposition that describes the data that he now observes. How is the subject to explain O? One hypothesis is that the person who claims to be his wife is actually a stranger: Label this hypothesis H_S. Another hypothesis is that this person really is his wife: Label this hypothesis H_W. Which hypothesis is better supported by his observations?

According to the Bayesian model, the first step in working out which hypothesis is better supported is to ask: Which hypothesis better explains the observed data? Or in other words, are the observed data more probable under the stranger hypothesis H_S or under the wife hypothesis H_W? The striking thing about these two particular hypotheses is that the observed data are clearly much more likely under the stranger hypothesis than under the wife hypothesis. It would be highly improbable for the subject to have the low autonomic response if the person really was his wife, but very probable indeed if the person were a stranger. Indeed, the difference in probability becomes more marked the more specific we imagine the observed data to be. If, for example, we suppose that what the subject unconsciously detects is a highly anomalous contrast between the high autonomic response he would expect to his wife and his low autonomic response occurring currently, then the stranger hypothesis will explain his observations much better than the wife hypothesis. So we conjecture that the person's subjective likelihood functions will make the following ratio very high:

$$\frac{P(O|H_S)}{P(O|H_W)} \tag{A}$$

This ratio does not by itself determine which hypothesis is better supported by the observed data. To determine this we have to know the prior probabilities of the two hypotheses. It would seem that a subject might give a very low prior probability to the stranger hypothesis H_S and a very high prior probability to the wife hypothesis H_W in view of the general implausibility of the first and the general plausibility of the second. So it would be reasonable to suppose that the subject might assign prior probabilities to the two hypotheses so as to make the following ratio very low:

$$\frac{P(H_S)}{P(H_W)} \tag{B}$$

Nonetheless, the crucial feature of the comparative form of Bayes' theorem is that the ratio of posterior probabilities

$$\frac{P(H_S|O)}{P(H_w|O)} \tag{C}$$

can still be high even when ratio (B) is low provided that the ratio (A) is sufficiently high. For example, if we suppose that the subject's prior probability $P(H_S)$ is 1/100 and $P(H_W)$ is 99/100 then the ratio (B) will be low: 1/99. But if we suppose that $P(O|H_S)$ is very high, say 999/1000, and that $P(O|H_W)$ is very low, say1/1000, then the ratio (A) will be very high, i.e., 999/1. In this case, the ratio of posterior probabilities (C) will also be high: 999/99. In other words, the posterior probability of the stranger hypothesis H_S will be more than 10 times greater than the posterior probability of the wife hypothesis H_W.

The general point here is that if the stranger hypothesis explains the observed data much better than the wife hypothesis, the fact that the stranger hypothesis has a lower prior probability than the wife hypothesis can be offset in the calculation of posterior probabilities. And indeed it seems reasonable to suppose that this is precisely the situation with the subject suffering from Capgras delusion. The delusional hypothesis provides a much more convincing explanation of the highly unusual data than the nondelusional hypothesis; and this fact swamps the general implausibility of the delusional hypothesis. So if the subject with Capgras delusion unconsciously reasons in this way, he has up to this point committed no mistake of rationality on the Bayesian model.

This account of the nature of the inferential processes which yield the delusional belief completes the first explanatory task we set ourselves. But of course everything we have said so far in this section applies to every patient who has suffered neuropsychological damage that has disconnected the face recognition system from the autonomic nervous system; and as we pointed out earlier, only some of these patients exhibit Capgras delusion. Others (those with ventromedial frontal lesions) are not delusional despite the presence of the same abnormal data that is, we argue, causally implicated in the genesis of the Capgras delusion. Why doesn't the presence of these abnormal data in the ventromedial patients result in delusion? How do these patients escape the incipient delusion?

We have argued that any subject with this neuropsychological disconnection will arrive at the belief that he is faced with a stranger through an abductive reasoning process that relies heavily on the fact that this hypothesis provides a better explanation of his highly unusual data than the rival hypothesis that the person really is his wife. However, after he has accepted the stranger hypothesis, new data relevant to this hypothesis will emerge that he should take into account; and these additional data should undermine his belief in the stranger hypothesis. For example, the subject might learn that trusted friends and family believe the person is his wife, that this person wears a wedding ring that has his wife's initials engraved in it, that this person knows things about the subject's past life that only his wife could know, and so on. Let us suppose that these further data can be formulated by the proposition O*. Surely, an application of abductive reasoning to these new data should lead the subject to lower his credence in the stranger hypothesis. For example, let P* be the subjective probability of a subject who has already incorporated the data O into his belief system. Then the comparative form of Bayes' theorem states:

$$\frac{P^*(H_S|0^*)}{P^*(H_W|0^*)} = \frac{P^*(H_S).\ P^*(O^*|\ H_S)}{P^*(H_W).\ P^*(O^*|\ H_W)}$$

Here employing the same kind of reasoning as before, one should be able to show that the subject will assign a very low posterior probability to H_S by comparison with H_W because even if the ratio of prior probabilities of the two hypotheses is high (supposing the subject gives a higher initial probability to H_S than to H_W), the ratio of likelihood probabilities will be very low indeed. The reason for this is that whatever the earlier observational data were, the wife hypothesis explains the new data O* much, much better than the stranger hypothesis and hence $P^*(O^*|\ H_W)$ is much higher than $P^*(O^*|\ H_S)$. In this case the wife hypothesis is much better supported by the new data than the stranger hypothesis. Our suggestion is that patients with ventromedial frontal damage reason in this way, and their taking into account the new evidence against H_S is the mechanism via which these patients avoid succumbing to a delusional belief in the longer term, even if this belief was initially entertained.

But how are we to explain the fact that Capgras patients, exposed to just the same data as the ventromedial patients (both the old abnormal data caused by the neuropsychological disconnection and the new data provided by wife, family, friends, and clinicians that contradicts the belief) respond differently to these new data? Why do they not reject the stranger belief on the basis of these new data that disconfirm it? What the deluded Capgras subject seems to be doing here is ignoring or disregarding any new evidence that cannot be explained by the stranger hypothesis. It is as though he is so convinced of the truth of the stranger hypothesis by its explanatory power that his conviction makes him either disregard or reject all evidence that is inconsistent with that hypothesis, or at least cannot be explained by the hypothesis.

Rejection of such evidence frequently takes the form of confabulation. Asked to explain how he know that the "stranger" is not his wife, a Capgras patient will often mention differences (which must of course be fictitious) between the physical appearance or characteristic behaviour of his wife and the "stranger" (for many examples see Coltheart & Turner, 2010, and other papers in this Special Issue).

So it seems as if the new information does not even enter the deluded subject's belief system as data that need to be explained (as distinct from needing to be explained away, via confabulation). It is a commonplace that scientists who are wedded to an explanatory theory have an irrational tendency to reject evidence that cannot be explained by their theory. The reaction of the deluded subject in response to the new information O* looks like a highly exaggerated and unreasonable version of the same tendency.

To be sure, it is sometimes reasonable to reject information that cannot be explained by the hypothesis one is committed to. And indeed the Bayesian framework explains how this can be so. Again, let P* be the probability function of a rational subject who has already incorporated the anomalous perceptual data O into his belief system. What credence should this subject give to the proposition O* before he actually learns it? The Bayesian model enables us to answer this question in terms of the theorem on total probability, which implies:

$$P^*(O^*) = P^*(H_S).\ P^*(O^*/\ H_S) + P^*(H_W).P^*(O^*/\ H_W)$$

(Here we assume for the sake of simplicity that H_W is the negation of H_S.) In other words, the credence that the subject should give to the information O* is a weighted average of the probability that the information is true under the two competing hypotheses. Assuming that the rational subject will take the wife hypothesis to be a much better explanation of the data O* than the stranger hypothesis, he'll give a low value to $P^*(O^*/\ H_S)$ and a high value to $P^*(O^*/Hw)$. For the sake of illustration, suppose he gives the first the value 1/100 and the second the value 90/100. However, when these probabilities are weighted by the probabilities that he assigns the two hypotheses, say $P^*(H_S) = 99/100$ and $P^*(H_W) = 1/100$, the previous formula implies the overall credence assigned to O* will be very low; indeed, it will be just less than 2/100. So even though the data O* would be much better explained by the wife hypothesis than the stranger hypothesis, the low credence that is given to the wife hypothesis at this stage means that the rational subject should not expect the observational proposition O* to be true.

Of course, this is the credence that a rational subject should give to the proposition O* *before* actually learning it. As we noted earlier, the Bayesian model presupposes that it is reasonable in suitable circumstances to accept the evidence of one's senses and the testimony of others. So, for example, when the ventromedial patient sees the woman wearing his wife's wedding ring and hears his friends and clinicians repeatedly tell him she is indeed his wife, it is reasonable for him to accept this information regardless of the fact that he earlier gave it low credence. It is precisely at this point that the Capgras patients differ from the ventromedial patients: The Capgras subjects are so much in the grip of the stranger hypothesis that they refuse to accept the evidence of their senses and the testimony of others. They fail to incorporate the new data into their belief systems when it is reasonable to do so. Although their abductive reasoning is faultless in response to the endogenous data caused by their neuropsychological impairment, they fail at a later stage to accept the exogenous information available to them through their senses and the testimony of others. This is the way in which they differ from the ventromedial patients, who do not suffer from this failure.

So we have arrived at an account of the phenomena we set out to explain. We have proposed that Capgras patients and ventromedial patients who are subject to the same neuropsychological impairment both initially favour the stranger hypothesis over the wife hypothesis. This piece of reasoning is a perfectly rational response to very abnormal data. In both sets of patients this reasoning results in the conscious belief "This is a stranger who looks like my wife". However, as time goes on, both kinds of subjects receive additional information, much of it in the form of the evidence of their senses and the testimony of others. The ventromedial subjects respond rationally to this extra information by revising the credence they give to the two hypotheses and settling on the wife hypothesis as the true hypothesis; so the delusional belief is rejected. In contrast, the Capgras subjects depart from rationality by rejecting this evidence: despite its seeming reliability, they irrationally ignore or discount the evidence on the basis of its incompatibility with the hypothesis to which they have become committed; so the delusional belief persists.

This account involves the conjecture that even the ventromedial patients initially experience the belief "This is not my wife" and only later abandon this belief in the face of contradictory evidence. We know of no studies that have provided evidence in support of or conflicting with this conjecture; but future research could certainly provide such evidence (for example, by confronting patients with their spouses immediately after the occurrence of the brain insult, and assessing spouse identification).

What we have done here is to flesh out a little a two-factor theory of delusional belief, which has been developing over the past decade (Coltheart, 2007; Coltheart et al., 2007; Langdon & Coltheart, 2000). In that theory, Factor 1 is the abnormality, which is responsible for the content of a delusional belief (and hence differs for different beliefs; the first factors for seven delusions are listed in Column 1 of Table 1; the first factor is what prompts the delusional belief. A delusional belief needs to be prompted in this way if it is to come to mind (something which occurs, we have suggested, via a process of Bayesian abductive inference); but when this happens the belief will ultimately be rejected unless Factor 2 is also present. This factor is, according to the two-factor theory, common to all forms of delusional belief. It has been rather vaguely described as "defective belief evaluation". We have been more specific about its nature: After Factor 1 has prompted an hypothesis about the endogenous data which prompts a delusional belief, new exogenous evidence emerges that is inconsistent with that belief, and the second factor is a failure of the system whose job it is to consider new evidence of this type so as to revise current beliefs.

The idea here is that Factor 1 is present in both Capgras and ventromedial patients, whereas Factor 2 is present only in Capgras patients. There is a little neuroanatomical support for these claims. In the case of Capgras delusion, Factor 1 is a disruption at some point in the neural pathway from the face recognition system to the autonomic nervous system. Nothing is known about which point in that pathway is damaged in Capgras patients, but the data from skin conductance studies of autonomic responding to familiar and unfamiliar faces by Capgras patients shows that it must be damaged at some point. For the same reason this pathway must also be damaged in the patients with ventromedial frontal lesions, and here we do have some evidence as to where this pathway is damaged. Tranel et al. (1995, pp. 431–432) consider that the pathway from face recognition to autonomic nervous system involves "triggering of central autonomic control nuclei from the ventromedial frontal cortices" and so if there is ventromedial frontal damage this triggering "would be precluded, and electrodermal skin conductance responses would not occur in response to the types of stimuli used in these experiments" (i.e., familiar and unfamiliar faces).

What about the neuroanatomical basis of Factor 2 in Capgras delusion? Coltheart (2007, pp. 10–11) reviewed a number of neuropsychological studies of patients with Capgras or other delusions, and pointed out that damage to the right frontal lobe has very commonly been reported in such studies. Hence, the ability to update the belief system on the basis of new evidence relevant to any particular belief may depend on the integrity of some region in the right frontal lobe. The ventromedial patients studied by Tranel et al. (1995) did not have damage to lateral regions of the right frontal lobe; their damage was to medial regions of both frontal lobes. We speculate therefore that what all seven delusions represented in Table 1 (and other delusions also) have in common is damage to some lateral region of right frontal cortex, a consequence of which is that subjects are impaired at revising preexisting beliefs on the basis of new evidence relevant to any particular belief.

An objection to this sweeping claim that immediately springs to mind is this. Surely odd beliefs of all kinds occur to all of us from time to time. If so, wouldn't someone who could not evaluate beliefs become delusional over time about all kinds of things? But that is not what the kinds of patients referred to in Table 1 are like: Their delusions are monothematic (confined to a single belief or set of related beliefs).

A response to this objection can be developed from the observations of Bisiach, Rusconi, and Vallar (1991). Their delusional patient AR, who had suffered a right hemisphere stroke that had paralysed her left arm, exhibited somatoparaphrenia in relation to that arm: She believed it to be her mother's. In the course of a neurological investigation, the patient received a standard assessment for vestibular dysfunction, irrigation of the left external ear canal with ice water. That abolished the delusion; after receiving this cold caloric left vestibular stimulation, the patient acknowledged that her left arm was hers. Two hours later, the delusion had returned.

Brain imaging studies have shown that cold caloric left vestibular stimulation produces activation of the right hemisphere, including regions of the right frontal lobe (Fasold et al., 2002; Lobel, Kleine, Le Bihan, Leroy-Willig, & Berthoz, 1998). If AR's ability to counter delusional belief via revising preexisting beliefs had been completely destroyed, nothing should be able to overcome the delusion. Instead, it seems plausible to argue here that the right frontal system responsible for such updating was impaired rather than abolished, and so could be recruited when there is abnormally high activation of the right frontal lobe, as is produced by the left cold caloric vestibular stimulation.

This hypothesis allows us to offer an explanation for why patients with Capgras and other delusions are delusional about only one topic. The odd thoughts that all of us have come and go, and because of their fleeting nature even a deficient belief updating system can prevent them from turning into delusional beliefs. But the failure of autonomic response to a spouse's face is omnipresent, and so the evidence for the stranger hypothesis is permanently powerful—too powerful to be overcome by a weakened belief updating system.

The hypothesis also allows us to say something about another feature of Capgras and other delusions: that they wax and wane. There are reports in the Capgras literature of patients who at some times believe the spouse to be a stranger and at other times have the correct belief about the spouse's identity. When patients first express some delusional belief, it is common for family, friends, and clinicians to challenge the belief, to assure the patient that it is false, and to offer various lines of evidence against it: These are the O* data we discussed earlier. If this campaign against the delusional belief is strong enough, and if the right frontal belief updating system is not too seriously impaired, the result may be that the patient can respond to the O* data by rejecting the delusional belief. Now there is no longer any need for others to campaign against the belief, and so the O* data, data inconsistent with the delusional belief, cease to be presented to the patient. But data consistent with the delusion—the data listed in Column 1 of Table 1—remain present. So the delusion returns.

A NOTE ON HELMHOLTZIAN UNCONSCIOUS INFERENCE

The idea that stimulus recognition and identification involves unconscious processes of abductive inference is of course far from new; it goes back at least as far as Helmholtz (1867/1910), and figures prominently in the theoretical work of Irvin Rock (1983). The information collected by the senses is inherently ambiguous. For example, when an object has an elliptically shaped retinal image, that might be because what is being viewed is an ellipse in the frontoparallel plane; but the observation is equally compatible with this object being circular but tilted. There are thus effectively an infinite number of questions to the answer: Given that I have this particular image on my retina, what must the world be like? Hatfield (2002, p. 116) commented on Helmholtz's approach to such issues as follows: "Helmholtz maintained that perception draws on the same cognitive mechanisms as do ordinary reasoning and scientific inference (1867/1910, 3: 28–29)", and he commented on Rock's approach as follows:

> "The most explicit recent analysis of unconscious inferences in perception is due to Irvin Rock (1983). Rock identified four sorts of cognitive operations at work in perception, [two of which were] (1) unconscious description, in the case of form perception (1983, ch. 3); (2) problem solving and *inference to the best explanation*, in the case of stimulus ambiguity or stimulus features that would yield unexplained coincidences if interpreted literally (1983, chs. 4–7)." (p. 125, emphasis added)

The similarity between these ideas about how perception works and the ideas about the genesis of delusional belief which we introduced with our quotations from William James and Brendan Maher at the beginning of this paper and which we have elaborated upon in our paper could hardly be clearer.

CONCLUSIONS

We have offered a general account of the seven delusions described in Table 1—which perhaps also applies to other forms of delusional belief too. The first step in the genesis of a delusional belief is the introduction into a person's unconscious (or conscious) mental life of some new and at present inexplicable observation O. These are the observations listed in Column 3 of

Table 1, and, at least for the seven delusions considered there, the source of the abnormal observation is the neuropsychological impairment given in Column 1.

The next step involves the patient seeking to explain the novel observation. This search involves discovering some hypothesis H about the world, which, if true, would make O very probable. (Of course, it is the facts described by the observation O rather than the mere occurrence of the observation that the hypothesis H must make probable.) There will be many possible potential states of the world such that, if any of these were actually true of the world, the facts described by O would be likely to obtain. The choice between these hypotheses that is part of the process of abductive inference is, we have suggested, done in a Bayesian manner that depends crucially on the likelihood function P(O|H), the (subjective) probability of O given the truth of H. No matter how unlikely a particular H is, this probability function may be higher for that H than for any other Hs no matter how much more plausible these other Hs are than the H which is adopted. So an H for which the conditional probability P(O/H) is particularly high can be assigned a very high value of the posterior probability P(H|O) even when P(H) is very low; and it is these posterior probabilities that control the adoption of hypotheses as beliefs.

But we have been at pains to emphasise that even when everything described in the previous paragraph occurs to someone, that person will not necessarily become delusional; these counterexamples are listed in Column 4 of Table 1. What is needed to create a full-blown delusional case is a second cognitive impairment, one that prevents new observations occurring after the initial adoption of the hypothesis as a belief from causing the rejection of that belief, as they ought to because they conflict with that belief. Our present account implies, though, that even for patients without this second impairment—patients in Column 4 of Table 1—the delusional belief will initially occur, but then be rejected. As we have noted, this is speculative: We would welcome further studies of the behavioural and phenomenological differences between these two groups of patients—for example, between Capgras patients and ventromedial patients—in the very early aftermath of neuropsychological damage.

We have largely used the Capgras delusion to work through this account, but the application of this account to at least some of the other delusions in Table 1—the Cotard and Frégoli delusions, for example—is readily apparent. What needs to be done next is to work through all these seven forms of delusion—and others—to determine whether or not a plausible two-factor account involving a Bayesian process of abductive inference can be spelled out for all.

REFERENCES

Binkofski, F., Buccino, G., Dohle, C., Seitz, R. J., & Freund, H. J. (1999). Mirror agnosia and mirror ataxia constitute different parietal lobe disorders. *Annals of Neurology, 47*, 553–554.

Bisiach, E., Rusconi, M. L., & Vallar, G. (1991). Remission of somatoparaphrenic delusion through vestibular stimulation. *Neuropsychologia, 10*, 1029–1031.

Brighetti, G., Bonifacci, P., Borlimi, R., & Ottaviani, C. (2007). Far from the heart far from the eye": Evidence from the Capgras delusion. *Cognitive Neuropsychiatry, 12*, 189–197.

Coltheart, M. (2007). The 33rd Bartlett lecture: Cognitive neuropsychiatry and delusional belief. *Quarterly Journal of Experimental Psychology, 60*, 1041–1062.

Coltheart, M., Langdon, R., & McKay, R. (2007). Schizophrenia and monothematic delusions. *Schizophrenia Bulletin, 33*, 642–647.

Coltheart, M., & Turner, M. (2009). Confabulation and delusion. In W. Hirstein (Ed.), *Confabulation: Views from neurology, psychiatry, neuroscience and philosophy* (pp. 173–188). Oxford, UK: Oxford University Press.

Copeland, J. (1993). *Artificial intelligence: A philosophical introduction*. Oxford, UK: Blackwell.

Ellis, H. D., Lewis, M. B., Moselhy, H. F., & Young, A. W. (2000). Automatic without autonomic responses to familiar faces: Differential components of covert face recognition in a case of Capgras delusion. *Cognitive Neuropsychiatry, 5*, 255–269.

Ellis, H. D., Young, A. W., Quayle, A. H., & de Pauw, K. W. (1997). Reduced autonomic responses to faces in Capgras delusion. *Proceedings of the Royal Society, Series B: Biological Science, 264*, 1085–1092.

Fasold, O., von Brevern, M., Kuhberg, M., Ploner, C. J., Villringer, A., Lempert, T., et al. (2002). Human vestibular cortex as identified with caloric stimulation in functional magnetic resonance imaging. *NeuroImage, 17*, 1384–1393.

Fodor, J. A. (1975). *The language of thought*. New York: Crowell.

Fodor, J. A. (1983). *The modularity of mind*. Cambridge, MA: MIT Press.

Fodor, J. A. (2000). *The mind doesn't work that way*. Cambridge, MA: MIT Press.

Fourneret, P., Paillard, J., Lamarre, Y., Cole, J., & Jeannerod, M. (2002). Lack of conscious recognition of one's own actions in a haptically deafferented patient. *Neuroreport, 13*, 541.

Hatfield, G. (2002). Perception as unconscious inference. In D. Heyer & R. Mausfeld (Eds.), *Perception and the physical world: Psychological and philosophical issues in perception* (pp. 113–143). New York: Wiley.

Heims, H. C., Critchley, H. D., Dolan, R., Mathias, C. J., & Cipolotti, L. (2004). Social and motivational functioning is not critically dependent on feedback of autonomic responses: Neuropsychological evidence from patients with pure autonomic failure. *Neuropsychologia, 42*, 1979–1988.

Helmholtz, H. L. (1867). *Handbuch der physiologischen Optik*. Leipzig: L. Voss. Reprinted 1910, with extensive commentary, in A. Gullstrand, J. von Kries, & W. Nagel (Eds.), *Handbuch der physiologischen Optik* (3rd ed.). Hamburg and Leipzig: L. Voss.

Hirstein, W., & Ramachandran, V. S. (1997). Capgras syndrome: A novel probe for understanding the neural representation of the identity and familiarity of persons. Proceedings of the Royal Society. *Series B: Biological Science, 264*, 437–444.

James, W. (1950). *Principles of psychology* (Vol. 2). New York: Henry Holt & Co. (Original work published 1890).

Langdon, R., & Coltheart, M. (2000). The cognitive neuropsychology of delusions. *Mind and Language, 15*, 184–218.

Lobel, E., Kleine, J. F., Le Bihan, D., Leroy-Willig, A., & Berthoz, A. (1998). Functional MRI of galvanic vestibular stimulation. *Journal of Neurophysiology, 80*, 2699–2709.

Magnifico, F., Misra, V. P., Murray, N. M. F., & Mathias, C. J. (1998). The sympathetic skin response in peripheral autonomic failure—evaluation in pure autonomic failure, pure cholinergic failure and dopamine-hydroxylase deficiency. *Clinical Autonomic Research, 8*, 133–138.

Maher, B. A. (1974). Delusional thinking and perceptual disorder. *Journal of Individual Psychology, 30*, 98–113.

Mandler, G. (1975). Consciousness: Respectable, useful and probably necessary. In R. Solso (Ed.), *Information processing and cognition: The Loyola symposium* (pp. 229–254). Hillsdale, NJ: Lawrence Erlbaum Associates, Inc.

Pearl, J. (1988). *Probabilistic reasoning in intelligent systems: Networks of plausible inference.* San Francisco: Morgan Kaufman.

Pylyshyn, Z. W. (Ed.). (1987). *The robot's dilemma: The frame problem in artificial intelligence.* Norwood, NJ: Ablex.

Ramachandran, V. S., & Blakeslee, S. (1998). *Phantoms in the brain: Human nature and the architecture of the mind.* London: Fourth Estate.

Rock, I. (1983). *The logic of perception.* Cambridge, MA: MIT Press.

Thagard, P. (2007). Abductive inference: From philosophical analysis to neural mechanisms. In A. Feeney & E. Heit (Eds.), *Inductive reasoning: Cognitive, mathematical, and neuroscientific approaches* (pp. 226–247). Cambridge, UK: Cambridge University Press.

Thagard, P., & Shelley, C. P. (1997). Abductive reasoning: Logic, visual thinking, and coherence. In M. L. Dalla Chiara, K. Doets, D. Mundici, & J. van Benthem (Eds.), *Logic and scientific methods* (pp. 413–427). Dordrecht, The Netherlands: Kluwer.

Tranel, D., Damasio, H., & Damasio, A. R. (1995). Double dissociation between overt and covert face recognition. *Journal of Cognitive Neuroscience, 7*, 425–432.

Turner, M., & Coltheart, M. (2010). Confabulation and delusion: A common monitoring framework? *Cognitive Neuropsychiatry, 15*(1/2/3), 346–376.

Vuilleumier, P., Mohr, C., Valenza, N., Wetzel, C., & Landis, T. (2003). Hyperfamiliarity for unknown faces after left lateral temporo-occipital venous infarction: A double dissociation with prosopagnosia. *Brain, 126*, 889–907.

COGNITIVE NEUROPSYCHIATRY
2010, 15 (1/2/3), 288–318

Confabulation, delusion, and anosognosia: Motivational factors and false claims

Ryan McKay[1,2] and Marcel Kinsbourne[3]

[1]*Institute for Empirical Research in Economics, University of Zürich, Zürich, Switzerland,* [2]*Centre for Anthropology and Mind, University of Oxford, Oxford, UK,* [3]*Department of Psychology, The New School, New York, USA*

False claims are a key feature of confabulation, delusion, and anosognosia. In this paper we consider the role of *motivational factors* in such claims. We review motivational accounts of each symptom and consider the evidence adduced in support of these accounts. In our view the evidence is strongly suggestive of a role for motivational factors in each domain. Before concluding, we widen the focus by outlining a tentative general taxonomy of false claims, including false claims that occur in clinical settings as well as more garden-variety false claims, and incorporating both motivational and nonmotivational approaches to explaining such claims.

Keywords: Anosognosia; Confabulation; Delusion; Motivational processes

Patients in neurological and psychiatric settings are known to make rather striking claims. Consider the following two examples:

1. "I am the left foot of God."
2. "My father is 95–96. My mother is 10 years younger so she is 85–86."

The first claim is striking because it is bizarre and grandiose, but also because the individual who made it was a brilliant mathematician who went on to win a Nobel prize (see Nasar, 1998). In contrast, the striking nature of

Correspondence should be addressed to Dr Ryan McKay, Centre for Anthropology and Mind, University of Oxford, 51–53 Banbury Road, Oxford OX2 6PE, UK. E-mail: ryantmckay@mac.com

RM was supported by a research fellowship as part of a large collaborative project coordinated from the Centre for Anthropology and Mind (http://www.cam.ox.ac.uk) at the University of Oxford and funded by the European Commission's Sixth Framework Programme ("Explaining Religion"). Thanks to Katerina Fotopoulou for valuable discussions, and to those who organised and participated in the Delusions and Confabulations workshop, held at Macquarie University in July 2007. We also acknowledge the helpful comments of two anonymous reviewers.

 DOI: 10.1080/13546800903374871

the second claim requires some context to appreciate. At the time he made this statement, this man's parents had been dead for years (and had died in their seventies—see Moscovitch, 1995, p. 228).

How are we to account for such claims? And how can we characterise them? According to the scientific literature, the first example is considered to reflect a *delusion* (David, 1999), whereas the second is a paradigmatic instance of *confabulation* arising in the context of memory impairment (Moscovitch, 1995). The problem from a theoretical perspective is that it is not clear what the distinctions are between these two classes of symptom, nor what the nature of the overlap is between them, if any. This is most obvious when one considers that certain patient presentations are thought of as involving delusion in some circles, and confabulation in others. An example is anosognosia, which involves unawareness or denial of disease or disability, in particular denial of left hemiplegia following right-hemisphere brain damage. Recent authors have explicitly characterised this condition as either delusion (e.g., Aimola Davies, Davies, Ogden, Smithson, & White, 2009; Davies, Aimola Davies, & Coltheart, 2005) or confabulation (e.g., Heilman, 2009; Hirstein, 2005).

One feature common to confabulation, delusion, and anosognosia is that each of these symptoms typically involves some sort of false public claim. There may be exceptions to this—for example, delusions are usually conceptualised as false beliefs (cf. Hamilton, 2007; Stephens & Graham, 2004), and beliefs can be kept private. On the other hand, it is typically because of the public declarations of deluded individuals that delusions attract clinical attention. Another exception involves the fact that delusions and confabulations might be, as it were, "serendipitously" true. A patient may lack access to his biographical information, yet by chance may confabulate the correct answer when asked his age. Such exceptions aside, false claims are a key feature of these disorders. Our primary aim in this paper is to consider the role of *motivational factors* in such claims. In the sections that follow we will discuss motivational accounts of confabulation, delusion, and anosognosia. Before concluding, we will widen the focus by outlining a tentative general taxonomy of false claims, including false claims that occur in clinical settings as well as more garden-variety false claims, and incorporating both motivational and nonmotivational approaches to explaining such claims.

MOTIVATIONAL ACCOUNTS

What *are* motivational factors? In essence, they are goal-directed states or processes such as desires and intentions: processes that generate and structure action (Bayne & Fernández, 2009). Bayne and Fernández (2009) contrast such "telic" processes with "thetic" processes that provide, or at least aim to provide, a veridical representation of the world. Whereas thetic states (aim to) represent the way the world is, telic states (insofar as they are representational) represent the way we would like the world to be.

A complication here stems from the fact that our ideal world might be a world in which we have accurate representations of reality. We therefore invoke a further distinction (although not much will turn on it here), a distinction between representations and metarepresentations:

- *Thetic representations* represent the way the world actually is. Example: "I believe that I am a poor athlete."
- *Telic representations* represent the way we would like the world to be. Example: "I wish that I were a great athlete."
- *Thetic metarepresentations* represent our thetic and telic representations. Examples: (1) "I believe that some of my beliefs are false (although I don't know which ones specifically)"; (2) "I believe that I like chocolate."
- *Telic metarepresentations* represent the kinds of thetic and telic representations we would like to have. Examples: (1) "I wish that all of my beliefs were true"; (2) "I wish that I liked broccoli."

On our definition, motivational accounts of symptoms at the interface of psychiatry and neurology (e.g., delusions, confabulations) are accounts of such symptoms that implicate the motivationally biased handling of evidence (Mele, 1997; see also Davies, 2009). In such accounts, the symptoms in question arise when telic factors figure unduly[1] in the formation of thetic representations (or metarepresentations). Moreover, the symptoms are viewed as conferring some kind of psychological benefit, and this is their *raison d'être*. In some instances the symptoms may be seen as reflecting efforts to disarm inner threats and to defuse tension. In other instances the putative goal may be to reduce confusion and ambiguity.

[1] What do we mean by "unduly"? An example may serve to clarify. Imagine that a scientist, motivated by a desire for certainty (see later), conducts an experiment to investigate which of two theories best explains a given phenomenon. She runs the experiment, but sadly the results she obtains are utterly equivocal. However, her desire for certainty is sufficiently strong that her consideration of her evidence is motivationally biased: instead of admitting that her data are completely inconclusive, she concludes that the evidence favours one theory over the other. This conclusion (a thetic representation) has stemmed from her desire for certainty (a telic factor: specifically a telic metarepresentation), both in the sense that this factor provided the original impetus for conducting the experiment and in the sense that this factor biased her handling of the evidence. It is only in the second sense, however, that the telic factor has figured *unduly* in the formation of the thetic representation.

In contrast, proponents of nonmotivational accounts do not view psychoneurological symptoms as having a *raison d'être*—at least not in the teleological sense. Rather, these symptoms are viewed as representing functionless—indeed, *dys*functional—departures from normal operation. This is the pure neuropsychological deficit perspective (note that an integrated motivational and deficit perspective is also possible; see later). From the purely deficit perspective the symptoms do, however, have a "reason for being" in the mechanical, aetiological sense—they stem from abnormalities in ordinary cognitive processes, underpinned by damage or disruption to the brain.

We turn now to a brief consideration of some recent evidence for motivational accounts of confabulation.

MOTIVATIONAL ACCOUNTS OF CONFABULATION

Broadly speaking, there are two main types of motivational account where confabulation is concerned. In the first place, a number of authors have suggested that some patients confabulate in order to conceal embarrassing gaps in their memories. This "gap-filling" hypothesis has a long history (e.g., Bonhoeffer, 1901), but to date there is very little evidence that the theory is valid, at least as a general account (see Schnider, 2008, for a review). Note, in any case, that this account only qualifies as "motivational" in our terms if individuals confabulate so as to conceal memory gaps from *themselves*. This is because attempts to conceal memory gaps from others need not involve any departure from rationality. Patients who are cognisant of their memory gaps may seek to influence the thetic representations of others with respect to these lacunae, but this goal does not require the motivationally biased handling of evidence. Note also that a purely gap-filling account need make no prediction regarding the *emotional valence* of confabulatory content. If patients are motivated by a desire to avoid revealing (to themselves?) the limitations of their memories, the key consideration should be to paper over embarrassing gaps with *plausible* content, whether positive or negative. Yet confabulations are frequently implausible (and indeed frequently *impossible*).

In contrast, other authors have claimed that confabulations are purposive constructions that function to embellish the situation of the patient (e.g., Conway & Tacchi, 1996). On this view, confabulations are compensatory not (or not merely) by virtue of their existence, but via their motivated content. Purely motivational variants explain both the existence and the content of confabulation in motivational terms. Integrated variants, on the other hand, incorporate a role for both motivational and nonmotivational factors. For example, Fotopoulou and colleagues (see Fotopoulou, 2010 this issue, for an overview) have suggested that self-serving confabulations are prominent because impairments in executive processes responsible for the inhibition of previously rewarded responses lead to the preferential selection of personally rewarding representations (e.g., memory representations). Whether pure or integrated, motivational accounts of the second type make specific predictions regarding the emotional valence of confabulations—that they should be *positively biased*, and in particular *more* positively biased than the memory distortions of healthy control participants. Fotopoulou and colleagues have tested these predictions in a number of systematic empirical investigations, two of which we outline here (see Fotopoulou, 2010 this issue, and Metcalf, Langdon, & Coltheart, 2010 this issue, for reviews of other recent studies, and for more thorough general treatments of the role of motivational factors in confabulation).

First, Fotopoulou, Conway, Griffiths, Birchall, and Tyrer (2007) investigated the provoked confabulations of a 60-year-old male patient ("LH") who had undergone surgical clipping of an anterior communicating artery (ACoA) aneurysm. A CT angiographic study performed 10 days postsurgery had revealed a large acute infarction within LH's left frontal lobe, including both the dorsolateral and ventromedial prefrontal cortex. On clinical examination 4 months postsurgery he presented as talkative, hyperactive, verbally disinhibited, amnesic, and densely anosognosic. LH's confabulations at this time appeared to be wishful and self-aggrandising. For example, he claimed that he was in a holiday resort and treated hospital staff accordingly. To substantiate this clinical impression of his confabulations, LH and five neurologically healthy age-, sex-, and education-matched control participants were each asked to describe a series of "self-defining" events, including high and low points of their lives, turning points, and earliest memories. The resulting protocols were coded for valence, and separate interviews held with participants' relatives and staff provided corroborating information for the reported memories. The authors found that the confabulations produced by LH in this paradigm were significantly more positively valenced than both his true memories and the memories of the control participants.

In a subsequent investigation (Fotopoulou et al., 2008), false memories were elicited in 10 severely amnesic confabulating patients, 10 healthy age- and education-matched controls, and four amnesic nonconfabulating controls. Control participants were asked to deliberately alter true self-referential memories in order to create false memories. Memory protocols drawn from interviews with these groups were later coded for valence: raters indicated, on a 7-point scale, whether self-representations in the confabulated events were positive/self-enhancing, or negative/self-diminishing, relative to the relevant self-representations in the corresponding "reality" (as gleaned, for confabulators, by information provided by relatives, staff, or medical files). The authors found that the false memories of the confabulating patients distorted previous experiences in a significantly more pleasant and self-enhancing manner than those of controls.

To summarise, two main classes of motivational explanation exist for confabulation. The first hypothesis, that patients confabulate to conceal gaps in their memories, has garnered little empirical support. The second hypothesis, however, that confabulations reflect the operation of processes that embellish the patient's situation, looks more promising. A series of studies are suggestive of a systematic positive bias in the emotional valence of confabulations. Importantly, there is evidence that such biases exceed those displayed by healthy control participants. Although evidence of a positive bias is consistent with a purely motivational account of confabulation, Fotopoulou and colleagues favour a more nuanced account that integrates both motivational factors and neuropsychological impairments.

MOTIVATIONAL ACCOUNTS OF DELUSION

The Capgras, Cotard, and Frégoli delusions

We begin this section by outlining motivational accounts of three intriguing delusions—the Capgras, Cotard, and Frégoli delusions. Consider, first, the Capgras delusion. Capgras patients believe that an impostor has replaced a person close to them. In an early formulation of this condition, Capgras and Carette (1924) described a young woman's impostor delusions as representing an attempt to veil incestuous desires for her father. The suggestion here seemed to be that in coming to believe that the object of her desire was actually a fraudulent impersonator of her father, the woman had found a way of rendering her desire acceptable (sexual desire is not so troubling if the object of desire is merely *impersonating* a family member). Converting an unacceptable desire into an acceptable desire was thus the proposed *raison d'être* of this woman's delusion.

Now consider Cotard syndrome, which can involve the conviction that one is dead or has ceased to exist (Cotard, 1882; Young & Leafhead, 1996). A motivational account of this condition can be found in Enoch and Ball (2001), who suggest that it may serve the protective function of reducing existential anxiety caused by awareness of mortality (cf. Becker, 1973; Greenberg, Pyszczynski, & Solomon, 1986). If one is already dead or does not exist, then one cannot fear death or the future cessation of existence (a kind of "you-can't-fire-me-because-I-quit" strategy). Such seems to be the spirit of Enoch and Ball's formulation.

Finally, consider the Frégoli delusion. Patients with this delusion believe that they are being followed about by a familiar person who is in disguise and thus unrecognisable (Davies & Coltheart, 2000; cf. Banov, Kulick, Oepen, & Pope, 1993). Collacot and Napier (1991; cited in Mojtabai, 1994) put forward a motivational account of this delusion. The case was a woman who had misidentified certain strangers as her deceased father. According to Collacot and Napier, the woman's delusion represented an attempt to fulfil a wish that her father still be alive. Transforming an intolerable reality into a desired reality was thus the proposed *raison d'être* of her delusion.

What are we to make of accounts such as these? One criticism is that some of these accounts can get very convoluted. The subject of the Capgras formulation just described, for example—the woman with the delusion about her father—also believed that impostors had replaced her mother, brother, uncle, and aunt (de Pauw, 1994). It would seem necessary, therefore, to have postulated additional incestuous fantasies if the theory in question was to hold. The Cotard and Frégoli formulations also seem rather convoluted. If you are afraid of death, why not adopt the belief that you are immortal? This seems a happier solution (and no less realistic) than to adopt the belief that you are already dead. If grief is intolerable, why not believe that your departed loved one is in heaven? This seems more comforting, and less confusing, than the belief that your loved one would follow you around in disguise. Of course, many people *do* believe in immortality and heaven, and many others have argued that telic factors figure unduly in the formation of such thetic representations. But this just underscores the point with regard to the Cotard and Frégoli delusions—if a culturally sanctioned belief system already provides the relevant psychological benefits, why seek these benefits in exotic beliefs that are likely to be opposed at every turn?

Whatever credibility these motivational formulations might have for the cases in question, they seem implausible as general theoretical accounts. The sexual desire formulation of Capgras, for example, seems hard-pressed to explain all reported cases. After all, impostor delusions have been reported for a range of animals including a dog (Raschka, 1981), a cat (Reid, Young, & Hellawell, 1993), a parrot (Somerfield, 1999), and a canary (Rosler, Holder, & Seifritz, 2001). There are also reports of cases involving inanimate objects such as tools and ornaments (see Ellis et al., 1996). A second example is that the wish fulfilment account of Frégoli delusion struggles to explain Frégoli cases where strangers are misidentified as familiar, but *hostile*, individuals. Proponents of motivational accounts might point out that their accounts are not intended as stock explanations, applicable to each and every occurrence of the delusions in question. But if motivational accounts are to be useful, they should at least be testable—not simply assembled ad hoc.

Interestingly, a single testable framework exists that may potentially explain all three of these delusions—a framework that is not motivational but purely neuropsychological. Briefly, the framework implicates disrupted connections between face-processing areas and the limbic system in the formation of these delusions (Ellis & Young, 1990; Langdon & Coltheart, 2000; Stone & Young, 1997; although see Hirstein, 2010 this issue, for an alternate interpretation). Such disruptions are thought to generate discrepancies between visual and autonomic familiarity data. In the case of Capgras delusion, visually familiar others may be rendered autonomically unfamiliar, an incongruence that the impostor belief may be generated to explain. In their original description, Capgras and Reboul-Lachaux (1923) related that their patient had developed a feeling of strangeness when viewing the faces of familiar people. So the conclusion that there are doubles is a judgement explained in part by emotional factors (which is not to say that emotion biases the patient's treatment of the unusual emotional data; see Mele, 2009). A study conducted by Ellis, Young, Quayle, and de Pauw (1997) provided empirical evidence consistent with this proposal. These researchers recorded skin-conductance responses (SCRs) while showing Capgras patients and control participants a series of predominantly unfamiliar faces, with occasional familiar faces interspersed. Whereas control participants showed significantly greater SCRs to familiar faces than unfamiliar faces, Capgras patients showed SCRs of equivalent magnitude to photographs of both types (see also Brighetti, Bonifacci, Borlimi, & Ottaviani, 2007; Hirstein & Ramachandran, 1997).

Young and colleagues (e.g., Wright, Young, & Hellawell, 1993; Young, 2000; Young & Leafhead, 1996; Young, Leafhead, & Szulecka, 1994) have suggested that a disjuncture between visual and autonomic data may be a causal feature of Cotard delusion as well as of Capgras delusion. The difference, they maintain, is a matter of the individual's prevailing attributional style. Whereas Capgras patients make external attributions for the incongruous data (e.g., "that woman is not my wife, she's a stranger who looks just like her—an impostor"), Cotard patients make internal attributions (e.g., "that woman looks like my wife but doesn't 'feel' like her—I must be dead").

The latter attribution, it must be said, seems rather unlikely—involving an extravagant logical leap. Ramachandran and Blakeslee (1998; see also Gerrans, 2000, 2002) favour a different proposal, that whereas Capgras delusion involves disruption to pathways underpinning the emotional component of face recognition, Cotard delusion involves a more global disconnection of *all* sensory areas from the limbic system. This would result in a fundamentally altered experience of the world, in light of which the belief that one has died might not seem so outlandish. Although on the face of it this proposal is perhaps more credible than the Young et al. attributional hypothesis, a recent study by McKay and Cipolotti (2007) found evidence consistent with the latter—namely, a pronounced internalising attributional bias in a patient with Cotard delusion. More research is needed here—in particular, it would be useful to investigate whether Cotard patients do in fact show deficits in autonomic arousal, and if so whether these deficits are restricted to facial stimuli or whether they involve a more global loss of autonomic responsiveness to all familiar stimuli.

Finally, the discrepant familiarity data framework can also be plausibly extended to the Frégoli delusion. Whereas the evidence outlined previously suggests that the Capgras delusion stems from a diminished affective response to known faces (visual familiarity in the absence of autonomic familiarity), Ramachandran and Blakeslee (1998; cf. Christodoulou, 1976, 1977; Feinberg & Keenan, 2005) proposed that the Frégoli delusion may be generated to explain a *heightened* affective response to *un*familiar faces (autonomic familiarity in the absence of visual familiarity). Although this specific hypothesis is yet to be investigated, the appeal of the neuropsychological familiarity data framework lies in its testability (where Capgras delusion is concerned, predictions have already been tested and confirmed), plausibility (in contrast to the rather extravagant motivational stories outlined earlier) and parsimony (three separate delusions are accommodated in a single framework). For these reasons, motivational accounts of these delusions have been rendered largely obsolete (although, given the neuropsychological disorder, the surface manifestations might well vary from case to case due to idiosyncratic motivational factors).

Before we move on, we wish to emphasise that the discrepant familiarity data theory is not without its own problems. Regarding Capgras, for example, some account needs to be given of the (variable) selectivity of impostor delusions. Although many Capgras patients believe that multiple others have been replaced by impostors (one of Ellis et al.'s, 1997, patients had "Capgras for virtually the entire town of residence", p. 1087), others misidentify just a single individual. Presumably the reason for this variability is that the extent of autonomic disruption is variable across patients. For patients with minor disruption, therefore, the discrepancy between visual and autonomic familiarity would only be significant for highly familiar others (those emotionally close to the patient), whereas more major disruptions would generate more widespread discrepancies ("virtually the entire town of residence"). However, given that the patients in the Ellis et al. study showed a diminished affective response to pictures of famous people, why did none of them claim that these were pictures of impostors?

A second problem concerns the claim that Capgras delusion implicates pathways underpinning the emotional component of *face* recognition. Some cases of Capgras do not involve face perception at all—for example, Reid et al. (1993) described the case of a blind woman with Capgras, and we have already noted that misidentification can occur for inanimate objects. Such cases call for explanations involving different recognition systems (see Ellis et al., 1996). We mention this fact not to discredit such accounts, but merely to show that neuropsychological accounts can also quickly become convoluted when the range of different patient presentations is taken into consideration. We are not sure, however, how a purely neuropsychological account would explain the case of a woman who believed that she was pregnant with an impostor foetus ... (Silva, Leong, Longhitano, & Botello, 1991).

Persecutory delusions

Motivational accounts need not be convoluted. And for some delusions they seem quite natural:

> Consider the delusion of erotomania (de Clérambault's delusion), in which the patient forms the belief that someone of higher social status is secretly in love with him or her ... This delusion quite obviously cries out for a motivational explanation ... (Bayne & Fernández, 2009, p. 13).

As we indicated earlier, however, if motivational accounts are to be accepted they must be tested empirically—not just constructed ad hoc. With respect to motivational accounts of delusions, the most systematic experimental work has focussed on persecutory delusions, and especially on the psychodynamically inflected motivational formulation of Bentall and colleagues (see, for example, Bentall & Kaney, 1996; Kinderman & Bentall, 1996, 1997; see also McKay, Langdon, & Coltheart, 2007a, who chart the evolution of this theory through increasingly complex conceptions).

Persecutory delusions are the most common delusional subtype. According to the classic psychodynamic conception, paranoid symptoms are occasioned by defensive attempts to escape intolerable feelings of shame and culpability by projecting them onto others (see McWilliams, 1994). Any sense of personal guilt or failure is transformed into dangers that threaten from outside, and the deluded individual assuages his or her sense of personal inadequacy at the cost of living in a world replete with hostile, malevolent agents (Adler, 1914/1929; Bell, 2003; Freud, 1895; Zigler & Glick, 1988). Notwithstanding differing conceptions of the *syntax* of the putative projective process (see McKay et al., 2007a), the formulation of Bentall et al. retains certain elements of this classic notion, particularly the idea that paranoid individuals impute malicious intentions to others so as to evade conscious awareness of negative self-representations. In brief, Bentall and colleagues have claimed that persecutory delusions are constructed defensively, for the preservation of explicit *self-esteem*. A key prediction of their model is that persecutory delusions will occur in association with discrepancies between *relatively* high measures of conscious, explicit self-esteem and *relatively* low measures of unconscious, implicit self-esteem.[2]

A number of studies have attempted to test this prediction. Kinderman (1994), for example, used an "emotion" version of the Stroop test (Stroop, 1935) to measure preconscious attentional biases to different word types. Participants in this task are required to name the colours of various words; because colour naming is typically slowed for emotionally salient words, response speeds can be used to index the degree to which the emotional salience of a word (or concept) has interfered with performance. Kinderman found that although persecutory deluded individuals rated positive personally descriptive adjectives as more self-relevant than negative adjectives, they showed an attentional bias (as indexed by degree of colour-naming interference) for the negative adjectives. According to Kinderman, this discrepancy reflected the operation of a defensive process associated with discrepancies between high explicit and low implicit self-esteem. Garety and Freeman (1999), however, have critiqued this interpretation of Kinderman's results. These authors noted that the persecutory deluded group in Kinderman's study did not differ from a depressed psychiatric comparison group in terms of explicit self-relevance ratings of negative adjectives. Garety and Freeman thus questioned the suggestion that Kinderman's persecutory deluded participants showed high self-esteem on the ratings task.

In a different attempt to demonstrate explicit/implicit self-esteem discrepancies in persecutory deluded individuals, Lyon, Kaney, and Bentall (1994) presented paranoid patients with two measures of *attributional style*. Attributional style refers to one's tendency to generate certain types of explanations for events—for example, one's tendency to regard events as being caused by oneself versus caused by external factors. One of the administered measures was a parallel form of the Attributional Style Questionnaire (ASQpf; Peterson et al., 1982), which functioned as a transparent (explicit) measure of attributional style. This questionnaire comprises brief descriptions of 12 hypothetical events. Half are positive events (e.g., "You become very rich") and half are negative (e.g., "You go out on a date and it goes badly"). Respondents are instructed to vividly imagine each event and to write down what they feel would be the major cause of each situation. They are then required to rate each cause along different attributional dimensions (e.g., internality–externality).

[2] Italicisation of *relatively* here denotes the "weaker" formulation of the Bentall et al. account (Garety & Freeman, 1999), whereby explicit self-esteem is high relative to implicit self-esteem (in the "stronger" formulation explicit self-esteem is high—and implicit self-esteem low—relative to that of healthy individuals). The weaker formulation provides for scenarios where persecutory delusions only partially fulfil their putative defensive function, and explicit self-esteem is not fully preserved.

The other measure Lyon and colleagues administered was the Pragmatic Inference Task (PIT; Winters & Neale, 1985), an opaque (implicit) measure of attributional style based on the original ASQ but presented as a memory test. Although persecutory deluded individuals displayed a self-serving attributional style on the ASQpf (being more inclined to take the credit for positive events and to attribute negative events to external factors), their responses on the PIT were decidedly non-self-serving (taking responsibility for negative events and attributing positive events to external factors). This seems quite a successful demonstration of an explicit–implicit discrepancy, albeit a discrepancy between explicit and implicit *attributions* rather than explicit and implicit self-evaluations. Unfortunately, however, attempts to replicate this finding have not been successful (Krstev, Jackson, & Maude, 1999; Martin & Penn, 2002; Peters, Day, & Garety, 1997).

The delusion-as-defence account of Bentall and colleagues holds that paranoid individuals are motivated to prevent conscious awareness of negative implicit self-representations. A successful test of this theory therefore requires elicitation of such implicit representations, which is a challenge methodologically. Two recent studies (McKay et al., 2007a; Moritz, Werner, & von Collani, 2006) have approached this problem by using the popular and influential Implicit Association Test (IAT; Greenwald, McGhee, & Schwartz, 1998).

The IAT is a computerised task designed to measure the relative strengths of automatic interconcept associations. In the crucial conditions of the task words from four different categories are flashed randomly onto the computer screen (e.g., *self* words, *other* words, *pleasant* words, and *unpleasant* words). Participants are instructed to press (say) a right key on the keyboard if the word is a *self* word (e.g., me, myself) or a *pleasant* word (e.g., freedom, rainbow) and to press a left key if the word is an *other* word (e.g., they, them) or an *unpleasant* word (e.g., vomit, murder) (for illustration see Table 1). Faster responding to a particular pairing of the concepts is assumed to index a stronger association between those concepts. The particular categories

TABLE 1
Sample items from one of the crucial conditions of an Implicit Association Test (IAT) for implicit self-esteem

Left key category label	*Sample items*	*Right key category label*
Other or unpleasant		Self or pleasant
	Myself	***
***	Vomit	
	Rainbow	***
***	Them	

Asterisks indicate correct responses.

described here feature in an IAT for implicit self-esteem, and were first investigated by Greenwald and Farnham (2000). These authors showed that the relative ease of making judgements when the *self* and *pleasant* categories are combined (in which case *other* is paired with *unpleasant*) can be used to index a participant's implicit self-esteem (individuals with higher implicit self-esteem should find categorisations easier when *self* and *pleasant* are paired than when *self* and *unpleasant* are paired).

In order to test the predicted association between persecutory delusions and explicit/implicit self-esteem discrepancies, both Moritz et al. (2006) and McKay et al. (2007a) administered the IAT for implicit self-esteem to persecutory deluded patients. Moritz et al. found that patients with schizophrenia (with or without current persecutory delusions) had lower implicit self-esteem than healthy control participants. Although the explicit self-esteem of their persecutory deluded patients was also markedly lower than that of the controls, it was higher than that of nonparanoid patients with schizophrenia. In the McKay et al. study, paranoid patients were found to have lower implicit self-esteem than healthy controls and remitted patients, in that the response advantage for the condition combining *self* and *pleasant* was significantly reduced for this group (see Figure 1). On two measures of explicit self-esteem, however, the persecutory deluded group did not differ significantly from the other groups once appropriate adjustments had been made for levels of comorbid depression. This was necessary since people who are depressed report low levels of explicit self-esteem.

The results of these two studies are consistent with the Bentall et al. suggestion that persecutory delusions are associated with a discrepancy between explicit and implicit self-esteem, and they accord with psychodynamic accounts of paranoia dating back to Freud (1895) and Adler (1914/1929).

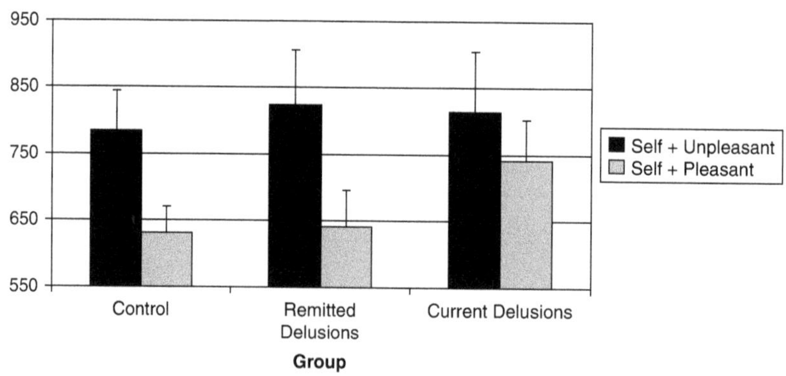

Figure 1. Results of the McKay et al. (2007a) IAT study. The bars show the mean response latencies of each experimental group for the two crucial IAT conditions (self/pleasant vs. self/unpleasant).

However, a more recent study by Vazquez, Diez-Alegria, Hernandez-Lloreda, and Moreno (2008) failed to find any evidence of a discrepancy between explicit and implicit measures of self-concept in patients with acute and remitted persecutory delusions. One of the explicit measures used here was a task requiring endorsement of self-relevant adjectives; the implicit measure comprised a free recall test of the same adjectives. More experimentation is clearly required to resolve the discrepancies between these studies.

Grandiose delusions

Although the notion that delusions are a defence against low self-esteem has been most systematically applied to persecutory delusions, the applicability of the idea to grandiose delusions is perhaps more obvious, as the latter typically appear more self-enhancing than persecutory beliefs (Smith, Freeman, & Kuipers, 2005). Zigler and Glick (1988) have suggested that the grandiose delusions observed in mania represent a "camouflaged depression", a proposal that accords with Jordan, Spencer, Zanna, Hoshino-Browne, and Correll's (2003) discussion of narcissistic grandiosity: "[N]arcissists are viewed as simultaneously holding positive conscious self-views while harbouring significant self-doubts at less conscious levels . . ." (p. 970). Using the IAT, Jordan et al. found that nonclinical participants with high explicit but low implicit self-esteem showed significantly more narcissism than individuals high in both explicit and implicit self-esteem (but see Campbell, Bosson, Goheen, Lakey, & Kernis, 2007). Given that grandiose delusions might be construed as involving "clinically significant narcissism", might one expect individuals with delusions of grandeur to show discrepancies between explicit and implicit self-esteem?

We know of only a single published study that has directly addressed this question to date, with negative results. Smith et al. (2005) administered explicit and implicit measures of self-esteem to individuals with grandiose delusions and healthy controls and failed to find any evidence of a self-esteem discrepancy in the grandiose patients. Implicit self-esteem here was gauged by measuring recall of low self-esteem words and by measuring the speed with which participants named the colours of depression-related words relative to neutral words.

A separate investigation by Lyon, Startup, and Bentall (1999), however, is worth considering in this regard. Adapting the methodology of their earlier investigation of persecutory delusions (already outlined; Lyon et al., 1994), Lyon et al. (1999) presented two measures of attributional style (the ASQpf as an explicit measure and the PIT as an implicit measure) to a group of nondelusional, manic patients, as well as to matched depressed and healthy controls. With a direct administration of the ASQpf, the manic patients showed evidence of a self-serving attributional style (i.e., internal attributions for positive events and external attributions for negative events). The response of these same individuals on the PIT, however, was similar to that of the depressed controls and dissimilar to that of the healthy controls, and decidedly nonself-serving (i.e., being more inclined to make internal attributions for negative events and external attributions for positive events).

The relevance of this study for investigations of self-discrepancies in grandiose delusions is arguable. On the one hand, these authors tested manic bipolar patients rather than patients with grandiose delusions (and their paradigm taps underlying attributions rather than self-evaluations—as did the earlier study by Lyon et al., 1994). On the other hand, grandiosity is clearly a feature of both presentations, and indeed inflated self-esteem or grandiosity is the first symptom listed in the DSM-IV's Criterion B for a Manic episode (American Psychiatric Association, 2000). Seen in this light, the results of the study are tantalising and suggest that further investigation into connections between delusional grandiosity and self-esteem discrepancies may be worthwhile—perhaps using suitable adaptations of the IAT.

Need for closure

A number of ingenious motivational accounts have been proposed to explain delusional beliefs. In some cases, such as with the Capgras, Cotard, and Frégoli delusions, a disparate collection of exotic and convoluted accounts has been more or less superseded by a single neuropsychological framework—although it is well to note that neuropsychological accounts can quickly become convoluted as well. What is key is that hypotheses should be framed in a testable fashion. The most systematic efforts to test motivational accounts to date have been seen in studies of persecutory delusions—although here too the evidence remains equivocal. Even if one accepts a defensive framework for delusions such as persecutory and grandiose delusions, however, many questions remain. One such question concerns the reasons for developing one delusion rather than another—if the aim is to preserve self-esteem, what explains why one patient develops grandiose delusions while another develops persecutory delusions? The former seem a more straightforward means of preserving self-esteem—but the latter are more common.

Perhaps the most robust evidence of motivational factors in the aetiology of delusions comes from investigations of a so-called "need for closure", a construct associated with a preference for certainty and predictability (Kruglanski, 1989). Individuals who are highly motivated to seek an explanation for anomalous experiences may prefer *any* explanation—even a deluded one—rather than none at all (Colbert & Peters, 2002). This suggestion parallels the gap-filling account of confabulation in that both explanations are *hedonically noncommittal*—neither makes any prediction regarding the emotional valence of confabulatory or delusional content (see Davies, 2009). Note that a need for closure is an epistemic motive—in our terminology it constitutes a telic metarepresentation, i.e., it represents a preference for any thetic representation of a given state of affairs rather than none at all.

What is the evidence for an association between delusions and need for closure? Colbert and Peters (2002) examined need for closure in nonclinical participants who were screened for delusion-proneness using the Peters et al. Delusions Inventory (PDI-21; Peters, Day, & Garety, 1996). They found that delusion-prone individuals (those scoring in the upper quartile on the PDI) scored significantly higher on need for closure than nondelusion-prone (lower quartile) individuals. Need for closure was assessed with the Need for Closure Scale (NFCS; Webster & Kruglanski, 1994), a self-report measure containing five subscales: desire for predictability, need for order, intolerance of ambiguity, decisiveness, and closed-mindedness. A subsequent study by Bentall and Swarbrick (2003) investigated need for closure in a clinical sample: patients with either current or remitted persecutory delusions were compared to healthy controls. Both patient groups scored higher on need for closure than the control group, although no difference was found between the two patient groups. This pattern was observed for the five distinct facets of need for closure.

Later studies have replicated the reported connections between delusions and need for closure—although not with all facets of the latter. Neuberg, Judice, and West (1997) had argued that the NFCS assesses two separate dimensions: a desire for simple structure represented by the desire for predictability, need for order, and intolerance of ambiguity subscales, and a preference for quick, decisive answers captured by the decisiveness subscale. McKay, Langdon, and Coltheart (2007b) found that patients with a history of persecutory delusions scored higher than healthy control participants on the first of these dimensions, but did not show evidence of greater decisiveness (the findings of other studies are consistent with this pattern; see Colbert, Peters, & Garety, 2006; Freeman et al., 2006). In fact, paranoid ideation has been found to be associated with greater *indecisiveness* in both clinical and nonclinical individuals (McKay, 2004).

What is the theoretical significance of this dissociation between decisiveness and a desire for simple structure? Individuals who desire simple structure dislike confusion, uncertainty, and ambiguity. By their very nature, however, decisions imply uncertainty—after all, a course of action is not certain if it requires a decision to be made. It may be, therefore, that whereas some individuals who desire "simple structure" make decisions quickly in order to terminate the stress of decision making and to achieve a sense of closure, others may avoid confronting the uncertainty that is part and parcel of any decision. Perhaps for the latter individuals, the uncertainty of a decision left unmade is preferable to uncertainty about the wisdom of a decision that *has* been made.

Avoidance is rarely an effective strategy for dealing with fear, however, so the latter group of people are likely to be somewhat dysfunctional—burdened with a strong aversion to ambiguity and uncertainty, yet unable to manage the inevitable uncertainties in life by making decisions to resolve them. In a speculative vein, one might conjecture that indecisive people fear the responsibility of making incorrect decisions, that they fear the *culpability* of a wrong choice. Continuing this speculation, one could contend that the link between indecisiveness and paranoia consists in the fact that they both provide dysfunctional means of avoiding (feelings of) culpability.

It may be that people high in paranoid ideation fear uncertainty and culpability, yet deal with these fears in dysfunctional ways—on the one hand by avoiding making conscious decisions, and on the other hand by automatically abrogating responsibility for negative events in their lives, attributing their misfortunes to the actions of malevolent others (Kinderman & Bentall, 1997). Although speculative, these ideas accommodate the finding of links between paranoid ideation and indecision on the one hand, and paranoid ideation and desires for simple structure on the other. Future research may demonstrate whether these suggestions can bear up under further empirical scrutiny.

MOTIVATIONAL ACCOUNTS OF ANOSOGNOSIA

We noted earlier that anosognosia, which involves the denial of manifest disability—particularly denial of left hemiplegia—has been variously characterised as delusional and confabulatory. Some historically prevalent accounts of anosognosic denial (e.g., Weinstein & Kahn, 1955) have held that it is employed defensively, to alleviate the distress occasioned by the unpleasant reality of disability. Such motivational accounts, however, have been subject to considerable criticism. In this section we briefly discuss two key criticisms of motivational accounts, and then consider evidence for such accounts.

Hemispheric asymmetry

A number of authors (e.g., Bisiach & Geminiani, 1991; Stone & Young, 1997) have highlighted a striking asymmetry in the expression of anosognosia for hemiplegia. Denial of hemiplegia is largely confined to cases of left-sided paralysis, and is seldom seen in right-sided paralysis. Such authors view this lateralisation as a major stumbling block for motivational accounts (there being no reason to suppose that right-sided paralysis should be any less upsetting than left-sided paralysis). It is true that this asymmetry would pose difficulties for a purely motivational account of anosognosia. But might such difficulties be bypassed through the adoption of an integrated motivational and neuropsychological deficit perspective?

Both Ramachandran (e.g., 1995; Ramachandran & Blakeslee, 1998) and Turnbull (e.g., Turnbull, Jones, & Reed-Screen, 2002; Turnbull & Solms, 2007) have offered such a perspective, putting forward motivational theories of anosognosia that incorporate damage to right-hemispheric mechanisms. Ramachandran has argued that the left hemisphere is the neurological locus of psychological defence, and has suggested that the left-hemispheric mechanisms that underpin defensive processes may be opposed by complementary right hemispheric mechanisms. Operating normally, these complementary mechanisms would constrain the influence of defensive processes on belief formation. If these mechanisms were damaged, however—perhaps by an aneurysm or accident—patients would be left without constraints on their capacities for psychological defence. This would permit the flagrant denials observed in anosognosia.

Whereas Ramachandran's explanation (1995; Ramachandran & Blakeslee, 1998) of anosognosia implicates a dysfunctionally enhanced capacity for managing negative emotions, Turnbull and Solms (2007) suggest that anosognosia involves an *impaired* ability to manage such emotions. Their proposal is that anosognosic patients fail to acknowledge their deficits because to do so would entail levels of aversive emotion that—because of damage to right-lateralised emotion-regulation systems—they could not tolerate. By incorporating damage to neurological structures that implement or constrain emotion regulation processes, accounts such as these defuse the asymmetry objection. If anosognosia results from an abnormality in the brain's management of negative emotions, an abnormality caused by damage to right-hemispheric mechanisms, then one would not expect left-hemispheric damage to result in anosognosia.

Selectivity

One problem for such accounts, however, is that patients with anosognosia for left hemiplegia may freely acknowledge other impairments (Cutting, 1978), and may in fact be overtly hypochondriacal with respect to even minor ailments (Bisiach & Geminiani, 1991; Kaplan-Solms & Solms, 2000). Some authors (e.g., Turnbull et al., 2002) argue that this disparity reflects a disparity in the perceived seriousness of the ailments in question. For example, hemiplegia represents a far greater threat to bodily integrity than minor complaints such as insomnia and back pain, or even medical conditions such as diabetes. The overt hypochondria regarding minor ailments might even be a dissimulative manoeuvre, a defensive attempt to shift the focus from the true underlying concern (Weinstein & Kahn, 1950). However plausible these suggestions are with respect to minor ailments, they seem less persuasive in situations where more serious conditions are concerned. Some patients, for example, are anosognosic for paralysis of the left leg while acknowledging left *arm* paralysis (Bisiach, Vallar, Perani, Papagno, & Berti, 1986). Accounts such as Turnbull's presumably need to assume that, at least for the patients in question, the former impairment poses a greater threat to bodily integrity than the latter.

Aimola Davies et al. (2009) note that a two-factor explanatory framework might incorporate motivational factors yet circumvent the selectivity issue. For example, anosognosia for a given impairment might require both (1) that the patient be unaware of this impairment, perhaps due to somatosensory loss or unilateral neglect; and (2) that the patient be unwilling or unable to acquire other evidence of the impairment. This account, which incorporates motivational processes as a potential second factor, evades the selectivity problem (somatosensory loss might affect the left leg but not the left arm), and also the asymmetry problem (the first factor might involve damage to primarily right-lateralised functions).

Evidence for motivational accounts

If anosognosic patients *are* motivated to prevent conscious awareness of their deficits, one might predict that they would show discrepancies between conscious and unconscious awareness of their disability, à la the Bentall et al. conception of persecutory delusions. The evidence available here is intriguing and mixed. Ramachandran (e.g., 1995; Ramachandran & Blakeslee, 1998) has carried out a range of simple and ingenious experiments to explore the possibility of tacit awareness of disability in anosognosia. In one experiment, he used a "virtual reality box", constructed of cardboard and mirrors, to present an anosognosic patient with the optical illusion that she was moving her paralysed left hand up and down to the rhythm of a metronome. This patient showed no sign of surprise, inconsistent with the hypothesis of tacit awareness of disability. A different experiment was also inconsistent with the notion of implicit awareness. Ramachandran presented left-hemiplegic patients with two water-filled cocktail glasses atop a large tray, and asked them to reach out and take the tray. Whereas nonanosognosic patients reached for the centre of the tray with their good right hand, anosognosic patients reached for the right side with their good hand—despite the fact that this strategy would have caused the glasses to topple. In a third experiment,

Ramachandran gave anosognosic patients the choice between performing a unimanual task for a small reward, or a bimanual task for a larger reward. Whereas nonanosognosic stroke patients chose the unimanual task, anosognosic patients repeatedly chose the bimanual task that they were in fact unable to perform. Although this result also seems inconsistent with the notion of tacit awareness of disability in anosognosia, Ramachandran notes that one of the patients in this experiment later spoke of performing the bimanual task successfully, *with both hands*. For Ramachandran, the unusual emphasis on "both hands" bespoke a degree of tacit awareness.

Turnbull et al. (2002) adduced a different form of evidence of implicit awareness. These authors analysed detailed notes from psychoanalytic therapy sessions with five anosognosic and nonanosognosic patients, all of whom had some degree of left-sided motor impairment (see Kaplan-Solms & Solms, 2000). They reported that anosognosic patients were more likely to experience emotional breakdowns at moments that were preceded by talk of loss, betraying some implicit awareness of their predicaments: "In some cases, the episodes led not only to a temporary tearfulness, but also to a fully-fledged (though short-lived) awareness of the paretic limb" (Turnbull et al., 2002, p. 72). In a more recent investigation, Nardone, Ward, Fotopoulou, and Turnbull (2007) used a dot probe paradigm to measure the emotional impact of different word types. In this task, participants pressed a keyboard key to quickly and accurately classify the colour of a red or blue dot probe flashed onto the computer screen. Presentation of each probe was immediately preceded by a word, which participants were instructed to ignore. Increased response latencies to particular word types are taken to indicate that those words are emotionally threatening. Nardone et al. used words related to disability (e.g., *crippled*, *immobile*, *paralysed*), and found that whereas nonanosognosic patients with severe motor impairments showed reduced latencies (i.e., facilitation) for disability-related words, anosognosic patients showed *increased* latencies (i.e., interference), suggestive of implicit awareness of their deficits.

It would be interesting to carry out additional investigations of this issue, perhaps utilising appropriate adaptations of the IAT. One way of accomplishing this would be to compare anosognosic and nonanosognosic individuals with hemiplegia for their relative ease of making judgements when (say) *self* and *disabled* categories are combined in an IAT (or, better still, an SC-IAT[3]). If anosognosic denial is implemented defensively, one might expect that the response advantage for a "*self* and *healthy* condition"

[3] Single Category Implicit Association Test (Karpinski & Steinman, 2006). Because the SC-IAT uses only a single attitude category (e.g., *self*) rather than pairs of complementary attitude categories (e.g., *self* vs. *other*), some of the ambiguity in test score interpretation is eliminated.

TABLE 2
Sample items from the first stage of a Single Category Implicit Association Test (SC-IAT) for self and healthy/disabled

Left key category label	*Sample items*	*Right key category label*
Disabled		Self or healthy
	Me	***
***	Paralysed	
	Mobile	***

Asterisks indicate correct responses.

(see Table 2) would be significantly reduced for anosognosic individuals relative to controls.[4]

Given the physical limitations of anosognosic patients, and the likelihood of comorbid visual neglect, adapting the IAT or SC-IAT in this manner would not be straightforward. But there seems no reason why careful experimental design could not circumvent these limitations. Pertinent modifications of the basic IAT paradigm might include the use of unimanual responses with the patient's unaffected hand, along with use of a dichotically presented auditory adaptation of the IAT or SC-IAT (see McKay, Arciuli, Atkinson, Bennett, & Pheils, in press).

Before we move on, we note that anosognosia for left hemiplegia may be accompanied by the disowning of the affected limb (somatoparaphrenia), and even by its personification as belonging to someone else—widely ranging from an existing person ("your hand"), through a dead person (a deceased husband) to an animal ("it's a monkey"; see also Hirstein, 2010 this issue). Extensive clinical experience shows that some degree of left neglect is consistently present, although varying greatly in severity (Feinberg, 2001). Since left neglect involves a biasing of attention rightwards, and withdrawal of attention from the left of space and body (Kinsbourne, 1977, 1993), the disowning and personification may be compensatory to the perplexing loss of familiarity with the affected limb. As the patients do not complain of these strange appendages or ask for them to be removed, it may be that the idiosyncratic labelling is metaphorical (Weinstein, 1991), in some way contributing to an adaptation to perplexing subjective bodily changes.

A TAXONOMY OF FALSE CLAIMS

We began this paper with two false claims, illustrative of delusion and confabulation, respectively. We finish by outlining a tentative taxonomy of

[4] The ideas outlined here have been developed collaboratively with Katerina Fotopoulou.

false claims—a taxonomy that incorporates claims such as these as well as more common, garden-variety false claims. Following McKay and Dennett (in press), we distinguish two broad categories: false claims that arise in the normal course of cognitive functioning and false claims that result from some kind of break (or congenital anomaly) in normal cognitive functioning. By "normal functioning" we refer not to some kind of statistical norm (e.g., not to the way a given individual *usually* functions), but rather to the adaptive functioning of cognitive systems throughout evolutionary history (see Millikan, 1993). The categories are overlapping rather than discrete, and they admit of intermediate subtypes.

Normal functioning: False claims that reflect design limitations

Evolution is not a perfect design process. In "designing" cognitive systems, evolution is subject to physical constraints (designs must be within the realm of physical possibility), economic constraints (beyond a certain level, system improvements may yield diminishing returns), historical constraints (the appropriate mutations must occur if selection is to act on them), and "topographical" constraints (selection cannot access optimal design solutions if it must cross fitness valleys to do so). Because evolution is an imperfect design process, the cognitive systems it has equipped us with are bound to be limited.

To give an example, Bayes' theorem specifies the optimal procedure for updating prior beliefs in the light of new evidence (see Coltheart, Menzies, & Sutton, 2010 this issue). If veridical belief is adaptive, then an organism cannot do better than to revise beliefs in accordance with the Bayesian prescription. No organism, however, can have perfect information—even in principle. So even flawless Bayesians will develop false beliefs, and such beliefs may provide the basis for false claims. These claims thus arise in the normal course of cognitive functioning, and can be accounted for without appeal to motivational factors or neuropsychological deficits. False beliefs, and consequent claims, may also stem from "ecologically rational" departures from Bayesian updating, departures that operate effectively given inevitable limitations of time and computational resources (see Gigerenzer & Goldstein, 1996).

Normal functioning: False claims that reflect design features

Not all false claims stem from design limitations—some actually reflect design *features*. The most obvious examples are false claims made with the deliberate intention to deceive. It has long been realised that individuals might increase their own relative fitness by disseminating false information to others. Indeed, modern humans are constantly bombarded with exaggerated and brazenly false claims—to cite just a single source, at the time of writing around 100 billion spam e-mails are sent every day. The false claims in such unsolicited messages are presumably not mistakes—they are motivated attempts to bring about false beliefs in the recipients.

Although individuals who disseminate false information to further their own interests need not believe their own false claims, a number of authors have argued that humans may be evolutionarily predisposed to form false beliefs in certain situations (e.g., Haselton & Nettle, 2006; Trivers, 1985; see McKay & Dennett, in press, for a detailed examination of such arguments). Such false beliefs may provide the basis for false claims. As an example, consider the domain of agency detection. In ancestral environments, the malevolent intentions of other agents (whether humans or animals) posed a great threat to survival. A plausible result is that humans gradually evolved cognitive mechanisms specialised for the detection of *agency*—what Barrett (2000) has termed "hyperactive agent-detection devices" (HADDs). As hyperactive agent detectors, we are biologically predisposed to make false positive errors in ambiguous contexts—imputing agency where there is none. Although such a bias would be adaptive in many scenarios, it might also have destructive consequences—perhaps underpinning accusations of witchcraft and sorcery, for example. Other consequences might include supernatural beliefs and their attendant claims. At present, the dominant evolutionary view of supernatural beliefs is that they are side effects of cognitive mechanisms adapted for other purposes—mechanisms such as HADDs (see Barrett, 2000; Guthrie, 1993).

A final point here is that we may be biologically equipped with tendencies to employ motivational processes "unduly" in certain scenarios. Such processes would distort veridical representations of reality, perhaps by appropriating executive resources (Turnbull & Solms, 2007). The result would be congenial false beliefs, for example unrealistically positive beliefs about one's children (see McKay & Dennett, in press). The congenial nature of such beliefs might feature in proximal explanations of their formation; an ultimate explanation, however, would reference their effects on biological fitness. Insofar as such false beliefs would give rise to false claims, therefore, the claims would reflect features of biological design.

Breakages: False claims with purely deficit explanations

The neuropsychological framework discussed in our earlier section on motivational accounts of delusion provides for an explanation of certain false claims (e.g., the claims of Capgras patients) in terms of breakages in normal cognitive functioning—breakages that entail disrupted connections between face-processing areas and the limbic system, for instance. Such cases represent dysfunctional departures from normal operation. Various authors have identified candidate neurocognitive defects potentially associated with a range of delusions. For instance, Frith and colleagues (Frith, 1992; Frith & Done, 1989; see Feinberg, 1978) have investigated the role of disrupted self-monitoring in the genesis of alien control delusions. Patients with these delusions believe that external agents such as gods or aliens control their actions. Frith and colleagues have proposed that neuropsychological disruption to "efference copies"—internal copies of motor signals, used to predict the sensory consequences of actions—undermines the normal sense that one has authored the actions. The suggestion is that beliefs about alien control are generated to explain this loss of a sense of agency.

Although it is nicely illustrative of a deficit approach to explaining delusion, it seems to us that the efference copy account is not without difficulties. Reefferent control of movement is highly conserved in evolution, from cockroach to fish to human. In humans it is integral to the accuracy of movements of the eyes, head, arms, and legs. If the operation whereby the efference copy is matched with exafferent feedback were lacking, patients would lack a sense of authorship for all of their actions, including the verbal acts by which they communicate their sense of being under alien control. Moreover, they would exhibit gross inaccuracies in guided movements, inaccuracies that have not been documented. An adjustment of the model seems to be called for.

Deficit accounts are also prominent where confabulation and anosognosia are concerned. For example, it has been suggested that confabulation results from a deficit in the strategic processes implicated in the controlled retrieval of memories (e.g., Burgess & Shallice, 1996; Conway & Tacchi, 1996). Levine's (1990) "discovery theory" suggests that anosognosia results when impaired somatosensory awareness of paralysis is coupled with cognitive impairments that prevent integration of other sources of evidence of paralysis (see Aimola Davies et al., 2009, for discussion).

Breakages: False claims that require integrated motivational and neuropsychological deficit explanations

One can envisage scenarios where premorbid motivational factors interact with neuropsychological deficits. In such cases neuropsychological damage yielding impairments in, say, language or memory functions, would be processed in a motivationally biased fashion, yielding false claims. Much as healthy individuals are prone to unrealistically positive self-evaluations and unrealistic optimism about the future (Taylor, 1989; Taylor & Brown, 1988), neuropsychological patients might underestimate and understate the extent of their impairments, and overestimate and overstate their prospects for recovery.

It is an open question whether the expression of such "positive health illusions" is on a continuum with the avowals and denials of severely anosognosic patients. In the example just considered, the neuropsychological damage is to nonmotivational cognitive components—language functions, for example. This is similar to the two-factor explanation proposed by Aimola Davies et al. (2009), and discussed earlier. The motivational processes operating in these examples are premorbid processes: whether they are ordinary, adaptive motivational processes or congenitally anomalous, exaggerated motivational processes, they are not themselves a direct result of the neuropsychological damage underpinning the first factor impairment. Their operation constitutes a "secondary reaction" to the new psychological reality brought about by the primary neuropsychological impairment (see Fotopoulou, 2010 this issue).

On accounts such as Ramachandran's (e.g., 1995; Ramachandran & Blakeslee, 1998) account of anosognosia, in contrast, the neuropsychological damage can be construed as affecting motivational structures—damage to neurological structures that constrain the implementation of psychological defences, for example (see, also, Fotopoulou's [2010 this issue] account of confabulation). Such breakage thus liberates or releases motivational processes: the motivational factor is itself a consequence of the neuropsychological damage, qualitatively and quantitatively distinct from the "positive illusions" of healthy people. Such accounts are thus genuinely "neuropsychodynamic" or "neuropsychoanalytic".

CONCLUSION

The nature and extent of overlap between the clinical concepts of *confabulation*, *delusion*, and *anosognosia* remains unclear. In this paper we have considered the role of motivational factors in each symptom. Although space considerations have precluded an exhaustive review of relevant studies in each domain, we hope to have conveyed a sense of the range of motivational theories available, and the types of evidence adduced in support of these theories. In our view the evidence is strongly suggestive of a role for motivational factors in each domain. We have put forward a taxonomy of false claims that incorporates both clinical and garden-variety variants. We suspect that the most comprehensive accounts of the false claims observed in clinical settings will occupy the final category of our taxonomy, integrating both motivational factors and neuropsychological deficits.

REFERENCES

Adler, A. (1929). Melancholia and paranoia. In A. Adler (Ed.), *The practice and theory of individual psychology.* London: Routledge & Kegan Paul. (Original work published 1914)

Aimola Davies, A. M., Davies, M., Ogden, J. A., Smithson, M., & White, R. C. (2009). Cognitive and motivational factors in anosognosia. In T. Bayne & J. Fernández (Eds.), *Delusion and self-deception: Affective and motivational influences on belief formation* (pp. 187–225). Hove, UK: Psychology Press.

American Psychiatric Association. (2000). *Diagnostic and statistical manual of mental disorders* (4th ed., Text revision [DSM-IV-TR]). Washington, DC: Author.

Banov, M. D., Kulick, A. R., Oepen, G., & Pope, H. G., Jr. (1993). A new identity for misidentification syndromes. *Comprehensive Psychiatry, 34*(6), 414–417.

Barrett, J. L. (2000). Exploring the natural foundations of religion. *Trends in Cognitive Sciences, 4*(1), 29–34.

Bayne, T., & Fernández, J. (2009). Delusion and self-deception: Mapping the terrain. In T. Bayne & J. Fernández (Eds.), *Delusion and self-deception: Affective and motivational influences on belief formation* (pp. 1–21). Hove, UK: Psychology Press.

Becker, E. (1973). *The denial of death.* New York: Free Press.

Bell, D. (2003). *Paranoia.* Cambridge, UK: Icon Books.

Bentall, R., & Swarbrick, R. (2003). The best laid schemas of paranoid patients: Autonomy, sociotropy and need for closure. *Psychology and Psychotherapy: Theory, Research and Practice, 76*(2), 163–171.

Bentall, R. P., & Kaney, S. (1996). Abnormalities of self-representation and persecutory delusions: A test of a cognitive model of paranoia. *Psychological Medicine, 26*, 1231–1237.

Bisiach, E., & Geminiani, G. (1991). Anosognosia related to hemiplegia and hemianopia. In G. P. Prigatano & D. L. Schacter (Eds.), *Awareness of deficit after brain injury: Clinical and theoretical issues* (pp. 17–39). Oxford, UK: Oxford University Press.

Bisiach, E., Vallar, G., Perani, D., Papagno, C., & Berti, A. (1986). Unawareness of disease following lesions of the right hemisphere: Anosognosia for hemiplegia and anosognosia for hemianopia. *Neuropsychologia, 24*, 471–482.

Bonhoeffer, K. (1901). *Die akuten Geisteskrankheiten der Gewohnheitstrinker: Eine Klinische Studie.* Jena, Germany: Gustav Fischer.

Brighetti, G., Bonifacci, P., Borlimi, R., & Ottaviani, C. (2007). "Far from the heart far from the eye": Evidence from the Capgras delusion. *Cognitive Neuropsychiatry, 12*(3), 189–197.

Burgess, P. W., & Shallice, T. (1996). Confabulation and the control of recollection. *Memory, 4*, 359–411.

Campbell, W. K., Bosson, J. K., Goheen, T. W., Lakey, C. E., & Kernis, M. H. (2007). Do narcissists dislike themselves "deep down inside"? *Psychological Science, 18*(3), 227–229.

Capgras, J., & Carette, P. (1924). Illusion de sosies et complexe d'oedipe. *Annales Medico-Psychologiques, 82*, 48–68.

Capgras, J., & Reboul-Lachaux, J. (1923). Illusion des sosies dans un delire systematise chronique. *Bulletin de la Societe Clinique de Medicine Mentale, 2*, 6–16.

Christodoulou, G. N. (1976). Delusional hyper-identifications of the Fregoli type: Organic pathogenetic contributors. *Acta Psychiatrica Scandinavica, 54*(5), 305–314.

Christodoulou, G. N. (1977). The syndrome of Capgras. *British Journal of Psychiatry, 130*, 556–564.

Colbert, S. M., & Peters, E. R. (2002). Need for closure and jumping-to-conclusions in delusion-prone individuals. *Journal of Nervous and Mental Disease, 190*(1), 27–31.

Colbert, S. M., Peters, E. R., & Garety, P. A. (2006). Need for closure and anxiety in delusions: A longitudinal investigation in early psychosis. *Behaviour Research and Therapy, 44*(10), 1385–1396.

Coltheart, M., Menzies, P., & Sutton, J. (2010). Abductive inference and delusional belief. *Cognitive Neuropsychiatry, 15*(1/2/3), 261–287.

Conway, M. A., & Tacchi, P. C. (1996). Motivated confabulation. *Neurocase, 2*, 325–339.

Cotard, J. (1882). Du délire des négations. *Archives de Neurologie, 4*, 150–170, 282–295.

Cutting, J. (1978). Study of anosognosia. Journal of Neurology. *Neurosurgery and Psychiatry, 41*, 548–555.

David, A. S. (1999). On the impossibility of defining delusions. *Philosophy, Psychiatry, and Psychology, 6*(1), 17–20.

Davies, M. (2009). Delusion and motivationally biased belief: Self-deception in the two-factor framework. In T. Bayne & J. Fernández (Eds.), *Delusion and self-deception: Affective and motivational influences on belief formation* (pp. 71–86). Hove, UK: Psychology Press.

Davies, M., Aimola Davies, A. M., & Coltheart, M. (2005). Anosognosia and the two-factor theory of delusion. *Mind and Language, 20*, 209–236.

Davies, M., & Coltheart, M. (2000). Introduction: Pathologies of belief. In M. Coltheart & M. Davies (Eds.), *Pathologies of belief* (pp. 1–46). Malden, MA: Blackwell Publishers.

De Pauw, K. W. (1994). Psychodynamic approaches to the Capgras delusion: A critical historical review. *Psychopathology, 27*, 154–160.

Ellis, H. D., Quayle, A. H., de Pauw, K. W., Szulecka, T. K., Young, A. W., & Kolkiewicz, L. A. (1996). Delusional misidentification of inanimate objects: A literature review and neuropsychological analysis of cognitive deficits in two cases. *Cognitive Neuropsychiatry, 1*(1), 27–40.

Ellis, H. D., & Young, A. W. (1990). Accounting for delusional misidentifications. *British Journal of Psychiatry, 157*, 239–248.

Ellis, H. D., Young, A. W., Quayle, A. H., & de Pauw, K. W. (1997). Reduced autonomic responses to faces in Capgras delusion. *Proceedings of the Royal Society of London: Biological Sciences, B264*, 1085–1092.

Enoch, M. D., & Ball, H. N. (2001). *Uncommon psychiatric syndromes* (4th ed.). London: Arnold.

Feinberg, I. (1978). Efference copy and corollary discharge: Implications for thinking and its disorders. *Schizophrenia Bulletin, 4*, 636–640.

Feinberg, T. E. (2001). *Altered egos.* Oxford, UK: Oxford University Press.

Feinberg, T. E., & Keenan, J. P. (2005). Where in the brain is the self? *Consciousness and Cognition, 14*(4), 661–678.

Fotopoulou, A. (2010). The affective neuropsychology of confabulation and delusion. *Cognitive Neuropsychiatry, 15*(1/2/3), 38–63.

Fotopoulou, A., Conway, M., Griffiths, P., Birchall, D., & Tyrer, S. (2007). Self-enhancing confabulation: Revisiting the motivational hypothesis. *Neurocase, 13*(1), 6–15.

Fotopoulou, A., Conway, M. A., Tyrer, S., Birchall, D., Griffiths, P., & Solms, M. (2008). Is the content of confabulation positive? An experimental study. *Cortex, 44*, 764–772.

Freeman, D., Garety, P. A., Kuipers, E., Colbert, S., Jolley, S., Fowler, D., et al. (2006). Delusions and decision-making style: Use of the Need for Closure Scale. *Behaviour Research and Therapy, 44*(8), 1147–1158.

Freud, S. (1895). Draft H. In J. Strachey (Ed.), *The standard edition of the complete psychological works of Sigmund Freud* (Vol. 1, pp. 206–213). London: Hogarth Press and the Institute of Psychoanalysis.

Frith, C. D. (1992). *The cognitive neuropsychology of schizophrenia*. Hove, UK: Lawrence Erlbaum Associates Ltd.

Frith, C. D., & Done, D. J. (1989). Experiences of alien control in schizophrenia reflect a disorder in the central monitoring of action. *Psychological Medicine, 19*, 359–363.

Garety, P. A., & Freeman, D. (1999). Cognitive approaches to delusions: A critical review of theories and evidence. *British Journal of Clinical Psychology, 38*, 113–154.

Gerrans, P. (2000). Refining the explanation of Cotard's delusion. *Mind and Language, 15*(1), 111–122.

Gerrans, P. (2002). A one-stage explanation of the Cotard delusion. *Philosophy, Psychiatry, and Psychology*, *9*(1), 47–53.
Gigerenzer, G., & Goldstein, D. G. (1996). Reasoning the fast and frugal way: Models of bounded rationality. *Psychological Review*, *103*(4), 650–669.
Greenberg, J., Pyszczynski, T., & Solomon, S. (1986). The causes and consequences of the need for self-esteem: A terror management theory. In R. F. Baumeister (Ed.), *Public self and private self* (pp. 189–212). New York: Springer-Verlag.
Greenwald, A. G., & Farnham, S. D. (2000). Using the Implicit Association Test to measure self-esteem and self-concept. *Journal of Personality and Social Psychology*, *79*(6), 1022–1038.
Greenwald, A. G., McGhee, D. E., & Schwartz, J. L. K. (1998). Measuring individual differences in implicit cognition: The implicit association test. *Journal of Personality and Social Psychology*, *74*(6), 1464–1480.
Guthrie, S. E. (1993). *Faces in the clouds: A new theory of religion*. Oxford, UK: Oxford University Press.
Hamilton, A. (2007). Against the belief model of delusion. In M. C. Chung, K. W. M. Fulford, & G. Graham (Eds.), *Reconceiving schizophrenia* (pp. 217–234). Oxford, UK: Oxford University Press.
Haselton, M. G., & Nettle, D. (2006). The paranoid optimist: An integrative evolutionary model of cognitive biases. *Personality and Social Psychology Review*, *10*(1), 47–66.
Heilman, K. M. (2009). Anosognosia for hemiplegia: A confabulatory state. In W. Hirstein (Ed.), *Confabulation: Views from neuroscience, psychiatry, psychology, and philosophy* (pp. 189–202). Oxford, UK: Oxford University Press.
Hirstein, W. (2005). *Brain fiction: Self-deception and the riddle of confabulation*. Cambridge, MA: MIT Press.
Hirstein, W. (2010). The misidentification syndromes as mindreading disorders. *Cognitive Neuropsychiatry*, *15*(1/2/3), 233–260.
Hirstein, W. S., & Ramachandran, V. S. (1997). Capgras syndrome: A novel probe for understanding the neural representation of the identity and familiarity of persons. *Proceedings of the Royal Society of London: Biological Sciences*, *264B*, 437–444.
Jordan, C. H., Spencer, S. J., Zanna, M. P., Hoshino-Browne, E., & Correll, J. (2003). Secure and defensive high self-esteem. *Journal of Personality and Social Psychology*, *85*(5), 969–978.
Kaplan-Solms, K. L., & Solms, M. (2000). *Clinical studies in neuropsychoanalysis: Introduction of a depth neuropsychology*. London: Karnac Books.
Karpinski, A., & Steinman, R. B. (2006). The Single Category Implicit Association Test as a measure of implicit social cognition. *Journal of Personality and Social Psychology*, *91*(1), 16–32.
Kinderman, P. (1994). Attentional bias, persecutory delusions and the self-concept. *British Journal of Medical Psychology*, *67*(1), 53–66.
Kinderman, P., & Bentall, R. P. (1996). Self-discrepancies and persecutory delusions: Evidence for a model of paranoid ideation. *Journal of Abnormal Psychology*, *105*(1), 106–113.
Kinderman, P., & Bentall, R. P. (1997). Causal attributions in paranoia and depression: Internal, personal, and situational attributions for negative events. *Journal of Abnormal Psychology*, *106*(2), 341–345.
Kinsbourne, M. (1977). Hemi-neglect and hemisphere rivalry. In E. A. Weinstein & R. P. Friedland (Eds.), *Hemi-inattention and hemisphere specialization* (pp. 41–49). New York: Raven Press.
Kinsbourne, M. (1993). Orientational bias model of unilateral neglect: Evidence from attentional gradients within hemispace. In I. H. Robertson & J. C. Marshall (Eds.), *Unilateral neglect: Clinical and experimental studies* (pp. 63–86). Hove, UK: Lawrence Erlbaum Associates Ltd.
Krstev, H., Jackson, H., & Maude, D. (1999). An investigation of attributional style in first-episode psychosis. *British Journal of Clinical Psychology*, *38*, 181–194.
Kruglanski, A. W. (1989). *Lay epistemics and human knowledge: Cognitive and motivational bases*. New York: Plenum.

Langdon, R., & Coltheart, M. (2000). The cognitive neuropsychology of delusions. *Mind and Language*, *15*(1), 183–216.

Levine, D. N. (1990). Unawareness of visual and sensorimotor defects: A hypothesis. *Brain and Cognition*, *13*, 233–281.

Lyon, H. M., Kaney, S., & Bentall, R. P. (1994). The defensive function of persecutory delusions: Evidence from attribution tasks. *British Journal of Psychiatry*, *164*(5), 637–646.

Lyon, H. M., Startup, M., & Bentall, R. P. (1999). Social cognition and the manic defense: Attributions, selective attention, and self-schema in bipolar affective disorder. *Journal of Abnormal Psychology*, *108*(2), 273–282.

Martin, J. A., & Penn, D. L. (2002). Attributional style in schizophrenia: An investigation in outpatients with and without persecutory delusions. *Schizophrenia Bulletin*, *28*(1), 131–142.

McKay, R., Arciuli, J., Atkinson, A., Bennett, E., & Pheils, E. (in press). Lateralisation of self-esteem: An investigation using a dichotically presented auditory adaptation of the Implicit Association Test. *Cortex*. doi: 10.1016/j.cortex.2009.05.004

McKay, R., & Cipolotti, L. (2007). Attributional style in a case of Cotard delusion. *Consciousness and Cognition*, *16*, 349–359.

McKay, R., & Dennett, D. (in press). The evolution of misbelief. *Behavioral and Brain Sciences.*

McKay, R., Langdon, R., & Coltheart, M. (2007a). The defensive function of persecutory delusions: An investigation using the Implicit Association Test. *Cognitive Neuropsychiatry*, *12*(1), 1–24.

McKay, R., Langdon, R., & Coltheart, M. (2007b). Jumping to delusions? Paranoia, probabilistic reasoning and need for closure. *Cognitive Neuropsychiatry*, *12*(4), 362–376.

McKay, R. T. (2004). *"Sleights of mind": Delusions and self-deception*. Unpublished PhD thesis, Macquarie University, Sydney.

McWilliams, N. (1994). *Psychoanalytic diagnosis: Understanding personality structure in the clinical process*. New York: Guilford Press.

Mele, A. R. (1997). Real self-deception. *Behavioral and Brain Sciences*, *20*(1), 91–136.

Mele, A. R. (2009). Self-deception and delusions. In T. Bayne & J. Fernández (Eds.), *Delusion and self-deception: Affective and motivational influences on belief formation* (pp. 55–69). Hove, UK: Psychology Press.

Metcalf, K., Langdon, R., & Coltheart, M. (2010). The role of personal biases in the explanation of confabulation. *Cognitive Neuropsychiatry*, *00*(00), 000–000.

Millikan, R. (1993). *White queen psychology and other essays for Alice*. Cambridge, MA: MIT Press.

Mojtabai, R. (1994). Fregoli syndrome. *Australian and New Zealand Journal of Psychiatry*, *28*, 458–462.

Moritz, S., Werner, R., & von Collani, G. (2006). The inferiority complex in paranoia readdressed: A study with the Implicit Association Test. *Cognitive Neuropsychiatry*, *11*(4), 402–415.

Moscovitch, M. (1995). Confabulation. In D. L. Schacter (Ed.), *Memory distortion: How minds, brains, and societies reconstruct the past*. Cambridge, MA: Harvard University Press.

Nardone, I. B., Ward, R., Fotopoulou, A., & Turnbull, O. H. (2007). Attention and emotion in anosognosia: Evidence of implicit awareness and repression? *Neurocase*, *13*, 438–445.

Nasar, S. (1998). *A beautiful mind*. New York: Simon & Schuster.

Neuberg, S. L., Judice, T. N., & West, S. G. (1997). What the Need for Closure Scale measures and what it does not: Toward differentiating among related epistemic motives. *Journal of Personality and Social Psychology*, *72*, 1396–1412.

Peters, E., Day, S., & Garety, P. A. (1997). From preconscious to conscious processing—where does the abnormality lie in delusions? *Schizophrenia Research*, *24*, 120.

Peters, E. R., Day, S., & Garety, P. A. (1996). The Peters et al. Delusions Inventory (PDI): New norms for the 21-item version. *Schizophrenia Research*, *18*, 118.

Peterson, C., Semmel, A., von Baeyer, C., Abramson, L. Y., Metalsky, G. I., & Seligman, M. E. P. (1982). The Attributional Style Questionnaire. *Cognitive Therapy and Research*, *6*(3), 287–300.

Ramachandran, V. S. (1995). Anosognosia in parietal lobe syndrome. *Consciousness and Cognition*, *4*(1), 22–51.

Ramachandran, V. S., & Blakeslee, S. (1998). *Phantoms in the brain: Human nature and the architecture of the mind*. London: Fourth Estate.

Raschka, L. B. (1981). The Capgras syndrome. *Canadian Journal of Psychiatry*, *26*(3), 207–208.

Reid, I., Young, A. W., & Hellawell, D. J. (1993). Voice recognition impairment in a blind Capgras patient. *Behavioural Neurology*, *6*, 225–228.

Rosler, A., Holder, G., & Seifritz, E. (2001). Canary Capgras. *Journal of Neuropsychiatry and Clinical Neurosciences*, *13*(3), 429.

Schnider, A. (2008). *The confabulating mind: How the brain creates reality*. Oxford, UK: Oxford University Press.

Silva, J. A., Leong, G. B., Longhitano, M., & Botello, T. E. (1991). Delusion of fetal duplication in a Capgras patient. *Canadian Journal of Psychiatry*, *336*, 46–47.

Smith, N., Freeman, D., & Kuipers, E. (2005). Grandiose delusions: An experimental investigation of the delusion as defense. *Journal of Nervous and Mental Disease*, *193*(7), 480–487.

Somerfield, D. (1999). Capgras syndrome and animals. *International Journal of Geriatric Psychiatry*, *14*, 892–894.

Stephens, G. L., & Graham, G. (2004). Reconceiving delusion. *International Review of Psychiatry*, *16*(3), 236–241.

Stone, T., & Young, A. W. (1997). Delusions and brain injury: The philosophy and psychology of belief. *Mind and Language*, *12*, 327–364.

Stroop, J. R. (1935). Studies of interference in serial verbal reactions. *Journal of Experimental Psychology*, *18*, 643–662.

Taylor, S. E. (1989). *Positive illusions: Creative self-deception and the healthy mind*. New York: Basic Books.

Taylor, S. E., & Brown, J. D. (1988). Illusion and well-being: A social psychological perspective on mental health. *Psychological Bulletin*, *103*, 193–210.

Trivers, R. L. (1985). *Social evolution*. Menlo Park, CA: Benjamin Cummings.

Turnbull, O. H., Jones, K., & Reed-Screen, J. (2002). Implicit awareness of deficit in anosognosia? An emotion-based account of denial of deficit. *Neuro-Psychoanalysis*, *4*, 69–86.

Turnbull, O. H., & Solms, M. (2007). Awareness, desire, and false beliefs: Freud in the light of modern neuropsychology. *Cortex*, *43*, 1083–1090.

Vazquez, C., Diez-Alegria, C., Hernandez-Lloreda, M. J., & Moreno, M. N. (2008). Implicit and explicit self-schema in active deluded, remitted deluded, and depressed patients. *Journal of Behavior Therapy and Experimental Psychiatry*, *39*, 587–599.

Webster, D. M., & Kruglanski, A. W. (1994). Individual differences in need for cognitive closure. *Journal of Personality and Social Psychology*, *67*(6), 1049–1062.

Weinstein, E. A. (1991). Anosognosia and denial of illness. In G. P. Prigatano & D. L. Schacter (Eds.), *Awareness of deficit after brain injury: Clinical and theoretical issues* (pp. 240–257). New York: Oxford University Press.

Weinstein, E. A., & Kahn, R. L. (1950). The syndrome of anosognosia. *Archives of Neurology and Psychiatry*, *64*, 772–791.

Weinstein, E. A., & Kahn, R. L. (1955). *Denial of illness: Symbolic and physiological aspects*. Springfield, IL: Charles C. Thomas.

Winters, K. C., & Neale, J. M. (1985). Mania and low self-esteem. *Journal of Abnormal Psychology*, *94*, 282–290.

Wright, S., Young, A. W., & Hellawell, D. J. (1993). Sequential Cotard and Capgras delusions. *British Journal of Clinical Psychology*, *32*(3), 345–349.

Young, A. W. (2000). Wondrous strange: The neuropsychology of abnormal beliefs. *Mind and Language*, *15*(1), 47–73.

Young, A. W., & Leafhead, K. M. (1996). Betwixt life and death: Case studies of the Cotard delusion. In P. W. Halligan & J. C. Marshall (Eds.), *Method in madness: Case studies in cognitive neuropsychiatry*. Hove, UK: Lawrence Erlbaum Associates Ltd.

Young, A. W., Leafhead, K. M., & Szulecka, T. K. (1994). The Capgras and Cotard delusions. *Psychopathology*, *27*(3–5), 226–231.

Zigler, E., & Glick, M. (1988). Is paranoid schizophrenia really camouflaged depression? *The American Psychologist*, *43*, 284–290.

COGNITIVE NEUROPSYCHIATRY
2010, 15 (1/2/3), 319–345

Delusion and confabulation: Mistakes of perceiving, remembering and believing

Robyn Langdon[1] and Tim Bayne[2]

[1]*Macquarie Centre for Cognitive Science, Macquarie University, Sydney, NSW, Australia,* [2]*Faculty of Philosophy, University of Oxford and St. Catherine's College, Oxford, UK*

This paper adopts an inclusive approach to the relationship between delusion and confabulation, according to which some symptoms might qualify as both delusional and confabulatory. Our initial focus is on the cardinal signs of delusions: incomprehensibility, incorrigibility, and subjective conviction. Setting aside post hoc (or secondary) confabulations—plausible rationalisations that might be generated by nonpathological belief formation processes—we focus on spontaneous memory-based confabulations which, we suggest, conform to the characterisation of delusions. After considering current accounts of the role of experience in delusion formation, we propose that spontaneous confabulations are located at (or towards) the "received" end of a "received-reflective" spectrum of delusions: the spontaneous confabulator simply receives and endorses as genuine the content of an apparent—yet implausible—memory experience. Underlying both spontaneous confabulations and other received delusions, we propose, is an inability to inhibit the prepotent tendency to upload and maintain experiential content (mnemonic or perceptual) into belief.

Keywords: Belief formation; Confabulation; Delusion; Memory pathology; Perceptual aberration; Psychosis.

INTRODUCTION

A number of symptoms that arise in the context of brain injury and psychiatric illness can be broadly termed "distortions of reality". These include, most obviously, delusions and hallucinations. Delusions are distortions of belief, whereas hallucinations are distortions of experience. A patient with schizophrenia who has the hallucinatory experience of hearing voices

Correspondence should be addressed to Robyn Langdon, Macquarie Centre for Cognitive Science, Macquarie University, NSW 2109, Australia. E-mail: robyn@maccs.mq.edu.au

 DOI: 10.1080/13546800903000229

that comment continually on her behaviour might believe that her voices do not originate from an unseen speaker and instead reflect dysfunctional brain process(es). Likewise, a patient with Lewy body dementia might attribute his vivid visual hallucinations to a disease of the brain. In addition to hallucination, a number of other distortions of reality have traditionally been contrasted with delusions. These include, most notably, anosognosia, or unawareness of brain injury or mental illness (see Davies, Aimola Davies, & Coltheart, 2005), and confabulation, traditionally referred to as a falsification of memory arising unintentionally in the context of organic memory impairment (e.g., Berlyne, 1972). Our focus in this paper, along with that of other contributors to this Special Issue, concerns the relationship between delusion and confabulation.

Researchers and clinicians have been discussing the relationship between delusion and confabulation since the time of Bonhoeffer, Kraepelin, and Bleuler in the early 1900s, if not earlier (Berrios, 1998). This fact, if nothing else, suggests that there is a consensus for locating confabulation and delusion in a shared conceptual space. There is little consensus, however, as to how that space ought to be carved up. Some (e.g., Kopelman, 2010 this issue) favour an *exclusive* picture, according to which no particular symptom could ever qualify as an instance of both delusion and confabulation; on this view, a patient could qualify as simultaneously delusional and confabulatory only by manifesting concurrent yet distinct symptoms, at least one of which was a delusion and at least one of which was a confabulation. We favour an *inclusive* approach to the relationship between delusion and confabulation: Some symptoms qualify as both delusional *and* as confabulatory. Delusion might, for example, comprise the broader set and encompass a narrower subset of confabulation, or vice versa, or the set of delusions and the set of confabulations might intersect. More specifically, we propose that a certain species of confabulation—spontaneous confabulation—qualifies as a delusion. We then turn to the question of exactly how existing accounts of delusion formation might apply to spontaneous confabulation. Our point of departure is to contrast two experience-based accounts of delusion formation. One might adopt an "explanationist" account according to which delusions are formed in an attempt to explain unusual experience, or one might adopt an "endorsement" account according to which delusions are formed by endorsing the content of unusual experience as veridical. We propose that both accounts apply to the explanation of delusions, and that all delusions lie somewhere on a "received/reflective" spectrum. At one pole of this spectrum are "received" delusions, formed solely via "endorsement processes" (i.e., those processes of delusion formation according to an endorsement account); at the other pole are "reflective" delusions, formed solely via "explanationist processes". (We employ the terms "received delusions" and "reflective delusions" because they capture the phenomenological qualities of delusions at the two ends of this spectrum.) We further propose that most delusions are hybrids—they arise from a combination of endorsement and explanationist processes. We then argue that there is a strong case to be made for thinking of spontaneous confabulation as a delusion that involves memory pathology and which lies at the received end of the spectrum. We conclude by considering the (endorsement) process(es) that contribute to the adoption and maintenance of received delusions (whether or not memory pathology is also present) and discuss what role memory and the passage of time might play in expanding the scope of received delusions.

ON THE DEFINING OF DELUSION AND CONFABULATION

In 1999, David wrote "On the Impossibility of Defining Delusions". He was lamenting the apparent intractable problem of defining delusion, as many clinicians have done over the years (see, e.g., Oltmanns, 1988; Smith, 1968; Spitzer, 1990). The situation is little changed today with the nature of delusion appearing to elude definition according to a set of necessary and sufficient criteria. Consider the definition of delusion found in the Diagnostic and Statistical Manual of Mental Disorders—4th edition (DSM-IV: American Psychiatric Association, 1994):

> A false belief based on incorrect inference about external reality that is firmly sustained despite what almost everyone else believes and despite what constitutes incontrovertible and obvious proof or evidence to the contrary. The belief is not one ordinarily accepted by other members of the person's culture or subculture (e.g. it is not an article of religious faith). (p. 765)

This definition is open to many objections: For one thing, it seems possible that a delusion could be true by accident, so to speak (e.g., the frustrated partner of a patient with delusional jealousy starts an affair); for another, many "loss of boundary" delusions (e.g., delusions of thought insertion and of thought broadcast) seem more about the interface between internal and external reality.

Despite these well-known difficulties in defining delusions, most of us would agree that there is such a thing as delusional belief; certainly those of us who work with delusional people usually know a delusion when we see one. (In saying this, we do not mean to imply that clinicians are infallible.) The cardinal signs that are employed by clinicians as tests for the presence of delusions are incomprehensibility, incorrigibility and subjective certainty. We can distinguish between two kinds of incomprehensibility: "sheer incomprehensibility" and "contextual incomprehensibility". The sheer content of some delusions—fantastical delusions—is such as to render them incomprehensible. The beliefs that one is dead despite being able to walk and talk

(Cotard delusion) or has no internal organs (a case of somatic delusion in schizophrenia: RL) or is being controlled telepathically by an alien from outer space (a classic example of alien control delusion in schizophrenia) or can see, despite the presence of bilateral damage to the occipital lobes which causes a form of cortical blindness (Anton's syndrome) qualify as incomprehensible in this sense. Mundane delusions, such as the persecutory delusion that one's neighbours are plotting against one or the delusion that one's partner is having an affair (delusional jealousy) or the grandiose delusion that one is a gifted composer (in circumstances where one has never played a musical instrument or studied music: RL), qualify as contextually incomprehensible. What renders these propositions unworthy of belief is not their content per se but the fact that the subject in question lacks sufficient evidence for them—or, more precisely, lacks the kind of evidence that would warrant the subjective conviction with which the belief is held. (Here, we can see that incomprehensibility is not completely independent of subjective certainty.) RL once observed a paranoid schizophrenic patient who was asked about the last time that the patient knew her neighbour was intending to hurt her. The patient replied by describing the irritating way in which the neighbour had intentionally jingled her keys in a provocative manner when walking in front of the patient. Incorrigibility concerns the persistence of the belief in the face of counterevidence and rational counterargument; the delusional patient cannot be corrected. Subjective certainty is a phenomenological feature of delusions. It involves a sense of self-evidence; it appears to the patient as though the truth has been directly revealed to them.

In light of these considerations, we adopt the following as our working definition of delusion: a belief which is implausible in light of general knowledge and/or the weight of evidence to hand (which ought normally to confer doubt), and which is adopted and maintained uncritically as true with unwarranted subjective conviction. Although the vast majority of beliefs that meet this definition will be false, this definition does allow a true belief to qualify as delusional. The central feature of delusions—which is only implicit in the above definition—is that they are *pathologies* of belief. Delusions involve malfunctions somewhere in the processes responsible for normal belief formation, where the processes of belief formation are taken to include perceptual processes. Wherever exactly in the processes leading up to belief fixation these malfunctions are located—and, as we will see, they might be located in different places in different delusions—it leaves the patient with a belief that is implausible in the light of general knowledge and at odds with the evidence that is in their possession (see Bayne & Fernández, 2008).

What about confabulation? The uses of this term are even more diverse than are references to delusion in the literature, and attempts to define confabulation have proven even more problematic (Berrios, 1998). Sometimes the term is used in a general sense to refer to instances of fabricated gap-filling that do not involve memory processing, strictly speaking (see, e.g., Hirstein, 2005). Much of the behaviour of perfectly healthy people is confabulatory in this sense. For example, in a classic experiment, Nisbett and Wilson (1977) asked shoppers to choose between pairs of nylon stockings. Although the stockings were identical to each other, the shoppers nevertheless tended to choose the rightmost pair. When asked to justify their choices, the shoppers appealed to illusory differences in colour or texture rather than admit that they had no inkling as to what had prompted their choice. This is a typical example of what we might call post hoc (or secondary: Gilboa & Moscovitch, 2002) confabulation—a fabricated justification for action concocted unintentionally in order to meet the need to present the world with a coherent account of what one is up to.

Post hoc confabulatory rationalisations of the kind generated by Nisbett and Wilson's (1977) shoppers also occur in delusional contexts, although in such cases the fabricated excuses are not typically as plausible as those reported by Nisbett and Wilson. When patients with anosognosia for hemiplegia are asked why they are not able to clap their hands or get out of bed, they will say such things as "I never produce noise", "I haven't clapped my hands because we are not at the theatre" or even "my left hand has gone for a walk" (Berti, Làdavas, Stracciari, Giannarelli, & Ossola, 1998; Venneri & Shanks, 2004). Bisiach (1988) reports a famous exchange in which a patient with somatoparaphrenia insisted that one of her arms was not hers but belonged to the (three-handed) doctor. These instances of post hoc confabulation occur in delusional contexts, but we do not regard them as delusions as such because they are not—or at least do not appear to be—produced by pathologies of belief formation. Arguably, one can account for these reports by appeal to the normal operations of the mechanisms responsible for the kind of post-hoc confabulation seen in Nisbett and Wilson's study and allowing for the constraints imposed by the content of the incorrigible delusional belief in those delusional contexts.

Confabulation, as inventive plausible story-telling, also occurs when there is a compulsion to fill a gap in memory; unintentional false eye-witness reports in healthy people are a case in point (see, e.g., Hanba & Zaragoza, 2007). Once again these kinds of plausible gap-filling or excuse-making, even though they might involve the generation of a false memory and fit within the broader spectrum of confabulation, do not qualify as delusional, since they are products of normal belief formation processes. The kind of confabulation that does qualify as delusional occurs when memory *pathology* is present. But here too further distinctions are needed, because the normal processes of reconstructive memory (see, e.g., Conway, 1996) and of inventive plausible story-telling to fill a gap in knowledge or memory (without any intention to deceive and often with a sense of doubt), can also occur when memory pathology is present as "provoked confabulation".

Kopelman (1987, 1999, 2010 this issue) proposes a distinction between "spontaneous" and "provoked" confabulation. Whereas spontaneous confabulation is just that, spontaneous, provoked confabulation (sometimes termed momentary since the confabulation is often fleeting) arises only in response to direct questioning. Just like nonbrain-damaged individuals, amnesic patients who produce provoked confabulations may be simply responding in a perfectly normal way to the questions that they face. Further, confabulators who only ever produce provoked confabulations in the context of memory testing tend not to express their memory-based guesses with that same conviction that causes spontaneous confabulators to try to leave the hospital to go to school despite being 36 years of age, for example. In saying this we do not mean to imply that the contrast between subjective conviction and its absence straightforwardly maps onto the contrast between spontaneous and provoked confabulation. An individual patient might, for example, sometimes spontaneously generate a confabulation and sometimes confabulate in response to direct probing, and do so, in each case, with subjective conviction. Turner and Coltheart (2010 this issue) describe, who, when asked about his movements the previous evening, responded by saying that he had been to a party where he had met a woman with a bee's head (a provoked confabulation, according to the mode of elicitation), and who later spontaneously said that he had to leave the testing session to attend a business meeting (a spontaneous confabulation). Both the provoked and the spontaneous confabulation were espoused with subjective conviction. Nevertheless, despite the practical difficulties with operationalising the spontaneous versus provoked distinction (see, e.g., Gilboa et al., 2006), we agree with Kopelman that it is conceptually important. This is because we think that it reflects the presence versus absence of pathological belief formation processes (in an individual patient) which associate phenomenologically with the presence versus absence of an unwarranted subjective conviction on espousal of the confabulation. So, provoked confabulation (in the absence of cooccurring spontaneous confabulation) seems not to qualify as a delusion, for there is nothing pathological about the belief formation processes involved, and the provoked confabulators do not really seem to believe what they say, at least not with the same subjective certainty that is characteristic of delusion.

That leaves us with spontaneous confabulation to consider, that kind of "persistent, unprovoked outpouring of erroneous memories" (Kopelman, 2010 this issue) which typically occurs in the context of frontal lobe pathology. We refer readers to Kopelman (2010 this issue) for a review of the various theories of spontaneous confabulation that have been developed over the years. For our own purposes, we adopt the following as our working definition of spontaneous confabulation: a mistaken memory which is generated spontaneously (with no intention to deceive) and which is adopted uncritically as true and with a degree of subjective conviction that is unwarranted in light of general knowledge and/or the evidence to hand (either or both of which ought to confer doubt). On the face of things, spontaneous confabulations show the three cardinal signs of delusion: incomprehensibility, incorrigibility, and subjective conviction. They involve implausible beliefs that are mistakenly accepted as true with unwarranted subjective conviction in light of the general knowledge and/or the weight of evidence to hand, either or both of which ought to confer doubt.

To some degree this entire paper constitutes a defence of the previous claim, but let us attempt to head off at the pass some objections to it before we proceed any further (see also Turner & Coltheart, 2010 this issue).

OBJECTIONS TO A CONCEPTION OF CONFABULATION AS DELUSION-LIKE

The first common objection is to claim that confabulations are not beliefs; they are instead fanciful narratives that are not truly believed and are not acted upon. Some might respond to this objection by saying that delusions are not beliefs either (see, e.g., Berrios, 1991), but we are not tempted to take this route as we are inclined to think that there are good reasons to regard delusions as beliefs, or at least as interestingly belief-like (Bayne & Pacherie, 2005). Although it is true that the expression of confabulation-based thoughts does not always lead to the kind of actions that one would expect if the patient really believed what she says, the same can be said for delusions. Finally, some treatments of spontaneous confabulation do require that patients be known to have acted on their confabulations (Schnider, von Daniken, & Gutbrod, 1996). Although both delusion and confabulation can involve a puzzling lack of action, in both cases this can—at least in principle—be explained by the presence of additional pathology. Further, confabulation-based beliefs often concern the past, and beliefs about the more distant past are less inclined to issue in direct action than are beliefs about the present.

A second objection to the proposal that spontaneous confabulation qualifies as delusional concerns the content of the states in question. One might argue that implausibility is characteristic of delusion, but is not necessarily a feature of spontaneous confabulation. But spontaneous confabulations, although often involving rearrangements of partial memory traces of mundane real events, can nevertheless be fantastic. Delusions similarly vary in the degree to which their content is incredible. At one end of the spectrum are fantastical delusions, whose content is widely at odds with commonsense conceptions of what can be (e.g., that there is a thermonuclear power-station inside one's stomach); at the other end are relatively prosaic delusions (e.g., of persecution and jealousy), whose contents—although not incredible per se—are unjustified in light of the evidence to hand. This same kind of contextual implausibility also occurs in spontaneous confabulation.

Another objection to the proposal concerns maintenance; delusions are fixed, whereas confabulations are said to be labile. Here too matters are more complicated than the objection assumes, as becomes apparent when one considers the two heuristics that are often applied in clinical contexts: (1) If it's fixed it's a delusion; and (2) if it involves memory pathology it's a confabulation. According to the first heuristic a patient should be considered delusional if she espouses a fixed mistaken belief even if that fixed mistaken belief concerns the past and involves memory pathology which, in her case, results in a consistent (i.e., fixed) conflation of degraded memory traces. But, according to the second heuristic, this patient should be called confabulatory since memory pathology lies at the heart of her problems. To put it another way, delusional fixity (at the level of phenomenology) need not be inconsistent with the presence of confabulatory memory pathology. Likewise, confabulatory lack of fixity (at the level of phenomenology) need not be inconsistent with the presence of delusional pathology. A lack of fixity in some delusional confabulators might, for example, simply reflect the severity of the memory pathology that is present and that cooccurs with the delusional pathology; in other words, these patients might simply forget from one moment to the next what they have mistakenly recalled and espoused with momentary delusional conviction.

A final objection to the proposal concerns the pathological contexts in which delusion and confabulation occur. It is sometimes said that confabulation arises in the context of neurological insult, whereas delusion arises in the context of "psychosis" (see, e.g., Gilboa & Moscovitch, 2002, for discussion). This contrast seems doubly flawed. Not only do delusions occur in the context of neurological insult (see, for reviews, Fricchione, Carbone, & Bennett, 1995; Nasrallah, 1992), but confabulation can also occur in the apparent absence of neurological insult—that is, in the context of so-called "functional psychosis". Nathaniel-James and colleagues (Nathaniel-James, Foong, & Frith, 1996; Nathaniel-James & Frith, 1996), for example, report confabulation elicited via a fable recall task in people with schizophrenia, the classic functional psychosis, whereas McKay, McKenna, and Baddeley (1995) describe a psychotic patient who confabulated memories of a nonexistent twin sister. Schizophrenic patients with "formal thought disorder" (a characteristic symptom of schizophrenia) can also spontaneously generate idiosyncratic and implausible statements about self and the world (see, e.g., Laws, Kondel, & McKenna, 1999) that appear strikingly similar to (phenomenologically speaking, that is) the confabulations of some neurological cases (see, e.g., Kopelman, Ng, & van den Brouke, 1997). More fundamentally though, the very contrast between the organic and the functional psychoses is of dubious coherence. Although schizophrenia—the classic functional psychosis—may not result from acquired neurological insult caused by exogenous factors, it clearly has a neurological basis of some kind (see, e.g., Jarskog, Miyamoto, & Lieberman, 2007). Thus, the attempt to differentiate between confabulation and delusion by simple appeal to the presence or absence of neurological insult does not appear to be viable.

In summary, we can see no good reason for rejecting the intuitively plausible claim that spontaneous confabulation qualifies as a delusion. But in saying this, we want to allow that there is a particular variant of confabulation that is generated spontaneously but does not qualify as delusional. Some confabulators who spontaneously generate their mistaken memories are quite prepared to retract their statements in the face of challenges and not because they have simply forgotten their confabulation, although this corrigibility might be difficult to establish when the memory pathology is severe. This kind of confabulation is delusion-like insofar as it is incomprehensible, but it departs from delusions insofar as it is corrigible. There might also be some doubt about whether such confabulations are held with subjective certainty. This kind of confabulation—call it "corrigible confabulation"—might result from damage to a "plausibility monitor", which would normally filter out implausible memories (see, e.g., Hirstein, 2005; Turner & Coltheart, 2010 this issue) and which the spontaneous confabulator can correct for (if no other damage is present) when alerted to the counterevidence by others. But it is just this ability to revise which is absent in delusional patients who seem impervious to arguments of plausibility.

Although there is much to be gained by considering the processes that make corrigible confabulation a kind of "partial delusional" case, our focus here will be on incorrigible spontaneous confabulations—what we will henceforward refer to as simply "spontaneous confabulations". In the following section, we consider whether the close conceptual fit between (incorrigible) spontaneous confabulations and delusions extends to any common process(es) of pathological belief evaluation/revision by way of discussion of the role of experience in delusion formation.

TWO ACCOUNTS OF THE ROUTE FROM EXPERIENCE TO BELIEF

Following Davies, Coltheart, Langdon, and Breen (2001) and Gold and Hohwy (2000), we can distinguish between two accounts of how beliefs can be grounded in experience: an *explanationist* account and an *endorsement* account (see also Bayne & Pacherie 2004a, 2004b). On the explanationist account, the delusion is formed in an attempt to explain an anomalous experience of some kind. On the endorsement account, the delusion is adopted because the unusual experience is taken "at face value", so to speak, and then maintained because of some resistance to over-riding "the evidence of one's own senses" (more on this later).

We can illustrate the distinction between these two accounts by considering the Capgras delusion, the delusional belief that a loved one has been replaced by a visually similar impostor. It is agreed on all sides to this (endorsement/explanationist) debate that the Capgras delusion involves a primary neuropsychological abnormality associated with the viewing of a loved one's face; what is debated is the representational content of the associated anomalous experience and the relationship between it, conscious reflection and the delusional belief. Proponents of the explanationist account of the Capgras delusion hold a "thin" or "coarse-grained" account of the content of the experience, according to which it represents the fact that something in general is not right, or perhaps that there is something wrong with the particular person being looked at ("something is wrong about that person in front of me"). According to the explanationist theorist, the patient reflects upon her experience and hits upon the Capgras hypothesis in order to make sense of this reasonably nonspecific experience. By contrast, those who propose an endorsement account of the Capgras delusion regard the anomalous experience as imbued with more precise and fine-grained representational content and, as a result, take it to have a more direct role in the fixing of the delusional content. They might suppose that the patient literally *experiences* the object of the delusion as unfamiliar, as a stranger. This experience of seeing a stranger is then accepted as veridical and the patient believes, on seeing the stranger, that the person in front of him or her *is* a stranger. The Capgras content is then but a simple—and perhaps spontaneous and unconscious—inference away, one that also takes account of the observed visual similarity between the stranger and the loved one and that the stranger states that he/she is the loved one and behaves as such.

Whereas the Capgras delusion lends itself reasonably well to either an explanationist or an endorsement account, some other misidentification delusions conform more naturally to an endorsement account. "Mirrored-self misidentification" delusion is like this. Patients with a mirrored-self misidentification delusion believe that the person one sees in the mirror is a stranger and not oneself. Breen, Caine, and Coltheart (2001) describe a patient with mirrored-self misidentification delusion who also had "mirror agnosia" (Binkofski, Buccino, Dohle, Seitz, & Freund, 1999). Mirror agnosia is a condition that causes a loss of the normal usage of mirror knowledge (and perhaps knowledge of other reflective surfaces), acquired in childhood, to mediate interactions with mirrors. When a person with mirror agnosia looks into a mirror, his experience is of seeing a man looking back at him through a window into another room and is not of seeing his own reflection. According to the endorsement theorist, the delusional patient with mirror agnosia then accepts his experience as veridical and reports seeing a stranger—a stranger who might look like him but cannot be himself, since he, the patient, is located on the other side of the window to the strange man.

We can further illustrate the endorsement account by considering another case of misidentification delusion, patient DH (Langdon, Cooper, Connaughton, & Martin, 2006). Following severe right frontotemporal brain damage, DH developed the delusional belief that a nursing sister in the hospital was his ex-partner. The ex-partner lived a distance from the hospital and she and the nurse were never seen together. DH's delusion was incorrigible. He might speak to his ex-partner on the phone in his room and then see the nurse soon after on the ward. Although such events seemed a little odd to DH, they were not odd enough to cast doubt on his belief. Testing revealed that DH had suffered impairments to both face and voice processing. In order to account for his delusion, Langdon and colleagues drew upon models of person recognition (see Lucchellia & Spinnler, 2008, for a review) to propose that mannerisms of the nurse that resembled those of the ex-partner activated the "primed" person identity node (PIN) of the ex-partner. PINs are the entry nodes to general biographical information about familiar persons and the sites at which cross-modal decisions of person familiarity are worked out by integrating information from visual processing of faces (involving activation of "face recognition units"; FRUs), as well as processing of voice and gait and other mannerisms. In the case of DH, Langdon and colleagues proposed that the ex-partner's PIN was already at a high level of resting activation because of the personal history between DH and his ex-partner. The ex-partner's PIN was further activated via the processing of mannerisms that resembled those of the ex-partner. With no inconsistent input from the processing of either face or voice, which might otherwise have cancelled out the increased activation of the PIN, triggered by the familiar mannerisms, the PIN of the ex-partner was sufficiently activated to cause the mistaken recognition of the nurse as the ex-partner. DH "saw" his ex-partner, an experience that directly gave rise to (and continued to reinforce) DH's delusional belief that his ex-partner was in front of him.

Although misidentification delusions of this type conform quite naturally to an endorsement account, the endorsement account does have its limitations, however. Persecutory delusions are a notable case in point. Even when an endorsement theorist highlights the role that aberrant experiences play in the formation of a persecutory delusion, the content of the endorsed anomalous experience is quite some distance from that of the delusion to which it gives rise (see Langdon, McKay, & Coltheart, 2008, for further discussion). Consider persecutory delusions, which are grounded in hearing loss, memory loss, or ideas of reference. With hearing loss, the initial endorsed experience might be of hearing "people speaking at lower than expected volumes". It is only after a chain of further reflection— "Why are people speaking softly? They must be whispering. Why are they whispering? They must want to hide things from me"—that the persecutory delusional theme begins to emerge. Likewise, with memory loss, the initial endorsed experience might be of a patient opening his top drawer expecting to see his wallet, only to see it missing. Having forgotten that he had earlier moved his wallet, the patient might naturally think, "Someone has moved my wallet". Having accepted this thought as true, the patient may then question others about moving his wallet, only to be met with denials. Similar incidents will eventually promote persecutory themes. With regard to ideas of reference, these thoughts arise when innocuous events (e.g., the location of a crumpled brown paper bag on the pavement) are experienced as having a special self-referential significance. Kapur (2003) suggests that such referential experiences are caused by dopamine hyperactivity and reflect aberrant states of self-referential salience that attach inappropriately to events that ought normally to be screened from attention. In other words, the initial aberrant experience, which might be endorsed to seed an eventual persecutory delusion, is of sensing a self-referential significance, say, on reading newspaper stories; only many further inferential steps, and a likely premorbid paranoid personality, will lead eventually to a persecutory delusional belief in a conspiracy that the patient needs to uncover. And, if one is not premorbidly paranoid, the experience of (say) sensing self-referential significance on seeing Kylie Minogue performing on TV might trigger a quite different chain of inferences: "She's secretly sending a message to me. Why? It must be because she secretly loves me"—leading eventually to de Clérambault's syndrome or erotomania. Other nonpersecutory delusional themes also appear resistant to a purely endorsement account. Even the "bees-in-the-head" delusion that Maher (1988) describes would seem to involve some postreflective explanation. Maher describes a woman with the delusion that her skull was filled with bees; autopsy examinations later revealed that she had suffered from a softening of the bones of the skull, with consequent pressure on the brain and likely tinnitus. But, taking the buzzing that one hears to be that of bees would seem to require inference of some kind beyond endorsement, although it may be an inference that occurs quite spontaneously and without conscious deliberation.

We therefore propose that all delusions lie somewhere on a "received/reflective" spectrum, the content of each delusion formed by a variable weighting of endorsement and explanationist processes. At one pole of this spectrum are purely "received" delusions like mirrored-self misidentification delusion, formed solely from endorsement processes; at the other pole are purely "reflective" delusions like persecutory delusions, which begin with an anxious worry and rumination and are formed by explanationist processes alone. Postexperiential inferential processes feature largely in reflective delusions, whereas received delusions come to consciousness fully formed. Perhaps most delusions are hybrids, formed from a combination of explanationist and endorsement processes. The Capgras delusion might be such a hybrid. Arguably, the Capgras delusion begins with an experience of there being a stranger in front of oneself. It is not until the patient also takes into account the behavioural and perceptual similarities between the loved one and his/her "impostor" that the fully formed impostor content arises. We also note here that we can see no principled objection to the proposal that a particular delusion in one patient might be relatively more received, whereas the very same delusion in another patient might be more reflective.

A number of points that arise from the preceding discussion bear highlighting before we consider implications of the explanationist and the endorsement accounts for further theorising about the adoption and the maintenance of a delusional belief (which includes spontaneous confabulation).

THE EXPLANATIONIST AND ENDORSEMENT ACCOUNTS COMPARED AND CONTRASTED

Although the question of where a particular delusion might fall on the received-reflective spectrum is an empirical matter that must be decided on a case-by-case basis, it is useful to consider how the explanationist and the endorsement accounts generally compare.

First, both the explanationist and the endorsement accounts are alike with regard to the role of inferential transitions in the formation of delusions; the two accounts differ only in where they locate such transitions in relation to experience. The explanationist account of the route from experience to a reflective delusion locates most of the inferential processing downstream of experience, in the processes of hypothesis generation and evaluation, whereas the endorsement account locates it upstream of experience, before the received delusion is endorsed.

The two accounts do differ, however, with regard to their explanatory strengths—and weaknesses. A strength of the endorsement account is that it offers an attractive explanation of the subjective certainty and the incorrigibility of delusions. Suppose, for example, that you are asked to explain why you believe the sky to be blue. You would likely look to the sky and return to your questioner a puzzled gaze, as if wondering how one could think otherwise. If other people were to challenge your belief and to tell you that the sky was a lovely shade of green, you would likely think them crazy, at least initially. But, so long as your belief-evaluation capacity is unimpaired, you will, we suspect, begin to question your own senses if everyone else were to consistently refer to the "green sky"; and if you have suffered such brain damage? Well then it must be everyone else who is a little crazy. Plausibility just doesn't seem to count, at least for the patient with a received delusion—certainly it doesn't count enough to dislodge beliefs that are directly (and constantly) reinforced by perceptual content.

In contrast, the explanationist theorist has a much harder job of accounting for the self-evident conviction that is a cardinal sign of delusion. Delusions that are more reflective than received are associated with a slower onset of delusional conviction. Compare, for example, our (relatively more) endorsement and our (relatively more) explanationist interpretations of the Capgras delusion. In the first case, the delusional conviction is present at the very instant the patient endorses her experience of seeing a stranger as veridical. Now consider a Capgras delusion formed largely via explanationist processes: in this case, the patient does not believe that a stranger is present when she first experiences a coarse-grained feeling of strangeness. She might be convinced that there is something strange going on, but in this she is not mistaken—after all, there *is* something strange going on, and this belief is plausible in light of her feeling of strangeness. Delusional conviction (that a stranger's presence explains her feeling of strangeness) only comes later and perhaps with a more gradual crystallisation of subjective certainty. Certainly a purely reflective delusion, like a hypochondrial delusion that begins solely with a mere worry (and not a conviction) about one's physical health, would seem to involve a much more gradual crystallisation of delusional conviction.

An associated point here is that delusions that are purely received are not accompanied by any awareness of a precipitating experience as an explanandum, and hence the patient will have no *sense* of themselves as adopting the delusional belief for explanatory reasons. By contrast, patients with delusions that have been formed following reflection upon a disturbing "thin" experience might have some awareness of the delusional belief *as* an explanation, and hence as requiring justification. So, the fact that a delusion is espoused as a self-evident, god-given truth with accompanying bafflement when confronted with others' disbelief is suggestive of the operations of largely endorsement rather than explanationist processes. A related observation is that the *specific* content of patients' delusions sometimes shifts under challenge, whereas the *general* delusional theme remains fixed. Perhaps the delusional theme is fixed and nonrevisable by way of a received delusional seed that is endorsed, whereas that postreflective elaboration which also occurs is more amenable to demands for justification and a compulsion to revise in light of counterevidence.

An associated strength of the endorsement account is that it explains quite nicely why delusional patients form beliefs with the thematic content that they do. This is because experiences with fine-grained content place more constraints on the received beliefs to which they naturally give rise than do experiences with coarse-grained content. By contrast, advocates of a purely explanationist account need to work much harder in order to explain the generation of the delusional content, for on such an account the gap between experiential content and delusional content is wider. If the Capgras patient simply has an experience that something is wrong, why does she then form the belief that her husband has been replaced by an imposter? After all, there are many (and presumably better) competing explanations for why something might be wrong, including that the patient has acquired some brain damage (see, e.g., Langdon & Coltheart, 2000; Stone & Young, 1997).

But the tables are turned when it comes to accounting for the content of the aberrant experience itself. Here, the endorsement theorist faces objections that the explanationist theorist evades. It is relatively unproblematic to think that perceptual experience might be able to convey the vague content "something is wrong", especially if we allow for the existence of somatosensory mechanisms which signal warning, but it is more controversial to suppose that perceptual experience might be able to represent that a seen object or person is unfamiliar (but see Pacherie, 2008). We might call this the "experiential encoding" problem: Can experiential content represent the kinds of high-level properties that endorsement approaches to delusion formation might require? Engaging with the experiential encoding problem raises some very tricky questions—questions that go beyond the scope of this paper. Our inclination is to adopt a rather liberal conception of the admissible contents of perceptual experience, according to which a fairly broad array of high-level properties can be encoded. Perceptual experience is not restricted to the representation of shape, colour, motion, and texture, but is in the business of informing us about the kinds of objects in our world. Consider Maher's example of the bees-in-the-head delusion. We might think of this delusion as falling more towards the received end of the spectrum if we suppose that it begins with the experiential content "Some *thing* is buzzing in my ears" rather than simply "I am hearing *a buzzing* in my ears". Although the former state falls short of encoding the full content of the bees-in-the-head delusion—the *thing* that causes the buzzing might be taken to be a computer chip or a radio rather than bees—it does lead to the delusional content rather more directly than a mere experience of buzzing might.

We turn now to consider implications of the contrast between the endorsement and the explanationist accounts for further theorising about the processes that contribute to delusional incorrigibility. We do so by way of discussion of the two-factor explanatory framework for delusions.

DELUSIONAL FIXITY

Two-factor theorists (Coltheart, 2007; Davies et al., 2001; Langdon & Coltheart, 2000) began by accepting Maher's (1974, 1988, 1999) suggestion that aberrant experience is at work in delusions by way of accounting for the formation of a specific delusional theme, but they proposed that some other process(es) (not involved in the generation of the aberrant experience) must also be present to account for the adoption and the maintenance of the delusional belief. There are a number of reasons for positing a second factor of this type, the most fundamental of which is that the aberrant experiences underlying certain delusions do not appear to suffice for those delusions (see, e.g., Coltheart, Menzies, & Sutton, 2010 this issue). Not all patients with mirror agnosia are delusional, for example; such patients may describe an experience of looking through a window into another room inhabited by a man who might look like them but who is located in a different point in space, but know that this cannot be so. Giving an account of what makes for the difference between the nondelusional and delusional cases of mirror agnosia is a matter of some importance as far as the two-factor theorist is concerned. Most importantly, for the purposes of this paper, the model of the second factor that she develops will be constrained by her conception of the role of experience in relation to the first factor which explains the delusional theme.

So, let's start by considering received delusions that have been formed solely via endorsement processes. On this account, the delusional patient simply endorses her experience as veridical: She believes what her senses tell her. This seems quite a natural thing to do. We all default to such believing, at least initially, because the content of perception has a special status (so long as we have no prior reason to suspect our senses); this is the factual datum that we rely upon from one moment to the next to navigate our world. Just to clarify, we are not concerned here with the processes via which we come to judge whether some encoded propositional content is sourced to perception or imagination, let's say (see Johnson, 1991, and Johnson, Hashtroudi, & Lindsay, 1993, for theorising about such processes); we are concerned instead with the notion that perceived content has a special status—an automatic default setting to be uploaded as belief and a natural resistance to belief revision. This special status might be functionally realised in a number of different ways, perhaps by way of an immediate routing to a special database (separate to that for reflective beliefs) or by way of a "tagging" process which tags certain beliefs as special, "perceived truths", which, by virtue of their source, bypass preliminary evaluation. Whichever processes operate here, the general idea is that perceived content acquires a special status which insulates against doubt. But sometimes we need to reevaluate and revise even our purely received beliefs, for our senses sometimes trick us. We may be alerted to such tricks and come to doubt our senses when an internal plausibility monitor alerts us to the apparent discrepancies before the upload is fully complete. Or, if our internal monitor fails, we may be alerted to our error by other people. When so alerted, we are then able to inhibit the special status of the (mis)perceived content so as to demote it into a "maybe it's true/maybe it's not" working space for critical evaluation of plausibility. We might encapsulate these ideas by saying that a two-factor theorist conceives of the second factor in a purely received delusion (or a received delusional seed) as a difficulty in inhibiting the prepotent tendency to endorse (mis)perceived content as veridical (Davies et al., 2001; see also Langdon & Coltheart, 2000, and Stone & Young, 1997, for similar ideas).

A potential challenge to this endorsement account of the second factor involves explaining why the patient does not form a new delusion whenever her senses trick her, as they do for all of us quite regularly (Davies et al., 2001; Fine, Craigie, & Gold, 2005). There are two lines of response here. First, one might argue that although new "delusion-like" received thoughts of this type do arise quite often in patients with a compromise of inhibitory control (of the type described above), aberrant perceptual experiences lead to the fixation of received delusions proper only when they are continuous and/or cannot be corrected by other experiences that concurrently provide counterevidence (Hohwy & Rosenberg, 2005). Second, one might argue that experiences differ with regard to their prepotent tendency to be endorsed. The aberrant experiences that give rise to received delusions might be more affectively laden; they might, for example, involve what have been called "existential feelings", such as sensations of familiarity and unfamiliarity, of significance and insignificance, and of reality and unreality (McLaughlin, 2008; Ratcliffe, 2004). It might be much harder to inhibit existential feelings from being uploaded into the belief-box, or to dislodge them from the belief-box once uploaded, than it is to demote in a similar way more affectively neutral perceptual content.

Inhibitory compromise, as discussed above, is unlikely to be the second-factor mechanism in delusions that are purely reflective, because in such cases there is no (mis)perceived content which has been endorsed immediately and mistakenly as true. Delusional conviction grows more gradually; perhaps feed by rumination and attentional biases. For purely reflective delusions we need to consider other sorts of cognitive mechanisms or motivational factors that might disrupt postreflective inference making in order to explain the adoption and persistence of the implausible reflective delusion (see, e.g., Turner & Coltheart, 2010 this issue). One might conceptualise these (explanationist) second-factor processes in "cold" terms, as per, for example, an excessive jumping to conclusions bias (combined with a normal confirmatory bias which helps to explain the maintenance of the delusion), or in "hot" terms, as involving a motivational bias of some kind (or one might conceptualise both sorts of factors coming into play). Of course, when delusions are formed and fixed via a hybrid of explanationist and explanatory processes, then the two-factor theorist will need to consider not only the influence of a compromise of inhibitory control, but also the possibility of a disruption to postreflective inferential processes.

Before turning to consider where spontaneous confabulations might fit with regard to the received/reflective spectrum of delusions, we acknowledge here that some readers might have noted a strong resonance between our received versus reflective delusions and Jaspers' (1963) distinction between primary and secondary delusions. Primary delusions were so-called because they were conceived to arise in consciousness as fully formed kinds of judgements or statements with no antecedent event or context which would render them psychologically understandable (at least to the common folk). Secondary delusions, in contrast, were deemed psychologically understandable by way of prior events or circumstances such as associated mood; delusional guilt arising in the context of depression is a classic example. There are certainly strong points of contact between our distinction and Jaspers', but a quick look at some classic examples of primary delusions reveals points of contrast between our taxonomy and his. A prime example here is the patient who looked at marble tables in a cafe and suddenly knew they meant the end of the world was coming (see, e.g., Arthur, 1964). This is often referred to as a primary delusional perception in which the perceptual experience is normal but with the interpreted meaning being abnormal. Maher (1999) has suggested that such primary delusions arise as hypotheses generated to explain abnormally heightened sensations of salience, in this instance, associated with the viewing of the marble tables; the patient reflects upon the marble tables as signifying something important and generates an hypothesis, in this case that they signify the end of the world, so as to explain the aberrant sense of self-referential significance. In other words, at least some primary delusions cry out for an explanationist account, and would thus qualify as largely reflective rather than received delusions in our taxonomy.

INTERIM SUMMARY

Thus far we have suggested that the spontaneous/provoked distinction in confabulation research might be augmented by a further distinction between those spontaneous confabulations that are corrigible and those that are not. We suggested that only incorrigible spontaneous confabulations show the cardinal signs of delusion: They are beliefs about the past that are implausible and yet adopted and maintained with an unwarranted subjective conviction in light of general knowledge and/or the evidence to hand, either or both of which ought normally to confer doubt. We then prefaced our consideration of whether this close conceptual fit between spontaneous confabulation and delusion might extend to any common process(es) by way of contrasting two experience-based accounts of delusion formation: an explanationist account, according to which delusions are formed in an attempt to explain unusual experiences, and an endorsement account, according to which delusions are formed by endorsing an unusual experience as veridical. In order to contrast the associated phenomenology, we referred to delusions that arise via explanationist processes as reflective and delusions that arise via endorsement processes as received. In contrast to an exclusive approach to adjudicating between the endorsement and the explanationist accounts, we proposed a received/reflective spectrum of delusions, with each delusion formed via a unique weighting of endorsement and postreflective explanation. To explain delusions that lie more towards the reflective end of the spectrum, we placed more weight on postreflective reasoning biases and impairments (although consider also motivational factors: McKay & Kinsbourne, 2010 this issue) or any combination to explain the failure to reject an implausible reflective delusion; we attributed this same failure in delusions at the received end to a difficulty with inhibiting the prepotent tendency to upload and maintain perceptual content into belief. We also highlighted the general strengths and weaknesses of the endorsement versus the explanationist accounts. We turn now to consider where spontaneous confabulation fits in the received/reflective scheme of things.

SPONTANEOUS CONFABULATION: RECEIVED OR REFLECTIVE?

So what of the underlying pathology in spontaneous confabulation? Metcalf, Langdon, and Coltheart (2007) proposed that the two-factor approach to delusion might be fruitfully applied to spontaneous confabulation. They likened spontaneous confabulations to bizarre monothematic delusions that arise when two neuropsychological deficits are present (Langdon & Coltheart, 2000). The first neuropsychological deficit, which explains the memory-based content, is an inappropriate recombination of degraded memory traces caused by a deficit in executive functioning; a second deficit must also be present to explain why the implausible apparent memory is adopted uncritically by the patient as genuine (and maintained, if memory pathology is not too severe). Metcalf and colleagues also considered the influence of a third factor (but not a deficit)—normal premorbid motivational biases, which were seen to play a role in prioritising which particular degraded memory traces might be retrieved and how these might be recombined so as to conform with a patient's sense of self (see also Conway, 1996, and Conway & Pleydell-Pearce, 2000, for discussion of the role of the self in reconstructive memory).

We can now expand on the Metcalf et al. (2007) proposal within the context of the received/reflective spectrum of delusions. Crucial to our account is the notion that spontaneous confabulation is a delusion at the received end of the spectrum with confabulated content coming to mind with an autonoetic feeling of reexperiencing or reliving the past (Tulving, 1985, 2002). The confabulator has the recollective experience of remembering "x" (which is typically mistaken) and simply endorses the (mis)recalled content uncritically as a genuine memory, despite its implausibility. Recalled content, we suggest, functions in much the same way that perceptual content does: Like perceptual content, it is sent directly to a belief box unless blocked en route; and just as perceptual content must be inhibited in order to be critically evaluated, so too must mnemonic content. It is precisely this capacity for doxastic inhibition that the incorrigible confabulator struggles to deploy, even when given reasons to do so.

This is not to say that postreflective processing is never engaged in recollection. Perhaps the spontaneous confabulator sometimes has very patchy memory experiences which come to mind in a piecemeal kind of way and, while endorsed (as received delusional primitives), trigger both reflection and further memory search. Consider, for example, delusions of alien abduction. Arguably, such delusions might be the final end-product of a chain of postreflective processing to make sense out of initial fragmentary memories of hypnogogic experiences that are endorsed (just like spontaneous confabulations). The individual unlikely begins with fully formed confabulation-based memories (as) of having been abducted by aliens, but with various spontaneous memory fragments of, e.g., waking up with paralysis, sensing an alien presence in the room, and so on. Individuals with such memory fragments, who are antecedently open to new age ideas, might then generate the alien abduction hypothesis in order to make sense of these memory fragments. That the hypothesis successfully "binds together" the individual's memory fragments gives it an initial hold (we borrow from Carr, 2010 this issue, here) which—with time, further reflection, further encoding, and further retrieval—comes to be recalled as a fully-fleshed-out memory experience of having been abducted by aliens. In other words, with the passage of time, what began as a loose array of fragmentary recollections coalesced into a fleshed-out mnemonic experience (as) of having been abduction by aliens, which in turn gave rise to and reinforced the delusion of having been abducted by aliens via the process by which received delusions are endorsed. Clancy (2005), for example, suggests that alien abductees are intelligent people who unwittingly create false memories from a mix of nightmares and culturally available scenarios (stories of extraterrestrials in films and on TV) and Clancy, McNally, Schacter, Lenzenweger, and Pitman (2002) have reported that people who recollect alien abduction experiences are more inclined than controls to incorrectly endorse unseen items (in the Deese/Roediger-McDermott paradigm) as falsely recalled or recognised and are more likely to report schizotypal traits like magical ideation (e.g., beliefs in reincarnation or that certain numbers have special powers).

Another example of a more reflective confabulation is provided by Moulin and colleagues (Moulin, Conway, Thompson, James, & Jones, 2005; O'Connor, Lever, & Moulin, 2010 this issue) who have described "recollective confabulation" in two patients with dementia and diffuse temporal lobe pathology. These patients reported persistent déjà vecu—the sensation of recollectively experiencing the present moment as if it has occurred before (as occurs in normal remembering) but in the absence of any access to a stored mental representation that could stand as the genuine memory. These patients would reflect upon their aberrant "remembering", which was endorsed uncritically as veridical, and would then entertain post hoc justifications and explanations, which, in time and with further reflection and re-remembering, came to be experienced as (false) memories.

We will consider whether any forms of spontaneous confabulation might qualify as purely reflective delusions in the next section, where we also want to speculate a little bit more about perception, memory, and delusion, and about the role of memory in expanding the scope of received delusions.

MEMORY, PERCEPTION, AND DELUSION

One of the objections to the endorsement account is the experiential encoding problem—the concern that perceptual experience might not be able to encode representations with the sort of high-level content—such as, "That man in front of me is a *stranger*"— that this account requires. A critic of our approach to spontaneous confabulation might likewise object that mnemonic experiences cannot encode high-level content, and that we are confusing ("thin") memory experiences with ("rich") beliefs that are formed consequent to reflection upon the memory experiences. What force this line of objection might have in the context of perception-based delusions (and we certainly grant that it has some force), it has less force in the current context. Arguably, memory experience can include a greater range of high-level contents, since what is retrieved and recollected is not (merely) the perceptual features of an encoded event, but those perceptual features plus the effects of cognitive processes, which were engaged at the time of encoding and which also come into play at the time of reconstructive retrieval (Conway, 1996), and which embellish and filter (see, e.g., Mitchell & Johnson, 2000).

Another asymmetry—of degree if not of kind—between memory and perception that bears on the proposal presented above is that the objects of memory are not publicly accessible in the way that the objects of perception tend to be. The person at whom the patient with Capgras delusion is looking can be seen by others, but the objects of a patient who is confabulating will not typically be available to the others' recollection. There is such a thing as joint reminiscing, but in many cases those with whom the confabulator is conversing simply will not be in a position to confirm or disconfirm a confabulation. (In some cases they might be able to disconfirm them in the general sense that those memories might be outlandish, but this will not apply in all cases.) Of course, mnemonic experience is not unique in this respect. The states represented by unusual experiences of a lack of agency in delusions of alien control are also private in that no-one else can experience your agency "from the inside".

Are there *purely* reflective confabulations? We think so. To illustrate, consider the persecutory memories of Jane and Jake. Due to her faulty memory mechanisms, Jane generates, and endorses as genuine, a memory of being persecuted by her neighbour. She "remembers" that her neighbour's reckless driving caused her to crash her car last year. Jake also believes that he was persecuted in a similar way by his neighbour last year, but he does not suffer from any memory impairment. He does, however, have a difficulty with discriminating between imagination and reality. He also has a bias towards avoiding the blame for negative events. A while ago he began ruminating on the reason for his car crash last year. He started to imagine that his neighbour might have been involved, and these episodes of imagining about the past and reflecting upon those imaginings gradually took on a delusional conviction. Unlike Jane, he didn't spontaneously recall seeing the neighbour in the other car when he crashed, he simply started entertaining such a thought about the past, and, after a period of time, this thought was no longer merely entertained but believed with a delusional certainty.

What this shows us is that the delusional content is unlikely to be the best basis for taxonomising delusions, not if our primary interest is the underlying pathology. Jane and Jake believe the same things, but are suffering from quite different pathologies. Jane is a delusional spontaneous confabulator suffering from a pathology of memory (plus an inhibitory failure which explains her uncritical adoption and persistence of the mistaken memory despite the contextual implausibility—perhaps her neighbour doesn't drive!) Jake is also delusional about the past but he has no memory pathology. And so, we might use Kopelman's term (1999, 2010 this issue), "delusional memory", to describe Jake's condition were this term not potentially confusing in the context of our advocating a distinction between received and reflective delusions (which may or may not involve memory pathology). In any event, this is not the sense of delusional memory which has been of primary interest to us in this paper, which is in Jane's sense of a received delusion about events last year.

Our story about Jake is of further interest because it highlights the effects of the passage of time. So, let's return to the idea that a confabulation might become more received with the passage of time (our example here was the alien abduction delusion). Might the same transition apply with regard to delusions that are not, strictly speaking, about the past? Consider the Capgras delusion. While we might allow that perceptual experience could deliver, on first viewing of the loved one, the delusional content, "The man in front of me is a stranger", we can hardly allow that perceptual experience could deliver, on first viewing of the loved one, the delusional content, "That man in front of me is an impostor pretending to be my husband". The impostor thought could only have come to mind after some postreflective inference making. But now let's think about what might happen the next day when the patient sees her husband again. Having encoded a memory of her first encounter with the impostor on the previous day, the patient's perceptual experience might now acquire the content "This is the impostor who was in my house yesterday". In other words, one might argue that the hybrid Capgras delusion becomes progressively more "received" with the passage of time.

SUMMARY AND CONCLUSIONS

We did not set out to develop a comprehensive model of pathological belief. Our aim was much more modest; we sought only to adopt an inclusive approach so as to explore the implications for both theories of delusion and theories of confabulation. After reviewing the difficulties with defining delusion according to a set of necessary and sufficient criteria we narrowed down our focus to consider the cardinal signs of delusion: incomprehensibility, incorrigibility, and subjective conviction.

We then turned to confabulation. Setting aside what we called post hoc confabulation—the kind of plausible rationalisation endemic in nonpathological belief formation but which can also arise in delusional contexts—we focused on spontaneous memory-based confabulation. Spontaneous confabulation involves an apparent memory which is generated spontaneously (with no intention to deceive) and which is accepted as true with a degree of subjective conviction that is unwarranted in light of general knowledge and/or the evidence to hand, either or both of which ought normally to confer doubt. We then narrowed our search still further by setting aside instances of corrigible confabulation, where the patient will retract the confabulation when encouraged to do so, so as to focus on the question of whether current models of delusion might illuminate incorrigible confabulation. Our point of departure was to contrast explanationist and endorsement accounts of the route from experience to delusional belief: in the former, the emphasis is on the explanation of a reflected upon, "thin" discordant experience, whereas, in the latter, the emphasis is on the doxastic reception of "thick" experience: the endorsement of the received experiential content as veridical. We suggested that incorrigible spontaneous confabulation might be located at (or towards) the received end of the received-reflective spectrum of delusions. On this account, the spontaneous confabulator simply endorses as genuine the content of an apparent—yet implausible—memory experience. Hence, we argued that underlying both incorrigible spontaneous confabulation and other instances of received nonmnemonic delusions is a compromised ability to inhibit the prepotent tendency to upload and maintain experience—be it perceptual or mnemonic—into belief.

If this proposal is on the right track, then patients with incorrigible spontaneous confabulations ought to show difficulties in exerting inhibitory control, bearing in mind that incorrigibility might be difficult to establish when the memory pathology is severe. Although such difficulties might not be domain general, it is likely that they would extend beyond the domain about which the patient is confabulating. Such patients may have difficulty denying the evidence of their senses when confronted with perceptual illusions or other distortions of experienced reality. They might even show a general difficulty in inhibiting beliefs in circumstances where they are required to reason about preexisting beliefs as if they were not true. Whether or not these hypotheses are borne out, we submit that the distinction between received and reflective delusions (formed and fixed via endorsement versus explanationist processes) has the potential to illuminate the interface between delusion and confabulation.

REFERENCES

American Psychiatric Association. (1994). *Diagnostic and statistical manual of mental disorders* (4th ed.). Washington, DC: Author.

Arthur, A. Z. (1964). Theories and explanations of delusions: A review. *American Journal of Psychiatry, 121*, 105–115.

Bayne, T., & Fernández, J. (2008). Delusion and self-deception: Mapping the terrain. In T. Bayne & J. Fernández (Eds.), *Delusions and self-deception: Affective influences on belief formation* (pp. 1–20). Oxford, UK: Psychology Press.

Bayne, T., & Pacherie, E. (2004a). Bottom-up or top-down?: Campbell's rationalist account of monothematic delusions. *Philosophy, Psychiatry, and Psychology, 11*, 1–11.

Bayne, T., & Pacherie, E. (2004b). Experience, belief, and the interpretive fold. *Philosophy, Psychiatry, and Psychology, 11*, 81–86.

Bayne, T., & Pacherie, E. (2005). In defence of the doxastic account of delusions. *Mind & Language, 20*, 163–188.

Berlyne, N. (1972). Confabulation. *British Journal of Psychiatry, 120*, 31–39.

Berrios, G. E. (1991). Delusions as "wrong beliefs": A conceptual history. *British Journal of Psychiatry, 159*, 6–13.

Berrios, G. E. (1998). Confabulations: A conceptual history. *Journal of the History of the Neurosciences, 7*, 225–241.

Berti, A., Làdavas, E., Stracciari, A., Giannarelli, C., & Ossola, A. (1998). Anosognosia for motor impairment and dissociations with patient's evaluation of the disorder, theoretical considerations. *Cognitive Neuropsychiatry, 3*, 21–44.

Binkofski, F., Buccino, G., Dohle, C., Seitz, R. J., & Freund, H.-J. (1999). Mirror agnosia and mirror ataxia constitute different parietal lobe disorders. *Annals of Neurology, 46*(1), 51–61.

Bisiach, E. (1988). Language without thought. In L. Weiskrantz (Ed.), *Thought without language* (pp. 464–484). New York: Clarendon Press/Oxford University Press.

Breen, N., Caine, D., & Coltheart, M. (2001). Mirrored-self misidentification: Two cases of focal onset dementia. *Neurocase, 7*, 239–254.

Carr, V. J. (2010). Beauty and belief: William James and the aesthetics of delusions in schizophrenia. *Cognitive Neuropsychiatry, 15*(1/2/3), 181–201.

Clancy, S. A. (2005). *Abducted: How people come to believe they were kidnapped by aliens.* Cambridge, MA: Harvard University Press.

Clancy, S. A., McNally, R. J., Schacter, D. L., Lenzenweger, M. F., & Pitman, R. K. (2002). Memory distortion in people reporting abduction by aliens. *Journal of Abnormal Psychology, 111*, 455–461.

Coltheart, M. (2007). The 33rd Bartlett Lecture: Cognitive neuropsychiatry and delusional belief. *Quarterly Journal of Experimental Psychology, 60*, 1041–1062.

Coltheart, M., Menzies, P., & Sutton, J. (2010). Abductive inference and delusional belief. *Cognitive Neuropsychiatry, 15*(1/2/3), 261–287.

Conway, M. A. (1996). Autobiographical knowledge and autobiographical memories. In D. C. Rubin (Ed.), *Remembering our past: Studies in autobiographical memory* (pp. 67–93). New York: Cambridge University Press.

Conway, M. A., & Pleydell-Pearce, C. W. (2000). The construction of autobiographical memories in the self-memory system. *Psychological Review, 107*, 261–288.

David, A. S. (1999). On the impossibility of defining delusions. *Philosophy, Psychiatry and Psychology, 6*, 17–20.

Davies, M., Aimola Davies, A., & Coltheart, M. (2005). Anosognosia and the two-factor theory of delusions. *Mind and Language, 20*, 209–236.

Davies, M., Coltheart, M., Langdon, R., & Breen, N. (2001). Monothematic delusions: Towards a two-factor account. *Philosophy, Psychiatry, and Psychology, 8*, 133–158.

Fine, C., Craigie, J., & Gold, I. (2005). Damned if you do; damned if you don't: The impasse in cognitive accounts of the Capgras delusion. *Philosophy, Psychiatry, and Psychology, 12*, 143–151.

Fricchione, G. L., Carbone, L., & Bennett, W. I. (1995). Psychotic disorder caused by a general medical condition, with delusions: Secondary "organic" delusional syndromes. *Psychiatric Clinics of North America, 18*, 363–378.

Gilboa, A., Alain, C., Stuss, D. T., Melo, B., Miller, S., & Moscovitch, M. (2006). Mechanisms of spontaneous confabulations: A strategic retrieval account. *Brain, 129*, 1399–1414.

Gilboa, A., & Moscovitch, M. (2002). The cognitive neuroscience of confabulation: A review and a model. In A. Baddeley, M. D. Kopelman, & B. Wilson (Eds.), *The handbook of memory disorders* (2nd ed., pp. 315–340). Chichester, UK: Wiley.

Gold, I., & Hohwy, J. (2000). Rationality and schizophrenic delusion. *Mind and Language, 15*, 146–167.

Hanba, J. M., & Zaragoza, M. S. (2007). Interviewer feedback in repeated interviews involving forced confabulation. *Applied Cognitive Psychology, 21*, 433–455.

Hirstein, W. (2005). *Brain fiction, self-deception and the riddle of confabulation*. Cambridge, MA: MIT Press.

Hohwy, J., & Rosenberg, R. (2005). Unusual experiences, reality testing and delusions of alien control. *Mind and Language, 20*, 141–162.

Jarskog, L. F., Miyamoto, S., & Lieberman, J. A. (2007). Schizophrenia: New pathological insights and therapies. *Annual Review of Medicine, 58*, 49–61.

Jaspers, K. (1963). *General psychopathology* (J. Hoening & M. Hamilton, Trans.). Manchester, UK: Manchester University Press.

Johnson, M. K. (1991). Reality monitoring: Evidence from confabulation in organic brain disease patients. In G. P. Prigatano & D. L. Schacter (Eds.), *Awareness of deficit after brain injury* (pp. 176–197). Oxford, UK: Oxford University Press.

Johnson, M. K., Hashtroudi, S., & Lindsay, D. S. (1993). Source monitoring. *Psychological Bulletin, 114*, 3–28.

Kapur, S. (2003). Psychosis as a state of aberrant salience: A framework linking biology, phenomenology, and pharmacology in schizophrenia. *American Journal of Psychiatry, 160*, 13–23.

Kopelman, M. (1987). Two types of confabulation. *Journal of Neurology, Neurosurgery, and Psychiatry, 50*, 1482–1487.

Kopelman, M. D. (1999). Varieties of false memory. *Cognitive Neuropsychology, 16*, 197–214.

Kopelman, M. D. (2010). Varieties of confabulation and delusion. *Cognitive Neuropsychiatry, 15*(1/2/3), 14–37.

Kopelman, M. D., Ng, N., & van den Brouke, O. (1997). Confabulation extending across episodic, personal, and general semantic memory. *Cognitive Neuropsychology, 14*, 683–712.

Langdon, R., & Coltheart, M. (2000). The cognitive neuropsychology of delusions. *Mind and Language, 15*, 184–218.

Langdon, R., Cooper, S., Connaughton, E., & Martin, K. (2006). A variant of misidentification delusion in a patient with right frontal and temporal brain injury. *Neuropsychiatric Disease and Treatment, 2*(Suppl. 3), 8.

Langdon, R., McKay, R., & Coltheart, M. (2008). The cognitive neuropsychological understanding of persecutory delusions. In D. Freeman, R. Bentall, & P. Garety (Eds.), *Persecutory delusions: Assessment, theory and treatment* (pp. 223–238). Oxford, UK: Oxford University Press.

Laws, K. R., Kondel, T. K., & McKenna, P. J. (1999). A receptive language deficit in schizophrenic thought disorder: Evidence for impaired semantic access and monitoring. *Cognitive Neuropsychiatry, 4*, 89–106.

Lucchellia, F., & Spinnler, H. (2008). A reappraisal of person recognition and identification. *Cortex, 44*, 230–237.

Maher, B. A. (1974). Delusional thinking and perceptual disorder. *Journal of Individual Psychology, 30*, 98–113.

Maher, B. A. (1988). Anomalous experience and delusional thinking: The logic of explanations. In T. F. Oltmanns & B. A. Maher (Eds.), *Delusional beliefs* (pp. 15–33). New York: Wiley.

Maher, B. A. (1999). Anomalous experience in everyday life: Its significance for psychopathology. *The Monist, 82*, 547–570.

McKay, R., & Kinsbourne, M. (2010). Confabulation, delusion, and anosognosia: Motivational factors and false claims. *Cognitive Neuropsychiatry, 15*(1/2/3), 288–318.

McKay, A. P., McKenna, P. J., & Baddeley, A. D. (1995). Memory pathology in schizophrenia. In R. Campbell & M. A. Conway (Eds.), *Broken memories: Case studies in memory impairment* (pp. 124–136). Cambridge, MA: Blackwell.

McLaughlin, B. (2008). Monothematic delusions and existential feelings. In T. Bayne & J. Fernandez (Eds.), *Delusions and self-deception: Affective and motivational influences on belief-formation* (pp. 139–164). Oxford, UK: Psychology Press.

Metcalf, K., Langdon, R., & Coltheart, M. (2007). Models of confabulation: A critical review and a new framework. *Cognitive Neuropsychology, 2*, 23–47.

Mitchell, K. J., & Johnson, M. K. (2000). Source monitoring: Attributing mental experiences. In E. Tulving & F. I. M. Craik (Eds.), *The Oxford handbook of memory* (pp. 179–195). New York: Oxford University Press.

Moulin, C. J. A., Conway, M. A., Thompson, R. G., James, N., & Jones, R. W. (2005). Disordered memory awareness: Recollective confabulation in two cases of persistent déjà vecu. *Neuropsychologia, 43*, 1362–1378.

Nasrallah, H. A. (1992). The neuropsychiatry of schizophrenia. In S. C. Yudofsky & R. E. Hales (Eds.), *American Psychiatric Press textbook of neuropsychiatry* (2nd ed., pp. 621–638). Washington, DC: American Psychiatric Association.

Nathaniel-James, D. A., Foong, J., & Frith, C. D. (1996). The mechanisms of confabulation in schizophrenia. *Neurocase, 2*, 475–483.

Nathaniel-James, D. A., & Frith, C. D. (1996). Confabulation in schizophrenia: Evidence of a new form. *Psychological Medicine, 26*, 391–399.

Nisbett, R. E., & Wilson, T. D. (1977). Telling more than we can know: Verbal reports on mental processes. *Psychological Review, 84*, 231–259.

O'Connor, Lever, C., & Moulin, C. J. A. (2010). Novel insights into false recollection: A model of déjà vécu. *Cognitive Neuropsychiatry, 15*(1/2/3), 118–144.

Oltmanns, T. F. (1988). Approaches to the definition and study of delusions. In T. F. Oltmanns & B. F. Maher (Eds.), *Delusional beliefs* (pp. 3–11). New York: Wiley.

Pacherie, E. (2008). Perception, emotion and delusions: The case of the Capgras delusion. In T. Bayne & J. Fernandez (Eds.), *Delusions and self-deception: Affective and motivational influences on belief-formation* (pp. 105–123). Oxford, UK: Psychology Press.

Ratcliffe, M. (2004). Interpreting delusions. *Phenomenology and the Cognitive Sciences, 3*, 25–48.

Schnider, A., von Daniken, C., & Gutbrod, K. (1996). The mechanisms of spontaneous and provoked confabulations. *Brain, 119*, 1365–1375.

Smith, A. C. (1968). Notes on difficulties in the definition of delusion. *British Journal of Medical Psychology, 41*, 255–259.

Spitzer, M. (1990). On defining delusions. *Comprehensive Psychiatry, 31*, 377–397.

Stone, T., & Young, A. (1997). Delusions and brain injury: The philosophy and psychology of belief. *Mind and Language, 12*, 327–364.

Tulving, E. (1985). How many memory systems are there? *The American Psychologist, 40*, 385–398.

Tulving, E. (2002). Episodic memory: From mind to brain. *Annual Review of Psychology, 53*, 1–25.

Turner, M., & Coltheart, M. (2010). Confabulation and delusion: A common monitoring framework? *Cognitive Neuropsychiatry, 15*(1/2/3), 346–376.

Venneri, A., & Shanks, M. F. (2004). Belief and awareness: Reflections on a case of persistent anosognosia. *Neuropsychologia, 42*, 230–238.

COGNITIVE NEUROPSYCHIATRY
2010, 15 (1/2/3), 346–376

Confabulation and delusion: A common monitoring framework

Martha Turner[1,2] and Max Coltheart[2]

[1]*Institute of Cognitive Neuroscience, University College London, London, UK,*
[2]*Macquarie Centre for Cognitive Science, Macquarie University, Sydney, Australia*

Confabulations and delusions both involve the production of false claims. Although they may have different types of content, they share several characteristics. For example, they are often held with considerable conviction and are resistant to counter evidence, they may be acted upon, and they may be accompanied by a lack of concern about the false claim or its implications. Confabulations and delusions may initially arise from failures in different systems (e.g., mnemonic vs. perceptual or affective). However, their shared characteristics raise the possibility that the monitoring deficits involved might be the same, resulting in failure to reject the confabulatory or delusional ideas. In this paper we will focus on the nature of these common monitoring deficits. Critically, we argue that monitoring in confabulation and delusion involves both unconscious and conscious processes. We propose that an unconscious process is responsible for tagging suspect content which needs to be checked for veracity by a separate set of conscious evaluative processes. Failure of these monitoring processes would allow ideas which ought to be checked and rejected to instead be uncritically accepted: This would result in the production of confabulations or delusions. Importantly, inclusion of both unconscious and conscious monitoring stages allows the model to account for both "endorsement" and "explanation" delusions, and both "primary" and "secondary" confabulations. Our hope is that this model may provide a theoretical framework to guide empirical investigation of the commonalities and differences between the conditions.

Keywords: Confabulation; Delusion; Monitoring.

Correspondence should be addressed to Dr Martha Turner, Institute of Cognitive Neuroscience, 17 Queen Square, London WC1N 3AR, UK. E-mail: martha.turner@ucl.ac.uk

We thank Paul Burgess, Asaf Gilboa, and William Hirstein for very helpful comments on an earlier version of this manuscript. Martha Turner is supported by an ESRC/MRC Postdoctoral Fellowship PTA037270085.

DOI: 10.1080/13546800903441902

INTRODUCTION

Historically, confabulation and delusion have nearly always been treated separately in the literature (Fotopoulou, 2010 this issue). The term "confabulation" has most often been used to refer to the production of false memories by patients suffering from amnesia, whereas the term "delusion" has been reserved for the false beliefs encountered in psychiatric conditions such as schizophrenia, and sometimes after neurological damage. However, in recent years, there has been an interest in highlighting the potential similarities between confabulatory and delusional syndromes (Hirstein, 2005).

The claims made by patients suffering from these conditions can vary greatly. A confabulating patient may claim that he is a hospital porter, when in fact he is an inpatient being treated for a brain injury. A patient with Capgras delusion may claim that his wife has been replaced by an identical looking imposter. A patient with delusions of control may claim that her actions are being controlled by an outside force. However, despite differences in content, confabulations and delusions share several characteristics. Given this, there seems reason to consider the possibility that similar mechanisms may be involved in their production and/or maintenance.

In this paper we first explore some similarities between confabulation and delusion that might inform understanding of the nature of any common mechanisms. We next explore the possibility that both confabulation and delusion might be accommodated within a "two-factor" explanatory model. In the two-factor model of delusion formation, a first factor determines the content of the delusion, and a second factor accounts for its adoption and maintenance, rather than rejection (Davies, Coltheart, Langdon, & Breen, 2001). In this paper we focus on the second factor of this model and propose that failures of both conscious and unconscious evaluation processes might be involved. We propose that although the first factor will differ between confabulation and delusion, a common set of second factor impairments may be involved in both disorders.

SIMILARITIES BETWEEN CONFABULATION AND DELUSION

The term "delusion" is usually used to describe false beliefs that are: (a) consistent over time, (b) held with conviction, and (c) implausible or bizarre. It is often argued that confabulations do not meet these criteria, and thus should be treated separately. However, detailed examination reveals many similarities (see also Langdon & Bayne, 2010 this issue).

Consistency

It is argued that delusional beliefs are typically consistent over time. Once a Capgras patient adopts the belief that, for example, his wife has been replaced by an imposter, his belief tends to persist, often causing considerable distress and disruption. Confabulations, on the other hand, can be fleeting and never repeated. Consider for example, confabulating patient GN, studied by one of us (MT). Following a ruptured anterior communicating artery aneurysm he claimed at various times that he was in hospital because he had been attacked by enemy aircraft when boarding a submarine, had problems relaxing since being shelled, had problems with his legs, and had been bitten by a rabbit. None of these claims were ever presented more than once. However, there are also several examples of confabulations that are stable over time. For example, Burgess and McNeil (1999) describe a patient who awoke every morning and dressed for work in the belief that he had to conduct a stock-take at a local shop. Downes and Mayes (1995) report patient WF, whose confabulation that he had had an argument with his father the day before (despite acknowledging that his father had died and that he had attended the funeral) was repeated on a daily basis, gaining "delusional strength" as time progressed. It is important to take into account here that confabulation is often associated with severe memory impairment, making it much less likely that the same false memory will be consistently produced. However, over the course of recovery, as memory functions gradually improve, confabulations may become more entrenched, and more "delusion-like" in terms of consistency.

Not only can confabulations be consistent over time, but delusions can be inconsistent over time. There are reports that delusions may come and go (Ellis, Luaute, & Retterstol, 1994; Mackie, Ebmeier, & O'Carroll, 1994), or even that they may change in content. For example, Wright, Young, and Hellawell (1993) describe a patient JH who experienced the Cotard delusion (the belief that he was dead) and the Capgras delusion in sequence. Consistency of belief, rather than being a distinguishing criterion, seems to be a continuum along which both confabulations and delusions can vary.

Conviction

Delusions are traditionally associated with strong conviction in the truth of the delusional belief (including acting upon the belief) and resistance to counterargument. In contrast, it is often argued that there may be considerable variability in conviction in confabulation: Indeed sometimes a confabulating patient will willingly abandon one false claim in favour of another, equally untrue, claim. But this is not always the case. Sometimes confabulating patients will vehemently defend their position, often acting upon their confabulations, or providing further supporting confabulations to back up their original false assertion. In these cases confabulation can strongly resemble delusional belief. Once again, amnesia may be a contributing factor. If confabulations are fleeting and then forgotten, it would be difficult to demonstrate conviction in the false claim. However, momentary confabulations may still be fiercely defended and associated with "momentary conviction" before being forgotten.

Delusions too may vary along this dimension: Levels of conviction in delusion are not always absolute, and may fluctuate over time (Garety & Hemsley, 1994). There may be moments of clarity when a patient acknowledges some doubt about the delusional belief, only to relapse into conviction moments later, just as also occurs in many confabulations. Furthermore, even in the face of apparent conviction, both confabulation and delusion may be paradoxically associated with a lack of emotional concern or lack of action. Why, for example, do some Capgras patients continue to live with people they believe to be imposters rather than reporting the disappearance of their spouse to the police? And why do some confabulating patients report strange and disturbing events but then return to what they were doing unperturbed?

Content

Definitions of delusion often include the criterion that the content is implausible, bizarre, or patently untrue (following Jaspers, 1963), but, in fact, the content of both delusions and confabulations can vary from the mundane to the bizarre. For example the belief that you can move your own arm, in itself, is not a bizarre claim (on the contrary this is the norm) yet anosognosia for hemiplegia (the belief of a patient with a paralysed arm that he can move this arm) is a delusion. Similarly, claiming that you need to attend a stock-take at a local shop is not in itself bizarre (especially when this had been your job for many years). In these cases it is the current situation which renders the claims unusual (paralysis or retirement due to illness). At the other end of the spectrum, however, are delusional beliefs that your wife has been replaced by an identical-looking imposter (Capgras delusion), or that alien beings are controlling your actions. Bizarre claims also occur in confabulation. For example, Damasio, Graff-Radford, Eslinger, Damasio, and Kassell (1985) report a patient who believed that he was a "space pirate" at the time of the Columbia space mission. Similarly GN claimed that he had met a woman with the head of a bee at a party he had attended the previous night. These types of claims, in both delusion and confabulation, are bizarre in themselves, involving distortion of semantic knowledge of the world.

Primary and secondary claims[1]

One further intriguing similarity between confabulation and delusion is that patients very often offer rationales for their initial claims when directly challenged. In some instances these secondary claims may be relatively simple rationalisations. For example, Mattioli, Miozzo, and Vignolo (1999) describe a confabulating patient who claimed that he had been for a swim in the lake the previous afternoon (a primary confabulation). When it was pointed out that it was January, he responded "but this is an especially mild January" (a secondary supporting claim). Similar examples can be found in delusional patients. For example, Frazer and Roberts (1994) describe a Capgras patient who claimed that she could tell the difference between her real son and the imposter because the imposter "had different coloured eyes, was not as big and brawny, and that her real son would not kiss her" (p. 557).

In other cases the secondary claim may take the form of a more elaborated false memory, and therefore comprise a confabulation in itself. In the confabulation literature this phenomena is referred to as "secondary confabulation" (Gilboa & Moscovitch, 2002). For example, Moscovitch (1995) described HW, whose primary confabulation was that he had been married for 4 months despite having four adult children. When asked how he had managed to produce four children in 4 months, he produced the secondary confabulation that they had been adopted. Examples of this type of secondary confabulation are also found in delusional patients. For example, a Capgras patient studied by one of us (MC) accounted for the presence of two imposters in his home (identical in appearance to his wife), by producing the elaborated secondary confabulation that he had rescued two girls being chased by a gang and had asked them in. He said that he was now unable to ask them to leave because every time he tried they burst into tears (of course this was in reality his wife's reaction to being asked to leave her own house).

The production of secondary claims is another fascinating similarity between confabulation and delusion (and is explored further in Coltheart & Turner, 2009; see also the discussion of Langdon & Bayne, 2010 this issue, on post hoc rationalising confabulations). However, we note here that secondary claims and confabulations differ in some important respects from the primary confabulations and delusions that are the main focus of this paper. This is because secondary claims serve the purpose of defending an initial claim and therefore appear to have different motivational characteristics (e.g., to convince either the listener or oneself that the

[1] Note that the distinction we are making here is not the same as the distinction between primary and secondary *delusions* (Jaspers, 1963).

memory or belief is justified). As such, these secondary claims may be associated with less conviction and more conscious reasoning processes than the primary claims. Therefore there is reason to propose that they may arise in different ways to the primary claims, and we explore this possibility further in the final section.

Summary

Kopelman (2010 this issue) emphasises that confabulation and delusion arise in different domains. Delusions arise most commonly in psychosis in patients who are often otherwise cognitively intact, whereas confabulation is overwhelmingly associated with neural damage, amnesia, and executive dysfunction. However, confabulations and delusions also share many characteristics: (1) they both involve the production of unsubstantiated claims; (2) these claims are produced without the intent to deceive the listener; (3) these claims are inadequately evaluated, leading to their adoption and maintenance rather than their rejection; (4) they may both vary along the continua of consistency, conviction, and bizarreness of content; (5) they are both associated with the production of secondary supporting claims; and (6) they may both coexist in the same patient. These similarities indicate that they may share at least some aetiological or maintaining factors. In the remainder of this paper, we explore the possibility that both confabulation and delusion are associated with impairments in a common set of processes involved in the monitoring and evaluation of thoughts, ideas, memories, and beliefs. We outline a model of these monitoring processes, and suggest that different types of delusion and confabulation, and the accompanying variations in consistency, conviction, and content, may result from different combinations of biases and impairments in this system.

THE TWO-FACTOR THEORY OF DELUSION

Maher (e.g., 1999) proposed an influential theory of delusion in which false beliefs arise as normal responses to unusual experiences. His is a single factor account, in that the unusual perceptual experience is sufficient in itself to produce a delusion. However, as noted by Langdon and Coltheart (2000) and Davies et al. (2001), this account predicts that everyone who has the same unusual experience should form a delusional belief about it. This is not the case. For example, Cahill, Silbersweig, and Frith (1996) created an unusual perceptual experience by distorting the sound of a speaker's voice. This manipulation induced delusional attributions in schizophrenic patients who experienced delusions ("It's an evil spirit speaking when I speak"), but not in healthy controls or in schizophrenic patients who were delusion-free ("You are distorting my voice with that box"). For this reason, two-factor theorists propose that two factors are involved in delusion formation. The first factor is a neuropsychological or other anomaly that determines the content of the delusion. However, a second factor is also necessary to explain why this delusional content is adopted and maintained as belief rather than rejected.

This type of account fits well with theories of confabulation, which commonly include both production and monitoring components (e.g., Burgess & Shallice, 1996; Gilboa & Moscovitch, 2002; Kopelman, 1999; Moscovitch & Melo, 1997). Metcalf, Langdon, and Coltheart (2007) have explicitly applied the two-factor model of delusion formation to confabulation. They suggested that the first factor in spontaneous confabulation (see Kopelman, 2010 this issue, for discussion of the distinction between spontaneous and provoked confabulations) is a retrieval impairment resulting in disrupted search and selection of memories from the autobiographical store. When combined with a second factor, which prevents accurate evaluation of the retrieved memories, confabulations are produced.

If this second factor, involving impaired evaluation, is indeed common to both confabulation and delusion, what form might it take? First factor impairments have been extensively documented (Davies, Aimola-Davies, & Coltheart, 2005; Davies et al., 2001), but the processes involved in the second factor have received less attention. Ellis (1994), Garety and Hemsley (1994), and Stone and Young (1997) have proposed variations of the two-factor theory in which the second factor is explained by an attribution or reasoning bias. However, attribution and reasoning biases alone seem unable to fully account for the characteristics of confabulation and delusion (Davies et al., 2001; Langdon & Coltheart, 2000). Reasoning processes are usually thought of as conscious, and yet conscious reasoning seems not to be involved at all in many delusions and confabulations. More often, delusional and confabulatory ideas seem to enter consciousness fully formed with the patients unaware of any prior unusual experience. Certainly the rest of us who are not delusional or confabulatory are not aware of consciously considering and then rejecting the kinds of bizarre thoughts that delusional and confabulating patients espouse. There seems good reason therefore to propose that unconscious as well as conscious processes are normally involved in the production and evaluation of thoughts, ideas, memories, and beliefs, and this distinction may be helpful in specifying the nature of the second factor.

UNCONSCIOUS AND CONSCIOUS PROCESSES IN MONITORING AND EVALUATION

Perhaps insights from confabulation theory might be helpful in specifying the second factor more clearly. Retrieval theories of confabulation tend not to characterise the evaluation or monitoring impairment as a single process, but instead as a set of processes. Gilboa and colleagues (Gilboa, 2010 this issue; Gilboa et al., 2006; Gilboa & Moscovitch, 2002), in particular, have proposed a model of strategic retrieval that explicitly proposes the existence of two postretrieval monitoring stages: one rapid and preconscious, which leads to a "feeling of rightness" (FOR), and the other conscious and elaborate, involving checking for inconsistencies, conflicting evidence, and compatibility with task requirements. Gilboa (2010 this issue) discusses this system only in the context of the memory domain. However, it seems plausible, and evolutionarily viable, that evaluation and monitoring systems might be domain-general rather than domain-specific.

In support of this proposal is the fact that confabulation, despite being a memory disorder occurring in the context of amnesia, is not restricted to distortions or errors specifically in *memory*. Confabulations can indeed involve confusions of memory, where traces of memories for real events become inappropriately conflated. For example, patient GN believed that he was in hospital in Toronto (where he had lived for many years), and his confabulations were frequently about real events, but confused in time or place. However, his other confabulations were not so obviously tied to memory; recall that GN also confabulated that he had met a woman who had a bee's head. This confabulation did not involve distortion of a true memory; instead it appeared to involve imagination. Similarly many confabulations are not accounts of things *past*, but are false claims about general concepts (e.g., GN also insisted that life insurance companies based their premiums on how many pairs of socks their customers had purchased recently, as people who were about to die would not buy new socks). Other confabulations may take the form of false claims about future events (what the patient will be doing tomorrow, or in a year's time). These examples demonstrate how difficult it is to cleanly distinguish memory retrieval from the production of other thoughts. Sometimes confabulations are not memories, but ideas or imaginings. Similarly delusions are sometimes new ideas, but may also be based on memories. We therefore propose that thoughts, ideas, memories, and beliefs (referred to in the remainder of this paper as "thoughts" for brevity), although they may all be produced in different ways, are likely to pass through the same set of monitoring processes. A model of this monitoring system may therefore be able to explain the failure to reject unsubstantiated thoughts in both confabulation and delusion.

A NEW MODEL OF CONFABULATION AND DELUSION

Figure 1 illustrates a model of the production and evaluation of thoughts applicable to both confabulation and delusion. We propose that delusional and confabulatory content may be provoked initially by an impairment in perceptual, affective, or mnemonic processing (the "first factor"). This impairment results in the production of an unusual or unsubstantiated

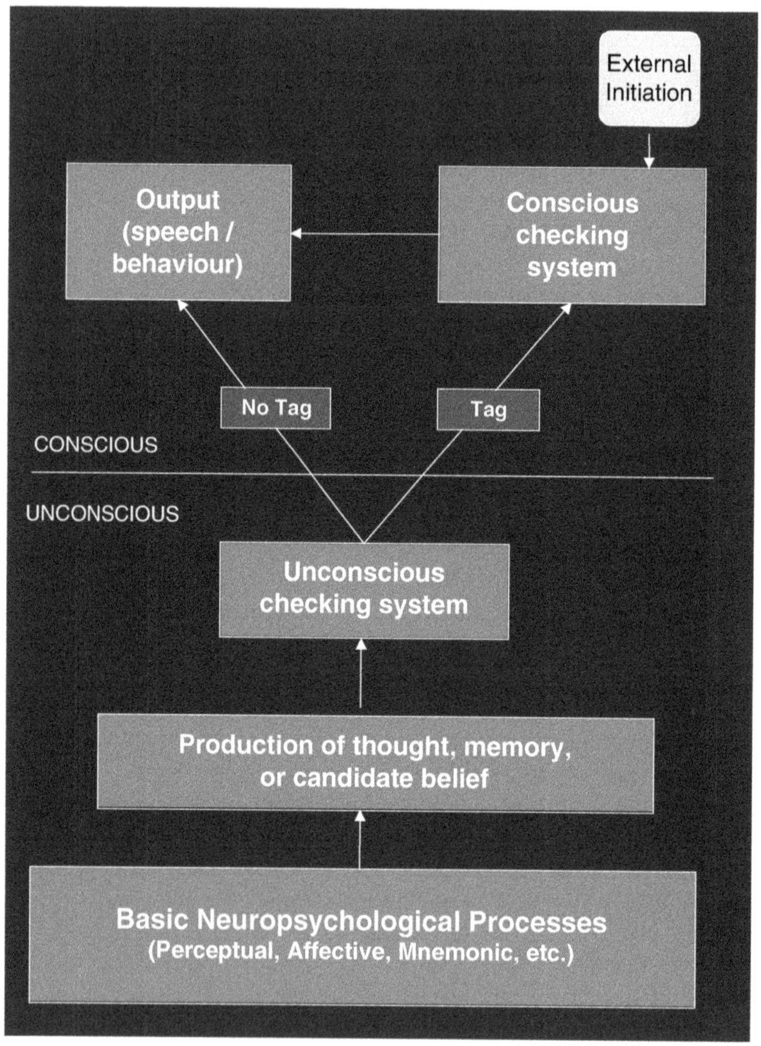

Figure 1. A model of the production and evaluation of thoughts, memories, and beliefs. [To view this figure in colour, please see the online issue of the Journal.]

thought, memory, idea, or candidate belief. Next we come to the evaluation stage (the "second factor"). Why are patients unable to use reasoning, or their knowledge of the world and "common sense" to reject their confabulatory or delusional thought? We think that the conviction and lack of doubt that confabulating and delusional patients often experience offers an important clue here. Maybe the checking system is not faulty; maybe it is never initiated, or at least part of it is never initiated.

Our point here is that patients often seem not to consciously check their thoughts in much the same way as most of us do not check our memory of what we did last night. It is simply experienced as incontrovertibly true. We only check when we have some doubt. Indeed it is economical only to check and evaluate thoughts about which there is some doubt, as reasoning and reality testing processes are time consuming and effortful. But where does this doubt come from? Like Gilboa and colleagues we think that there are two components to the evaluation process—one unconscious and one conscious. Specifically, we propose that there is an unconscious checking system which, in the nondelusional population, "tags" thoughts that require extra conscious checking. This "tagging" is accompanied by the normal experience of doubt. However, in delusional and confabulating patients this unconscious checking system fails, resulting in an absence of doubt, which we argue confers an inappropriate feeling of conviction. In the absence of doubt the patients then feel no necessity to consciously check their thoughts. However, we propose that conscious evaluative and reasoning processes, even if they are not initiated internally (by the unconscious checking system), may also be initiated externally (e.g., when a claim is challenged by a third party). In many patients these conscious reasoning processes will also be biased or impaired. In the remainder of the paper we speculate on some of the candidate processes that may be involved at each stage of this model, and show how the model might explain the production and maintenance of different types of confabulation and delusion.

The first factor: Determining the content of delusions and confabulations

According to the two-factor theory it should be possible to identify a first factor that is responsible for the specific content of the delusion. In many bizarre delusions this takes the form of a neuropsychological impairment. In Capgras delusion, for example, there is argued to be a disconnection between the face recognition system and the limbic system that results in a reduced affective response to familiar faces (Ellis & Lewis, 2001). A Capgras patient recognises the face of his wife, but does not have the usual emotional response that would accompany this recognition. This affective anomaly then determines the content of the Capgras delusion: that the wife has been replaced by an imposter. First factor neuropsychological impairments have also been proposed for several other monothematic delusions (Davies et al., 2001, 2005; Turner, Shores, Breen, & Coltheart, 2009) and for some of the delusions typical of schizophrenia, including alien control, thought insertion, thought broadcasting, and delusions of reference (Davies & Coltheart, 2000; Davies et al., 2001; Langdon & Coltheart, 2000), although the account also allows for nonneuropsychological first factors (e.g., Davies, 2009; Langdon & Coltheart, 2000; McKay, Langdon, & Coltheart, 2009).

More recently the two-factor approach has been extended to include mnemonic first factor impairments, in order to accommodate confabulation. Metcalf et al. (2007) suggest that the first factor in confabulation is a retrieval deficit resulting in impaired search and selection of memories from the autobiographical episodic memory store. However, the nature of the impairment is relatively unspecified beyond this. A first factor impairment should be able to explain the content of the delusion or confabulation. Thus, the first factor in confabulation cannot simply be amnesia, as this would indicate only the absence of accurate memories, rather than the presence of false memories. Instead, we suggest the following, more specific, possibility for the first factor impairment in confabulation. In confabulation we suggest that there is damage to, or loss of the ability to use, contextual and source information associated with memories, imaginings, and ideas. This information would include temporal and spatial context that is used to bind fragments of a memory trace into a coherent event memory, and source information used to distinguish real memories from imaginings. This explanation then allows us to predict the nature of the accounts that are produced by confabulating patients: They should be traceable either to inaccurately conflated elements of true memories, or to inaccurately conflated elements of imaginings, ideas, and memories. Mundane confabulations would result from contextual impairments involving temporal and spatial information about real memories (when fragments of true memories from different episodes would be incorrectly conflated, or memories from previous time periods would be experienced as "current", e.g., Schnider, 2008), whereas bizarre confabulations would result from disorganised retrieval in which elements of imagination and memory were incorrectly conflated.

The two-factor account argues that the content of most confabulatory or delusional thoughts is largely determined by specific impairments in perceptual, affective, or mnemonic processing of the type summarised here (as well as being influenced by a range of personal, affective, attributional, and motivational factors; see Fotopoulou, 2010 this issue; Langdon & Coltheart, 2000; McKay & Kinsbourne, 2010 this issue; Metcalf, Langdon, & Coltheart, 2010 this issue). Confabulation is a specific disorder that arises in the context of memory impairment, and its content will be determined by failures in strategic retrieval processes. On the other hand, delusions result from a range of specific affective, perceptual, or other anomalies that similarly determine their content. Therefore, delusions and confabulations are initially produced via different mechanisms. However, despite being triggered by different first factor impairments, we propose that confabulations and delusions share failures in a common set of evaluation and monitoring processes (the second factor), which allow these thoughts to be accepted and maintained rather than being rejected, and it is this argument we develop in the remainder of the paper.

The second factor: Failure to reject the unsubstantiated thought

Although we have argued that the variation in content across confabulations and delusions may be explicable in terms of the nature of a first factor impairment, this sort of impairment is not sufficient to explain why delusions or confabulations are accepted and maintained. Why does the patient not immediately reject the thought as illogical, and why are delusions and confabulations so resistant to counterevidence? Most accounts of evaluation and monitoring processes have characterised them as conscious and effortful. However, several authors have raised the possibility that unconscious processes might also be involved (e.g., Bell, Halligan, & Ellis, 2006; Coltheart, 2005; Gilboa & Moscovitch, 2002; Schnider, 2001). We agree that there are strong reasons to think that the evaluation process involves an unconscious stage. First, it seems unlikely that every thought that we produce is consciously evaluated and checked for consistency. This would be too demanding on resources, and everyday experience tells us that we only devote effort to consciously checking thoughts we feel some doubt about. When you are telling someone how many children you have, you do not consciously check the answer that springs to mind for consistency with the available evidence, logic, and plausibility. Rather, the information is experienced as true, is associated with conviction, and is resistant to challenge. We propose that confabulations and delusions are experienced in the same way, and that this is because they pass a preconscious "check" that fails to associate them with doubt.

The unconscious checking system

We propose that the role of this unconscious checking system is to "tag" thoughts that require extra conscious checking. The presence of a tag gives rise to the experience of doubt, and these thoughts are referred to the conscious evaluation system for further work. However, the lack of a tag enables thoughts to bypass the conscious evaluation system, and to directly affect speech or other behaviour. We suggest that, in many cases, delusional and confabulatory thoughts are not tagged with doubt as they should be by this unconscious system, and that this abnormal absence of doubt explains why confabulations and delusions are accompanied by such unwarranted conviction.

We note that an alternative function for an unconscious system of this type is inhibition, or suppression of thoughts (e.g., Schnider, 2001, 2008). In this scenario, inhibited or suppressed thoughts would be produced but never reach consciousness. However, we think it unlikely that this is a routine function. Our reasoning is as follows: The problem we have to address is to explain why we are not all consciously aware on a day-to-day basis of considering and rejecting bizarre thoughts of the type that are produced by confabulating and delusional patients. There are two possible solutions to this: The first is that in normal individuals they are suppressed preconsciously, so that they never reach awareness. The second is that they are not produced by normal individuals in the first place. In the case of delusions and confabulations we find the second scenario more plausible. Therefore, we suggest that thoughts of the type involved in delusions and confabulation are only produced when they are warranted or provoked in some way. In the case of the patients discussed here, they result from a range of first factor impairments. Therefore, we do not include a suppression mechanism in our unconscious monitoring system, but instead argue that all of these thoughts reach consciousness in some form, either tagged with doubt or untagged, and that the abnormality in delusional and confabulating patients is that these thoughts are produced at all. They may be *consciously* rejected at a later stage. But this is a rather different concept to most accounts of preconscious inhibition or suppression.

We now turn to consider on what basis the unconscious checking system might operate, and speculate on candidate processes that might result in a thought being tagged as doubtful and referred to conscious monitoring processes for further work.

Novelty. First, it may be that any *new* thought or combination of thoughts that has not previously arisen would be tagged with doubt. Memories that have been previously retrieved, thoughts that have previously been produced, and beliefs that have previously been espoused might be passed by this system as already having been evaluated, whereas new thoughts would be tagged for checking. In this case the tagging system might work on a simple familiarity basis, just tagging any novel thoughts or novel combinations of thoughts for checking. If this process failed, novel and potentially bizarre thoughts would be "passed" as if they were commonly produced, everyday claims. This account would also predict that thoughts (even if they were bizarre) that had been produced and passed through the system many times would become less likely to be tagged by virtue of repetition and reconsolidation.

Conflict. An alternative possibility is that the "doubt" tag results from conflict or discrepancy associated with a thought that is detected unconsciously. The system may detect elements within a thought that do not fit together (e.g., elements of memories that mark them as derived from different episodes). Alternatively the system may detect elements that do not fit with previous knowledge or a preexisting "belief system" (e.g., it may detect conflicts with long established information from the semantic store). Or the system may detect a mismatch between a thought and information that is being received from other senses (e.g., the thought that you are moving your arm and the visual input that it is not moving).

Insufficiency. Another, related, possibility is that the unconscious checking system may tag insufficiency rather than conflict. In this scenario, thoughts that are not backed up with sufficient supporting evidence might be tagged for further checking. This would mean that any thought arising purely from imagination, without supporting contextual information to identify it as externally generated, would be tagged for checking. This would be equivalent to an early unconscious reality monitoring check (Johnson & Raye, 2000). An "insufficient" tag would pick up not only pure imaginings, but also fragments of information derived from external experience, but lacking sufficient supporting elements. The latter would include fragments of genuine memory traces, fragments of perceptual experiences, and partial or degraded ideas and beliefs. In the absence of a tag, fragments of ideas, or ideas purely derived from imagination, would acquire the same status as fully formed beliefs based on a range of evidence.

Lack of input. Related to the idea of insufficiency is the possibility that the unconscious checking system might tag *lack* of relevant input, or information that is expected but missing. This type of tag would alert consciousness to a lack of information from a relevant system. For example, any thought that was presented to the tagging system with missing or degraded expected input from either the affective system (e.g., in Capgras patients), or the mnemonic system (e.g., in amnesia), or the proprioceptive system (e.g., in paralysis) would be identified as dubious and referred for conscious checking. The conscious checking system would then be required to actively initiate a search for this missing information. This type of check might play a particular role in cases where delusion and confabulation is associated with lack of awareness of deficit, as the lack of information coming from a particular system never becomes conscious. In this case it would be easy to be unaware that you have memory difficulties, that your affective responses to people are distorted, or that you are paralysed or even blind (Anton's syndrome).

Bayesian approaches to unconscious checking. Recent work on Bayesian models of human cognition may be important for the concept of an unconscious checking system. In these models brain systems are arranged hierarchically such that prediction errors emitted by lower level systems become the input for higher level systems. At the same time, feedback from higher level systems provides "prior beliefs" by which the lower level systems may operate (e.g., Friston, Kilner, & Harrison, 2006; Kveraga, Ghuman, & Bar, 2007). The unconscious checking system we have described would be conceptually similar to the lower level system in a hierarchical Bayesian model, which should generate prediction errors when the content of a thought is doubtful. In confabulating and delusional patients, prediction errors that *should* be generated may be missing.

Note the distinction between this account and that of Corlett, Fletcher, and colleagues (e.g., Corlett, Krystal, Taylor, & Fletcher, 2009; Corlett et al., 2007; Fletcher & Frith, 2009), who argue that delusions and hallucinations in schizophrenia may result from the *presence* of *incorrect* prediction errors, which patients then have to explain. Theirs is a single factor account, in that the presence of false prediction errors generates the unusual experience on which the delusion is based. By contrast our current discussion concerns a second factor which might be common to more than one type of delusion and confabulation. In our approach, the lack of a prediction error, when a prediction error should be present, might characterise failure of a rapid, unconscious monitoring system to identify a thought as requiring further conscious checking. Furthermore, Corlett et al.'s account relates to delusions that result from a conscious reasoning process (sometimes known as "explanation" delusions), which are rather different from the type of conditions we have been discussing so far. We return to the distinction between explanation delusions and other types of delusion and confabulation in the final section.

Summary. We have argued in this section that the failure of an unconscious checking system to "tag" a candidate thought would result in it being passed into consciousness with a lack of doubt. This absence of doubt would endow the thought with a subjective feeling of conviction, meaning that conscious evaluation or checking processes would not be initiated. This subjective feeling of conviction can be dramatic. A nice example is provided by Young and Leafhead (1996) in their description of patient JK, who was suffering from Cotard delusion—the belief that she was dead. Upon questioning she admitted that she could feel her heart beat, that she could sense hot and cold, and that she could feel when her bladder was full. When it was pointed out to her that surely these sensations were evidence that she was alive, she responded that since she had these feelings even though she was dead, they clearly were not evidence of being alive. Even when logical inconsistencies are acknowledged by the patient, this may not be enough to shake the sense of conviction associated with the thought. Young (1998) reports that "if you ask [the Capgras patient] 'what would you think if I told you my wife had been replaced by an imposter' you will often get answers to the effect that it would be unbelievable, absurd, an indication that you had gone mad. Yet these patients will claim that nonetheless, this is exactly what has happened to their own relative" (p. 37). We propose that this conviction might be the result of failure of an unconscious checking system.

It remains to be seen which of the candidate processes raised here (novelty, conflict, insufficiency, and lack of input) or indeed other processes we have not discussed, might be involved in unconscious checking of thoughts. It may be that some of these tagging processes are domain specific, i.e., relate only to the mnemonic, affective, or some other domain. Indeed, as the conscious reasoning, evaluation, and problem-solving operations involved in the conscious checking system are assumed to be domain-general, this might go some way to explaining monothematicity in some delusions and confabulations.

Unconscious processing is of course difficult to investigate, but there are methodologies available that might be used to shed light on the nature of the processes involved at this stage. For example, the relationship between the unconscious checking system and somatic markers seems a promising area for investigation. Patients with ventromedial frontal lobe damage often exhibit impulsive behaviour, and lack the skin conductance response (SCR) that is found in normal controls shortly before making disadvantageous choices on gambling tasks. This is assumed to reflect reduced or absent somatic markers: affective responses that are used to govern and inhibit behaviour (Damasio, 1996). The ventromedial frontal lobe is also considered to be a critical lesion site for confabulation (Gilboa & Moscovitch, 2002; Turner, Cipolotti, Yousry, & Shallice, 2008b). Somatic markers may therefore be implicated in the operation of an unconscious tagging system that associates thoughts with doubt, and skin conductance responses may be used to investigate this type of process (see also Gilboa, 2010 this issue, for discussion of the relationship between FOR and somatic markers). Other methodologies may also offer means of investigating unconscious processing. For example, there is some ERP evidence that an early electrophysiological signature associated with controlling false alarms in memory output in controls may be missing in patients with ventromedial prefrontal cortex (VMPFC) lesions (Gilboa, Alain, He, Stuss, & Moscovitch, 2009; see also

Schnider, Valenza, Morand, & Michel, 2002, for ERP evidence of preconscious suppression in controls). It is possible that this early processing stage, which is missing in patients, might be associated with preconscious tagging of the type we have proposed to be missing in confabulating and delusional patients.

We have spent some time discussing the result of failures in the unconscious checking system. But what would happen if this system was working? According to the model outlined here, a first factor impairment in combination with a functioning unconscious checking system would lead to some sense of doubt or unease about the thought. The result of this feeling of doubt, we propose, would be to search for a rational explanation using conscious evaluation of the thought and reasoning processes. It is this conscious evaluation and reasoning stage we describe next.

The conscious checking system

The conscious checking system is needed to explain why delusional and confabulatory patients are unable to use logic, reasoning and contradictory evidence to reject the false thought. Although patients with a malfunctioning unconscious checking system may not spontaneously initiate conscious checking, it should still be possible to initiate conscious checking from an outside source, for example when a relative confronts the patient about their confabulation or delusion and tries to provide them with counterevidence. In less severe patients, a functioning or partly functioning tagging system may initiate the conscious monitoring system directly, when the sense of doubt associated with a thought would prompt a search for supporting information or an alternative explanation. In either case, a functioning conscious checking system should allow the implausible thought to be rejected, whereas an impaired conscious checking system might result not only in perpetuation of the original thought, but also sometimes in its elaboration.

Several conscious reasoning, monitoring, checking, and evaluation processes have been discussed in the confabulation and delusion literature. These are all normal processes that we use every day, but which may be impaired in patients with delusions or confabulations. We propose that all of these processes are likely to be involved in the conscious checking system, and we discuss them next. In addition, several factors may influence the operation of these conscious checking processes, and these are discussed separately.

Reasoning. The most frequently discussed component of any conscious checking or evaluation system is the ability to reason, and reasoning biases in delusions have been extensively reviewed by Garety and Freeman (1999) and Langdon and Coltheart (2000). In brief, the evidence suggests that patients with delusions may have difficulty with inductive reasoning tasks involving the probabilistic assessment of hypotheses. Specifically, some patients show a "jumping-to-conclusions" reasoning style, in which they make rapid and overconfident judgements based on too little evidence. Stone and Young (1997) have interpreted this as a bias towards observational adequacy (the willingness to revise beliefs in accordance with what is observed) rather than conservativeness (avoiding change to one's existing belief system). In conjunction with a malfunctioning unconscious checking system this data-gathering bias would mean that patients would not seek enough alternative information to enable them to reject the feeling of conviction that accompanies their false belief, contributing to the maintenance of a delusion.

Interestingly, in contrast to inductive reasoning tasks, logical deductive reasoning tasks have been reported to be intact in delusional patients (Kemp, Chua, McKenna, & David, 1997). Bentall and Young (1996) have also reported that delusional patients appear not to have any difficulty in deciding how to go about testing hypotheses. Furthermore, when all information is provided to delusional patients (and their data-gathering bias is externally overcome) reasoning can be normal (Garety & Freeman, 1999). Delusional beliefs therefore can persist, even in the face of apparently intact deductive reasoning. According to our model, reasoning about a delusion or confabulation most often occurs in the context of some first factor neuropsychological impairment, and sometimes also in the presence of an abnormal feeling of conviction arising from failure of an unconscious checking system. It is possible that in some circumstances this combination may make the resulting delusions and confabulations "immune" to reasoning to some extent, even when reasoning abilities are intact.

Source and reality monitoring. Impairments in source and reality monitoring have been implicated in the production and maintenance of delusions and confabulations (Johnson & Raye, 2000). Source and reality monitoring refers to the ability to identify either the source of a memory (when and where it was encountered), or the reality of a memory or thought (whether it represents an externally derived, experienced event, or an internally generated, imagined event). We have already discussed unconscious reality or source monitoring processes as potentially being part of the unconscious checking system. However, there are also conscious source and reality monitoring processes, and these processes are the ones measured by typical source and reality monitoring experiments. For example, participants may be asked to identify in which of two sessions they encountered a particular piece of information (source monitoring) or which of a list of stimuli they previously saw and which they only imagined (reality monitoring). These tasks require a conscious search for contextual information associated with an event.

Failures of conscious source and reality monitoring may arise for several different reasons. First, as with reasoning failures, these processes may simply never be initiated. However, if they are initiated, either internally or via an external prompt, failures may occur at several levels. At the most basic level they may arise because the contextual information itself is unavailable. If the first factor impairment in confabulating patients is a loss of the ability to associate memory and thought fragments with contextual information which identifies their source, then reality monitoring processes will be severely impaired. Also at the bottom-up level, failures may result if confabulatory or delusional thoughts are unusually vivid or salient, as they are more likely to be mistaken for real, reliable experiences. At the top-down level, reality and source monitoring impairments may also arise from a data-gathering bias similar to that described previously, where insufficient information is sought before making a decision. This may involve a criterion setting impairment, in which a lax criterion is used to approve thoughts as genuine, or in which patients have difficulty adjusting their criterion in a context-relevant way. Alternatively, some sources of information may be incorrectly weighted as more salient than others. This type of monitoring failure may be involved when information that supports the implausible thought is treated as more salient than conflicting information, creating a confirmation bias.

Failures in conscious source and reality monitoring therefore seem likely candidates in the maintenance of confabulatory and delusional thoughts. Reality monitoring impairments are known to be associated with schizophrenia (e.g., Brebion et al., 2000), and have recently also been associated with anosognosia for hemiplegia (Jenkinson, Edelstyn, Drakeford, & Ellis, 2009). There is also evidence that confabulating patients have difficulty with source and reality monitoring tasks. For example, they are impaired at recalling correct source information associated with genuine event memories, and also produce false source information associated with confabulated memories (Ciaramelli & Ghetti, 2007). Furthermore, in reality monitoring experiments confabulating patients exhibit a bias towards identifying imagined events as externally derived (Johnson, O'Connor, & Cantor, 1997; Turner et al., 2008a). Further research is required to assess (a) the underlying reason for these monitoring impairments (whether they arise from bottom-up or top-down failures), and (b) the extent to which conscious source and reality monitoring deficits might be involved in the maintenance of other types of delusions.

Plausibility judgements. Related to both general reasoning processes and source and reality monitoring is the ability to judge whether thoughts are plausible in the context of your everyday knowledge about the world. This is often the most striking failure in cases of bizarre delusion and confabulation, as most of us would immediately identify the thought that, for example, a woman could have a bee's head, as implausible. Some confabulating and delusional patients seem unable to do this. The process of making a plausibility judgement depends on a deliberative evaluation of a thought in the light of other supporting memories or knowledge, and a search for consistency with previous experience. Again this process may fail for several reasons. First, it may simply not be initiated, because of the conviction associated with failure of the unconscious checking system. However, if challenged externally, this process should still be initiated. In some cases, plausibility judgement processes seem to be intact, but the delusional belief seems immune. For example, Startup (1997) reported that schizophrenic patients were well able to identify descriptions of others' delusional beliefs as indicative of mental illness, yet were unable to apply these standards to their own experiences. In other cases, plausibility reasoning itself may be disordered (e.g., Moritz et al., 2009), and patients may be unable to detect internal contradictions or conflicts with prior experience and general knowledge.

Theory of mind. Theory of mind is the ability to attribute mental states (beliefs, intents, desires, knowledge, etc.) to oneself and others, and to understand that others have beliefs, desires, and intentions that are different from one's own. As such it includes the ability to take on board the views of other people, and incorporate them into your reasoning process. One striking aspect of many confabulations and delusions is the lack of awareness by the patient that other people find their claims bizarre and unbelievable. As an example, take the following exchange with confabulating patient GN, conducted at his hospital bedside:

Examiner: What did you do this morning?
GN: This morning I got up, made myself a cup of coffee, did some work around the house, then came over here. Then I went back, and went to the National archive centre, where they were having a gunfight.
Examiner (audibly surprised):They were having a gunfight?
GN: Yes, they had a full-scale battle over there this morning.
Examiner: What was happening there? Are you pulling my leg?
GN: Well they were going to try and take over the, you know the archives, and the library.
Examiner: Who were?
GN: The ... er ... oh god ... the ... er ... the communists.
Examiner: Did that *really* happen this morning?
GN: Yes. It happens virtually about, anywhere from one to four Saturdays a month.
Examiner: Really?
GN: Yes. They're always going in there and trying to take it over.

Patient GN, previously a highly successful and intelligent man, showed no awareness that his claims seemed extraordinary to the Examiner.

This type of failure might also result in inability to acknowledge that someone else might have important information that should be taken into account, for example your doctor. Loss of the ability to consider another person's viewpoint would critically affect your ability to reason objectively as it restricts the information available to you. Chris Frith and colleagues propose that the human ability to share representations of the world is built upon two factors: an automatic empathic response where our representations of the world become aligned with those of the person with whom we are interacting, and a forward modelling process which enables us to predict the actions of others and use prediction errors to correct and refine our representations of the mental states of the person with whom we are interacting (Frith, 2007). Delusional and confabulating patients may have difficulty realigning their representations of the world with those of others, meaning that their reasoning processes are based only on egocentric representations (see also Hirstein, 2005; Langdon & Coltheart, 2001; Langdon, Coltheart, Ward, & Catts, 2001, for discussion of similar ideas).

Processes that influence the conscious checking system. Any conscious reasoning, reality and source monitoring, or plausibility evaluation process is likely to be effortful and demanding on resources, and would be dependent on a wide range of other supporting abilities and functions. Therefore, failures in conscious checking processes may be due, in part, to impairments in other systems necessary for their operation. For example, factors such as general intellectual decline and general comprehension impairment would obviously impact upon the ability to conduct complex reasoning and evaluation operations. Memory impairment would also have a significant impact. If the long-term semantic and episodic stores are degraded or inaccessible, patients will be unable to retrieve past regularities of personal experience, or semantic knowledge about the world, and therefore will not be able to use such information in their evaluation processes. Personality, experience, and one's preexisting belief system will also doubtless affect conscious reasoning and evaluation processes, as would affective state and motivational factors. However, the contributions of sustained attention and working memory seem particularly important for conscious checking, and we now turn to discuss these capacities in more detail.

One reason for failure on any effortful evaluation task might be the inability to hold multiple pieces of information "online" at one time in order to compare them. An inability to integrate multiple pieces of information, and to switch between different pieces of information held in working memory, would significantly disrupt the ability to evaluate a thought in the light of alternative knowledge, experience, or points of view. For example, a

Capgras patient with difficulties of this type would not be able to assess his belief that his wife was not who she appeared to be in the light of his doctor's explanation, the reactions of those around him, and previous knowledge of the plausibility of someone being replaced by an identical-looking imposter. If patients struggle to keep more than one piece of information online, this would explain difficulties in detecting conflict with other information, and the reliance on the current contents of consciousness. Patients would simply not be able to use alternative sources of evidence to negate their claims.

The idea that working memory and attentional deficits might contribute to delusions and confabulations is not new (Gilboa, 2010 this issue; Gilboa et al., 2006; Hirstein, 2005), and there is already some data to suggest that they may predict the course of recovery in some delusions (Aimola, 1999, described in Davies et al., 2005).Working memory and attentional deficits would also explain several features of the clinical presentation of delusions and confabulations. First, such deficits would explain the bias towards focusing on current stimuli when forming a belief, rather than on the weight of previous experience. Many confabulatory (and some delusional) thoughts appear to be "stimulus driven" and often based on some aspect of the immediate surroundings. Working memory and attentional deficits would also help to explain cases in which delusional or confabulating patients fleetingly accept the impossibility of their claim, but minutes later return to it as if it had never been challenged. Stuss and Benson (1986) for example provide the following example from a patient with anosognosia:

> When his hemiplegia was demonstrated to him he would accept the obvious fact and repeat the examiner's statement concerning the cause of the disability, but within minutes, if asked whether he had any disability, would adamantly deny hemiplegia. (p. 111)

Summary. We propose that a conscious checking system is responsible for a range of effortful reasoning, evaluation, and monitoring processes, and suggest that these processes will be heavily influenced by attentional and working memory function. The anatomical basis of these disparate functions is likely to be complex, but previous evidence suggests that conscious monitoring and evaluation processes may be associated with the right lateral prefrontal cortex (Coltheart, 2009; Corlett et al., 2007; Shallice, 2001, 2006).

In patients with delusions and confabulations conscious checking processes may fail for one of three reasons: (1) They are intact but not spontaneously initiated because of failure of the unconscious checking system; (2) they are intact and subsequently initiated by external triggers, but the strength of conviction stemming from the failed unconscious checking system is such that the delusional or confabulatory thoughts are "immune" to conscious reasoning; or (3) conscious checking processes are impaired themselves. These three alternatives could all account for the maintenance of a delusion or confabulation produced preconsciously. However, conscious reasoning processes could also, of themselves, lead to the production of a delusion: These would be those delusions that arise from a conscious search to explain some unusual experience, and we turn now to discussion of this phenomenon.

TWO ROUTES TO DELUSION AND CONFABULATION

An important result of the inclusion of both unconscious and conscious processes in this model is that it allows two routes to the production of delusions or confabulations. In the first, a delusional or confabulatory thought may be produced and passed unconsciously, and present as a fully formed memory or belief. This route would account for the majority of primary claims in confabulation and monothematic neurological delusions. In these cases the first factor perceptual, affective or mnemonic anomaly is not consciously experienced. A Capgras patient, for example, is not aware of the lack of emotional response to his wife, and a confabulating patient is not aware of his memory impairment. In these cases, we suggest that what reaches consciousness is an already formed, but basic, proposition. For example, in Capgras delusion what reaches consciousness would be the already formed thought "that person is not my wife", rather than an experience of reduced affective response. In confabulation, what reaches consciousness would be an incorrect memory. As the thought is generated and passes through the unconscious checking system before it ever reaches consciousness, the confabulatory or delusional thought seems to arise fully formed instead of being a consciously reasoned explanation for an unusual experience that the patient can report. Therefore, conscious reasoning and explanatory processes are not involved in determining the content of these types of basic thought (although they may be involved in elaborating them later). This is equivalent to the "endorsement" (Bayne & Pacherie, 2004), "expression" (Fine, Craigie, & Gold, 2005), "representational" (Davies & Coltheart, 2000), or "received" (Langdon & Bayne, 2010 this issue) account of delusions.

In contrast, other forms of delusion and confabulation appear to result from an experience that the patient is aware of. In these cases the delusion or confabulation may be produced by a second route, involving the conscious reasoning system in an attempt to explain an unusual experience. Conscious anomalous experiences may play a greater role in some of the delusional systems typical of schizophrenia. For example, this is likely to be the case when a heightened sense of significance is assumed to play the role of the first factor, and delusions of reference may result from a conscious reasoning process. In terms of our model, we would explain such cases as caused by disturbances in conscious reasoning processes which are put into place in an attempt to explain unusual experiences. This process would be equivalent to the "explanation" (Bayne & Pacherie, 2004; Fine et al., 2005), "attributional" (Davies & Coltheart, 2000), or "reflective" (Langdon & Bayne, 2010 this issue) account of delusions.

This view is also consistent with the account of delusional belief offered by Coltheart, Menzies, and Sutton (2010 this issue). They propose that in some forms of delusion (such as the seven delusions they list in their Table 1, which include Capgras, Frégoli, and Cotard delusions), the abnormality of cognition generated by a neuropsychological impairment is an unconscious one, and the abductive reasoning processes applied to this abnormality in an effort to explain it are also unconscious: Here, the delusion arises in consciousness fully fledged. But in other forms of delusion such as delusions of reference and of persecution, the delusional belief seems to arise from a process of conscious reflecting upon, and conscious reasoning about, some conscious experience which precedes the delusion.

As well as producing "explanation", delusions, conscious reasoning processes would also be responsible for the secondary claims and secondary confabulations discussed earlier, which serve to justify or support a primary confabulation or delusion. These may result from either intact or impaired conscious reasoning processes. For example, we described earlier the case where confabulating patient HW, having claimed that he had four adult children despite having only been married 4 months, produced the secondary claim that they were adopted. Our model would explain this by proposing that the faulty unconscious checking system produced a force of conviction that was too strong for him to be able to reject his confabulation. However, his intact conscious reasoning system had to find a way out of the logical problem his claim posed; hence, his plausible secondary claim. Faulty conscious reasoning systems, by contrast, would produce more bizarre secondary claims. For example, Bisiach (1988) reports the famous case of an anosognosic patient who "reasoned" that his doctor had three hands:

> Examiner: Whose hand is this?
> Patient: Your hand
> (The examiner then places the patient's hand between his own two hands)
> Examiner: Whose hands are these?
> Patient: Your hands
> Examiner: How many of them?
> Patient: Three
> Examiner: Ever seen a man with *three* hands?
> Patient: A hand is the extremity of an arm. Since you have three arms it follows that you must have three hands.

Finally, conscious processes would also be responsible for the elaboration (plausible if this system is intact and implausible if it is not) of primary delusions and confabulations. The thoughts that reach consciousness in these cases are likely to be fairly low level (for example "that is not my wife" in Capgras delusion). However, these may later be elaborated by conscious processes. This elaboration may flesh out the initial claim (perhaps creating the common explanation that the person in front of the patient is an imposter), or involve the production of background stories to support them (e.g., the account described earlier about the rescue of the two girls, identical in appearance to the patient's wife, who came to stay).

Delusions and confabulations produced by conscious reasoning processes are likely to have different characteristics to those produced via the unconscious route. For example, they are likely to be associated with less conviction and to be more amenable to modification. Garety and Freeman (1999) have reported that delusional patients are more likely than controls to switch hypotheses when given potentially contradictory information. This seems in contrast to the typical conviction associated with primary delusions and confabulations. However, it is in keeping with the behaviour associated with secondary claims and confabulations, which are often more willingly abandoned or modified than the primary claims which they defend. We believe that the model outlined here can offer an explanation for this variation in conviction by virtue of the suggestion that they are produced by two different routes. Primary confabulations and delusions produced by the unconscious route would be associated with failure of an unconscious tagging system, conferring an inappropriate feeling of conviction. However, consciously reasoned delusions, secondary claims, and elaborations deriving from conscious reasoning processes would not be associated with failure of an unconscious checking system, and would therefore be associated with less conviction than primary delusions and confabulations.

The existence of two routes to the production of confabulation and delusion also allows us to account for variation in consistency, with those delusions and confabulations produced by the unconscious route likely to be more consistent, more resistant to change, and less likely to be abandoned or adjusted in response to questioning, than those produced by the conscious route. However, it is important to note that consistency will also be influenced by the nature of the first factor. For example, the first factor impairment in confabulation is argued to be an impairment in strategic memory retrieval, which will result in the production of a wide range of different "memories". In contrast, the first factor impairment in Capgras delusion will lead to the production of a single, specific claim.

We have spent much time discussing the effects of impairments to the unconscious and conscious checking systems. We conclude therefore with two examples, which we suggest might illustrate the successful application of these checking systems. In both cases, the patients appear to have a first factor impairment which might lead to Capgras delusion. In the first case (studied by MC), the patient is in the early stages of recovering from his delusion, and appears to be employing conscious checking processes to control his interpretation of his experience.

> Examiner: What has made you realise that they're just imaginations? People telling you that?
> Patient: No it's just myself that's done it. I've started going through it, and seeing what could possibly happen and what couldn't happen. That was wrong, that couldn't happen. Even though it has happened it couldn't. Mary couldn't suddenly disappear from the room, so there must be an explanation for it. So then I try and work out what ... She [the imposter] knows me way back. The lady knows me way back. She could say things that happened 40 years ago, and I wonder where she gets them from. And then I worked it out and I've wondered if it's Mary all the time. It's nobody else.

In this patient, conscious and unconscious checking processes were presumably impaired during the acute stage of his delusion, to enable it to take hold. However, despite the continued presence of the first factor impairment, it appears that conscious checking processes are now being implemented to the extent that he is able to challenge the thought that the woman in his house is not his wife. It is difficult to speculate on whether unconscious checking processes might still be impaired in this patient. However, it seems plausible that this could be the case, but that he is able to use conscious checking processes (initiated by challenges from outside) to challenge the feeling of conviction associated with his experience. The resolution of delusions and confabulations is fascinating but poorly understood, and it remains unclear what factors might control the recovery process, even when the brain lesion remains constant, and in the continued presence of the first factor impairment.

However, first factor neuropsychological impairments are not always accompanied by checking impairments, even in the acute stages. Our second example (an extract from a patient studied by Nora Breen and Mike Salzberg, reproduced here with permission) seems to demonstrate the successful application of checking processes to a first factor impairment, enabling this patient (who had had temporal lobe surgery for relief of epilepsy) to avoid developing a Capgras-type delusion. Instead a functioning unconscious checking system and intact conscious checking processes enable her to describe the thought in "as if" terms, rather than as belief.

> Interviewer: After the operation, did you notice any change?
> Patient: Yes, the first thing I noticed was Mum, when she walked in the room, it was just a ... it was cardboard ... an image, if that's the right word ... it was like a picture of her, but it wasn't her ... it's hard to, I can't sort of explain it 'cause it ... inside ... it's hard.
> Interviewer: Right. It looked like a real person, did it?

Patient: Oh, yeah. There's Mum walking in the room.
Interviewer: Right. So you knew it looked like your Mum, but ...
Patient: Whether personality or what I don't know, but she was different, something was different about her
Interviewer: Did she look different or ...?
Patient: She ... I don't know ... so you can look different by expression or ... just through feeling, you can look different by, you know, doing your hair or whatever, but it wasn't different in that way, it was of having the different *inside* of her, I can't sort of explain it ....
Interviewer: Right is it that you *felt* different towards her?
Patient: I wouldn't have a clue because I'm just laying there and Mum's walked in the room ... well, this picture of Mum ... and started talking but it was only a picture of her but it didn't feel like her.
Interviewer: Right. OK.
Patient: Just didn't feel like her.
Interviewer: How did that feel to you?
Patient: Scary .... Has their lifestyle changed? Have I changed? Have they changed in a funny sort of way? I don't know. It's weird and it gets confusing.

CONCLUSIONS

In this paper we have drawn on the two-factor approach to propose a new model of confabulation and delusion. Specifically we have argued that the second factor must involve both unconscious and conscious processes, and proposed a monitoring framework consisting of (a) an unconscious checking system that either "tags" suspect thoughts as requiring extra conscious evaluation, or "passes" such thoughts, thus conferring conviction, and (b) a conscious checking system that enables elaborative and effortful evaluation of thoughts in the light of alternative evidence. Delusions and confabulations, we argue, will be maintained by impairments in one or both of these systems.

Importantly, the inclusion of unconscious and conscious evaluation systems allows for two routes to the development of confabulations or delusions: (1) an unconscious route where thoughts are produced and approved preconsciously. These then pass into consciousness fully formed and conferred with conviction by virtue of lack of a "doubt tag"; or (2) a conscious route where delusions or confabulations arise from conscious reasoning processes aimed at explaining unusual events or experiences. This model therefore allows for variation in the *content* of delusions and confabulations (in terms of differences in the type of first factor impairment), for variation in *conviction* (with conviction conferred by a impaired unconscious checking system) and for variation in *consistency* (in terms of both the nature of the first factor impairment, and mode of production, unconscious or conscious). The model also allows for development of a confabulation or delusion over time, as the systems are likely to operate in cyclical ways, with delusional and confabulatory thoughts becoming self-perpetuating as they cycle through interpreting new inputs. For example, repeated production of the same delusional or confabulatory thought will make it less likely to be tagged as doubtful, thus increasing conviction and increasing the salience of any other supporting information which might be considered by the conscious reasoning system.

At this stage our model is of course speculative. We have suggested processes that might contribute to the functioning of the unconscious and conscious checking systems. However, further investigation is necessary to establish exactly how they might operate, and how the component processes may dissociate in different patients. Our hope, however, is that the model provides an overarching framework within which to investigate similarities and difference between the two conditions. Our expectation is that different combinations of impairments may be able to explain the production and maintenance of both delusions and confabulations.

REFERENCES

Bayne, T., & Pacherie, E. (2004). Bottom-up or top-down? Campbell's rationalist account of monothematic delusions. *Philosophy, Psychiatry, and Psychology, 11*, 1–11.

Bell, V., Halligan, P. W., & Ellis, H. D. (2006). Explaining delusions: A cognitive perspective. *Trends in Cognitive Sciences, 10*, 219–226.

Bentall, R. P., & Young, H. F. (1996). Sensible hypothesis testing in deluded, depressed and normal subjects. *British Journal of Psychiatry, 168*, 372–375.

Bisiach, E. (1988). Language without thought. In L.Weiskrantz (Ed.), *Thought without language*. Oxford, UK: Oxford University Press.

Brebion, G., Amador, X., David, A., Malaspina, D., Sharif, Z., & Gormon, J. M. (2000). Positive symptomatology and source-monitoring failure in schizophrenia: An analysis of symptom-specific effects. *Psychiatry Research, 95*, 119–131.

Burgess, P. W., & McNeil, J. E. (1999). Content-specific confabulation. *Cortex, 35*, 163–182.

Burgess, P. W., & Shallice, T. (1996). Confabulation and the control of recollection. *Memory, 4*, 359–411.

Cahill, C., Silbersweig, D. & Frith, C. (1996). Psychotic experiences induced in deluded patients using distorted auditory feedback. *Cognitive Neuropsychiatry, 1*, 201–211.

Ciaramelli, E., & Ghetti, S. (2007). What are confabulators' memories made of? A study of subjective and objective measures of recollection in confabulation. *Neuropsychologia, 45*, 1489–1500.

Coltheart, M. (2005). Conscious experience and delusional belief. *Philosophy, Psychiatry and Psychology, 12*, 153–157.

Coltheart, M. (2009). The neuropsychology of delusions. *Manuscript in preparation.*

Coltheart, M., Menzies, P., & Sutton, J. (2010). Abductive inference and delusional belief. *Cognitive Neuropsychiatry, 15*(1/2/3), 261–287.

Coltheart, M., & Turner, M. S. (2009). Confabulation and delusion. In W. Hirstein (Ed.), *Confabulation: Views from neuroscience, psychiatry, psychology and philosophy*. Oxford, UK: Oxford University Press.

Corlett, P. R., Krystal, J. H., Taylor, J. R., & Fletcher, P. C. (2009). Why do delusions persist? *Frontiers in Human Neuroscience, 3*, 12.

Corlett, P. R., Murray, G. K., Honey, G. D., Aitken, M. R., Shanks, D. R., Robbins, T. W., et al. (2007). Disrupted prediction-error signal in psychosis: Evidence for an associative account of delusions. *Brain, 130*, 2387–2400.

Damasio, A. R. (1996). The somatic marker hypothesis and the possible functions of the prefrontal cortex. *Philosophical Transactions of the Royal Society of London, Series B: Biological Sciences, 351*, 1413–1420.

Damasio, A. R., Graff-Radford, N. R., Eslinger, P. J., Damasio, H., & Kassell, N. (1985). Amnesia following basal forebrain lesions. *Archives of Neurology, 42*, 263–271.

Davies, M. (2009). Delusion and motivationally biased belief: Self deception in the two-factor framework. In T. Bayne & J. Fernandez (Eds.), *Delusion and self deception: Affective and motivational influences on belief formation*. Hove, UK: Psychology Press.

Davies, M., Aimola Davies, A., & Coltheart, M. (2005). Anosognosia and the two-factor theory of delusions. *Mind and Language, 20*, 209–236.

Davies, M., & Coltheart, M. (2000). Introduction: Pathologies of belief. *Mind and Language, 15*, 1–46.

Davies, M., Coltheart, M., Langdon, R., & Breen, N. (2001). Monothematic delusions: Towards a two-factor account. *Philosophy, Psychiatry, and Psychology, 8*, 133–158.

Downes, J. J., & Mayes, A. R. (1995). How bad memories can sometimes lead to fantastic beliefs and strange visions. In R. Campbell & M. A. Conway (Eds.), *Broken memories: Case studies in memory impairment*. Oxford, UK: Blackwell.

Ellis, H. D. (1994). The role of the right-hemisphere in the Capgras delusion. *Psychopathology, 27*, 177–185.

Ellis, H. D., & Lewis, M. B. (2001). Capgras delusion: A window on face recognition. *Trends in Cognitive Sciences, 5*, 149–156.

Ellis, H. D., Luaute, J. P., & Retterstol, N. (1994). Delusional misidentification syndromes. *Psychopathology, 27*, 117–120.

Fine, C., Craigie, J., & Gold, I. (2005). The explanation approach to delusion. *Philosophy, Psychiatry, and Psychology, 12*, 159–163.

Fletcher, P. C., & Frith, C. D. (2009). Perceiving is believing: A Bayesian approach to explaining the positive symptoms of schizophrenia. *Nature Reviews Neuroscience, 10*, 48–58.

Fotopoulou, A. (2010). The affective neuropsychology of confabulation and delusion. *Cognitive Neuropsychiatry, 15*(1/2/3), 38–63.

Frazer, S. J., & Roberts, J. M. (1994). Three cases of Capgras' syndrome. *British Journal of Psychiatry, 164*, 557–559.

Friston, K., Kilner, J., & Harrison, L. (2006). A free energy principle for the brain. *Journal of Physiology (Paris), 100*, 70–87.

Frith, C. D. (2007). *Making up the mind: How the brain creates our mental world.* Oxford, UK: Blackwell.

Garety, P. A., & Freeman, D. (1999). Cognitive approaches to delusions: A critical review of theories and evidence. *British Journal of Psychiatry, 38*(2), 113–154.

Garety, P. A., & Hemsley, D. R. (1994). *Delusions: Investigations into the psychology of delusional reasoning*. Oxford, UK: Oxford University Press.

Gilboa, A. (2010). Strategic retrieval, confabulations and delusions: Theory and data. *Cognitive Neuropsychiatry, 15*(1/2/3), 145–180.

Gilboa, A., Alain, C., He, Y., Stuss, D. T., & Moscovitch, M. (2009). Ventromedial prefrontal cortex lesions produce early functional alterations during remote memory retrieval. *Journal of Neuroscience, 29*(15), 4871–4881.

Gilboa, A., Alain, C., Stuss, D. T., Melo, B., Miller, S., & Moscovitch, M. (2006). Mechanisms of spontaneous confabulations: A strategic retrieval account. *Brain, 129*, 1399–1414.

Gilboa, A., & Moscovitch, M. (2002). The cognitive neuroscience of confabulation: A review and a model. In A. D. Baddeley, M. D. Kopelman, & B. A. Wilson (Eds.), *The handbook of memory disorders* (2nd ed., pp. 315–342). London: Wiley.

Hirstein, W. (2005). *Brain fiction: Self-deception and the riddle of confabulation*. Cambridge, MA: MIT Press.

Jaspers, K. (1963). *General psychopathology*. Manchester, UK: Manchester University Press.

Jenkinson, P. M., Edelstyn, N. M. J., Drakeford, J. L., & Ellis, S. J. (2009). Reality monitoring in anosognosia for hemiplegia. *Consciousness and Cognition*, *18*, 458–470.

Johnson, M. K., O'Connor, M., & Cantor, J. (1997). Confabulation, memory deficits, and frontal dysfunction. *Brain and Cognition*, *34*, 189–206.

Johnson, M. K., & Raye, C. L. (2000). Cognitive and brain mechanisms of false memories and beliefs. In D. L. Schacter & E. Scarry (Eds.), *Memory, brain and belief*. Cambridge, MA: Harvard University Press.

Kemp, R., Chua, S., McKenna, P., & David, A. (1997). Reasoning and delusions. *British Journal of Psychiatry*, *170*, 398–405.

Kopelman, M. D. (1999). Varieties of false memory. *Cognitive Neuropsychology*, *16*, 197–214.

Kopelman, M. D. (2010). Varieties of confabulation and delusion. *Cognitive Neuropsychiatry*, *15*(1/2/3), 14–37.

Kveraga, K., Ghuman, A. V., & Bar, M. (2007). Top down predictions in the cognitive brain. *Brain and Cognition*, *65*, 145–168.

Langdon, R., & Bayne, T. (2010). Delusion and confabulation: Mistakes of perceiving, remembering and believing. *Cognitive Neuropsychiatry*, *15*(1/2/3), 319–345.

Langdon, R., & Coltheart, M. (2000). The cognitive neuropsychology of delusions. *Mind and Language*, *15*, 184–218.

Langdon, R., & Coltheart, M. (2001). Visual perspective-taking and schizotypy: Evidence for a simulation-based account of mentalising in normal adults. *Cognition*, *82*, 1–26.

Langdon, R., Coltheart, M., Ward, P. B., & Catts, S. V. (2001). Visual and cognitive perspective taking impairments in schizophrenia: A failure of allocentric simulation? *Cognitive Neuropsychiatry*, *6*(4), 241–269.

Mackie, J., Ebmeier, K. P., & O'Carroll, R. E. (1994). An MRI, SPECT and neuropsychological study of a patient presenting with Capgras syndrome. *Behavioural Neurology*, *7*, 211–215.

Maher, B. A. (1999). Anomalous experience in everyday life: Its significance for psychopathology. *The Monist*, *82*, 547–570.

Mattioli, F., Miozzo, A., & Vignolo, L. A. (1999). Confabulation and delusional misidentification: A four year follow-up study. *Cortex*, *35*, 413–422.

McKay, R., & Kinsbourne, M. (2010). Confabulation, delusion, and anosognosia: Motivational factors and false claims. *Cognitive Neuropsychiatry*, *15*(1/2/3), 288–318.

McKay, R., Langdon, R., & Coltheart, M. (2009). "Sleights of mind": Delusions and self deception. In T. Bayne & J. Fernandez (Eds.), *Delusion and self deception: Affective and motivational influences on belief formation*. Hove, UK: Psychology Press.

Metcalf, K., Langdon, R., & Coltheart, M. (2007). Models of confabulation: A critical review and a new framework. *Cognitive Neuropsychology*, *24*, 23–47.

Metcalf, K., Langdon, R., & Coltheart, M. (2010). The role of personal biases in the explanation of confabulation. *Cognitive Neuropsychiatry*, *15*(1/2/3), 64–94.

Moritz, S., Veckenstedt, R., Randjbar, S., Hottenrott, B., Woodward, T. S., von Eckstaedt, F. V., et al. (2009). Decision making under uncertainty and mood induction: Further evidence for liberal acceptance in schizophrenia. *Psychological Medicine*, *39*, 1821–1829.

Moscovitch, M. (1995). Confabulation. In D. L. Schacter (Ed.), *Memory distortion: How minds, brains and societies reconstruct the past*. Cambridge, MA: Harvard University Press.

Moscovitch, M., & Melo, B. (1997). Strategic retrieval and the frontal lobes: Evidence from confabulation and amnesia. *Neuropsychologia*, *35*, 1017–1034.

Schnider, A. (2001). Spontaneous confabulation, reality monitoring, and the limbic system—a review. *Brain Research: Brain Research Reviews*, *36*, 150–160.

Schnider, A. (2008). *The confabulating mind: How the brain creates reality.* Oxford, UK: Oxford University Press.

Schnider, A., Valenza, N., Morand, S., & Michel, C. M. (2002). Early cortical distinction between memories that pertain to ongoing reality and memories that don't. *Cerebral Cortex, 12*, 54–61.

Shallice, T. (2001). Deconstructing retrieval mode. In M. Naveh-Benjamin, M. Moscovitch, & H. Roediger (Eds.), *Perspectives of human memory and cognitive aging: Essays in honour of Fergus Craik.* New York: Psychology Press.

Shallice, T. (2006). Contrasting domains in the control of action: The routine and the non-routine. In Y. Munakata & M. Johnson (Eds.), *Attention and performance XXI: Processes of change in brain and cognitive development.* New York: Oxford University Press.

Startup, M. (1997). Awareness of own and others' schizophrenic illness. *Schizophrenia Research, 26*, 203–211.

Stone, T., & Young, A. W. (1997). Delusions and brain injury: The philosophy and psychology of belief. *Mind and Language, 12*, 327–364.

Stuss, D. T., & Benson, D. F. (1986). *The frontal lobes.* New York: Raven Press.

Turner, M., Burgess, P., Cipolotti, L., Frith, C., Gilbert, S., Shallice, T., & Simons, J. (2008a). Confabulation, reality monitoring and the inferior medial PFC: Converging evidence from lesion and functional imaging studies. *Journal of the International Neuropsychological Society, 14*(Suppl. 2), 67–68.

Turner, M. S., Cipolotti, L., Yousry, T. A., & Shallice, T. (2008b). Confabulation: Damage to a specific inferior medial prefrontal system. *Cortex, 44*, 637–648.

Turner, M. S., Shores, A., Breen, N., & Coltheart, M. (2009). Déjà vecu for news events but not personal events: A dissociation between autobiographical and non-autobiographical episodic memory processing. *Manuscript in preparation.*

Wright, S., Young, A. W., & Hellawell, D. J. (1993). Sequential Cotard and Capgras delusions. *British Journal of Clinical Psychiatry, 32*, 345–349.

Young, A. W. (1998). *Face and mind.* Oxford, UK: Oxford University Press.

Young, A. W., & Leafhead, K. M. (1996). Betwixt life and death: Case studies of the Cotard delusion. In P. W. Halligan & J. C. Marshall (Eds.), *Method in madness: Case studies in cognitive neuropsychiatry* (pp. 147–171). Hove, UK: Psychology Press.